Creating Synthetic Emotions through Technological and Robotic Advancements

Jordi Vallverdu
Universitat Autònoma de Barcelona, Spain

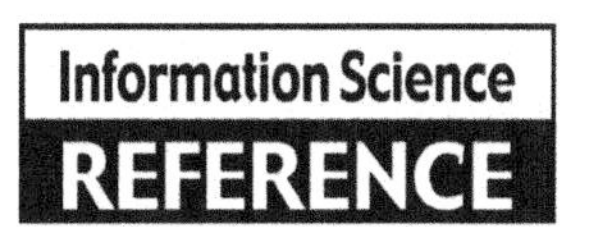

Managing Director:	Lindsay Johnston
Senior Editorial Director:	Heather A. Probst
Book Production Manager:	Sean Woznicki
Development Manager:	Joel Gamon
Development Editor:	Development Editor
Acquisitions Editor:	Erika Gallagher
Typesetter:	Jen McHugh
Cover Design:	Nick Newcomer, Lisandro Gonzalez

Published in the United States of America by
Information Science Reference (an imprint of IGI Global)
701 E. Chocolate Avenue
Hershey PA 17033
Tel: 717-533-8845
Fax: 717-533-8661
E-mail: cust@igi-global.com
Web site: http://www.igi-global.com

Library of Congress Cataloging-in-Publication Data

Creating synthetic emotions through technological and robotic advancements /
Jordi Vallverdu, editor.
p. cm.
Summary: "This book compiles progressive research in the emerging and groundbreaking fields of artificial emotions, affective computing, and sociable robotics that allow humans to begin the once seemingly impossible task of interacting with robots,systems, devices, and agent"-- Provided by publisher.
Includes bibliographical references and index.
ISBN 978-1-4666-1595-3 (hardcover) -- ISBN 978-1-4666-1596-0 (ebook) -- ISBN 978-1-4666-1597-7 (print & perpetual access) 1. Emotions. 2. Artificial intelligence. 3. Robots. I. Vallverdz, Jordi.
QP401.C68 2012
612.8'232--dc23

2012002110

British Cataloguing in Publication Data
A Cataloguing in Publication record for this book is available from the British Library.

Table of Contents

Detailed Table of Contents

Affective computing has proven to be a viable field of research comprised of a large number of multidisciplinary researchers, resulting in work that is widely published. The majority of this work consists of emotion recognition technology, computational modeling of causal factors of emotion and emotion expression in virtual characters and robots. A smaller part is concerned with modeling the effects of emotion on cognition and behavior, formal modeling of cognitive appraisal theory and models of emergent emotions. Part of the motivation for affective computing as a field is to better understand emotion through computational modeling. In psychology, a critical and neglected aspect of having emotions is the *experience* of emotion: what does the content of an emotional episode look like, how does this content change over time and when do we call the episode emotional. Few modeling efforts in affective computing have these topics as a primary focus. The launch of a journal on synthetic emotions should motivate research initiatives in this direction, and this research should have a measurable impact on emotion research in psychology. In this paper, I show that a good way to do so is to investigate the psychological core of what an emotion is: an *experience*. I present ideas on how computational modeling of emotion can help to better understand the experience of emotion, and provide evidence that several computational models of emotion already address the issue.

This paper gives a historical review of Kansei-based media technologies in Japan. Kansei is a Japanese word, the meaning of which covers sensibility, sentiment, emotion, and feeling. Kansei research started in the field of music, because music is the most acceptable of the arts to computer science. In the 1990s, the applications of Kansei machine vision became widespread in many industrial fields, including electronic production, automobile manufacture, steel-making, the chemical industry, the food industry, and office appliances, among others. Kansei technologies are also applied to human interface systems, including the field of brain science, for human communication.

Human intelligence requires decades of full-time training before it can be reliably utilised in modern economies. In contrast, AI agents must be made reliable but interesting in relatively short order. Realistic emotion representations are one way to ensure that even relatively simple specifications of agent behaviour will be expressed with engaging variation, and those social and temporal contexts can be tracked and responded to appropriately. We describe a representation system for maintaining an interacting set of durative states to replicate emotional control. Our model, the Dynamic Emotion Representation (DER), integrates emotional responses and keeps track of emotion intensities changing over time. The developer can specify an interacting network of emotional states with appropriate onsets, sustains and decays. The levels of these states can be used as input for action selection, including emotional expression. We present both a general representational framework and a specific instance of a DER network constructed for a virtual character. The character's DER uses three types of emotional state as classified by duration timescales, keeping with current emotional theory. We demonstrate the system with a virtual actor. We also demonstrate how even a simplified version of this representation can improve goal arbitration in autonomous agents.

It is hypothesized here that two classes of emotions exist: driving and satisfying emotions. Driving emotions significantly increase the internal activity of the brain and result in the agent seeking to minimize its emotional state by performing actions that it would not otherwise do. Satisfying emotions decrease internal activity and encourage the agent to continue its current behavior to maintain its emotional state. It is theorized that neuromodulators act as simple yet high impact signals to either agitate or calm specific neural networks. This results in what we can define as either driving or satisfying emotions. The plausibility of this hypothesis is tested in this paper using feed-forward networks of leaky integrate-and-fire neurons.

Recognition and analysis of human emotions have attracted a lot of interest in the past two decades and have been researched extensively in neuroscience, psychology, cognitive sciences, and computer sciences. Most of the past research in machine analysis of human emotion has focused on recognition of prototypic expressions of six basic emotions based on data that has been posed on demand and acquired in laboratory settings. More recently, there has been a shift toward recognition of affective displays recorded in naturalistic settings as driven by real world applications. This shift in affective computing research is aimed toward subtle, continuous, and context-specific interpretations of affective displays recorded in real-world settings and toward combining multiple modalities for analysis and recognition of human emotion. Accordingly, this paper explores recent advances in dimensional and continuous affect modelling, sensing, and automatic recognition from visual, audio, tactile, and brain-wave modalities.

Theories of cognitive processes, such as decision making and creative problem solving, for a long time neglected the contributions of emotion or affect in favor of analysis based on use of deliberative rules to optimize performance. Since the 1990s, emotion has increasingly been incorporated into theories of these cognitive processes. Some theorists have in fact posited a "dual-systems approach" to understanding decision making and high-level cognition. One system is fast, emotional, and intuitive, while the other is slow, rational, and deliberative. However, one's understanding of the relevant brain regions indicate that emotional and rational processes are deeply intertwined, with each exerting major influences on the functioning of the other. Also presented in this paper are neural network modeling principles that may capture the interrelationships of emotion and cognition. The authors also review evidence that humans, and possibly other mammals, possess a "knowledge instinct," which acts as a drive to make sense of the environment. This drive typically incorporates a strong affective component in the form of aesthetic fulfillment or dissatisfaction.

Chatterbox Challenge is an annual web-based contest for artificial conversational systems, ACE. The 2010 instantiation was the tenth consecutive contest held between March and June in the 60th year following the publication of Alan Turing's influential disquisition 'computing machinery and intelligence'. Loosely based on Turing's viva voca interrogator-hidden witness imitation game, a thought experiment to ascertain a machine's capacity to respond satisfactorily to unrestricted questions, the contest provides a platform for technology comparison and evaluation. This paper provides an insight into emotion content in the entries since the 2005 Chatterbox Challenge. The authors find that synthetic textual systems, none of which are backed by academic or industry funding, are, on the whole and more than half a century since Weizenbaum's natural language understanding experiment, little further than Eliza in terms of expressing emotion in dialogue. This may be a failure on the part of the academic AI community for ignoring the Turing test as an engineering challenge.

A psychological experiment was conducted to straightforwardly investigate the effects of polite behaviors expressed by robots in Japan, using a small-sized humanoid robot that performed four types of behaviors with voice task instructions. Results of the experiment suggested that the subjects who experienced "deep bowing" motion of the robot felt it more extrovert than those who experienced "just standing" motion. Subjects who experienced "lying" motion of the robot felt the robot less polite than those who experienced the other motions. Female subjects more strongly feeling the robot extrovert replied for the task instruction from the robot faster, although no such trend was found in the male subjects. However, the male subjects who did not perform the task felt the robot less polite than the male subjects who performed the task and the female subjects who did not perform the task.

Preface

"SUBSUMING OR EMBODYING EMOTIONS?"

STILL...WHAT IS A SYNTHETIC EMOTION?

There is a question with which I'm usually faced when I give talks on emotions and cognitive systems: "what is a synthetic emotion?" Everybody knows about feeling and emotion, but the doubts start when one tries to understand the bodily meaning, evolutionary reasons, or physiological details of emotions, and even more, what is the relationship between emotions and machines? Another important aspect is that the kind of audiences interested on the field of artificial emotions is very broad: AI experts, engineers, electronic artists, neurologists, robot producers, game programmers, computational theoreticians, psychologists....and despite their interest on how to relate emotions, social interaction, and intelligence (or intelligent task-solving designs), there has never been a clear idea about the history and highlights of this very short historical research field. The author of this preface can understand this confusion; emotions have not been completely implemented into the analysis or design of cognitive entities. And even in these cases in which something like *emotions* have been taken into account, they have been added to the system, instead of being the structural backbone of the cognitive system.

As a consequence of all the previously explained, it can be affirmed that the research on artificial emotions has two main and limited interests:

a. recognize and imitate human emotions;
b. consider the benefits of a emotion-like architecture or functioning (neural nets) for a cognitive system.

The truth is that the high complexity of the cognitive brain processes makes impossible to think about, emulate, or even to simulate those activities. Nevertheless, it is obvious that at the end, the real goal of the research on artificial emotions is to create machines that are able to feel. Not to feel as human beings, in the same way that airplanes don't fly like birds...but much faster and carrying heavy things, like cargo aircrafts. The future of synthetic emotions cannot be to design human-like robots able to interact in human environments, or AI programs with advanced cognitive skills as a consequence of some implemented emotional architecture. Machines will need to have emotions in order to survive, to fulfil the deep meaning of human existence, to know and to feel fine with this (partially) satisfied emotion. Allow the preface to explain briefly how this author thinks this process can start.

SUBSUMING OR EMBODYING EMOTIONS?

There is a very important problem (or, better, pending question) in the current research on artificial emotions: when one looks at the bibliography on this topic, they can observe a common tendency to consider emotions like something added to the artificial cognitive systems, but never natural or prewired to them. In most of published research on artificial emotions, the situation is like this: "well…if we implement an emotional-drive mechanism this machine will work better" or "with emotion recognition and expression this robot will perform better human interactions," because those artificial systems are not considered *autonomous entities*. Instead, those devices are designed as machines that perform tasks or run programs, even evolutionary ones, but they are never considered as real entities. Emotions are then subsumed into some secondary conceptual layer. Human physical structure determines whole behaviour: what can be thought, what can be touched or felt, where to go, and so on. Only thanks to extended instruments (telescope, computers, cars...) can humans go beyond the limits imposed by natural evolution. Even in the case of extended parts of human minds and bodies, people still project their physical structure over them, or human emotional nature. People live for several things: be loved, feel good, satisfy physical necessities, avoid pain, understand one's surrounding nature….and humans are driven by these intentional directions. Although all throughout man's lives, he tries to minimize pain and maximize pleasure, he cannot choose pain or pleasure: the body is prewired in these modes. Man cannot escape from hunger, fear, or future death. Perhaps humanity can learn to assume some emotional moods thanks to symbolic processes (death is nothing, because I can only feel me while I'm alive, as Epicurus said), but even in that case, the discussion is about emotions inside cognitive-processed behaviours. Any social activity involves several types of emotional regulations. If the aim is to understand at which point this is important, look at people with Asperger's syndrome or autism, and it is apparent how emotions are absolutely necessary for *normal* human daily activity: from performing scientific research (so often in coordinated teams) to social interactions (friendship, relationship, hobbies, ….).

Despite all the previous statements, this author can understand the reason of the lack of understanding, that is, denial of emotions into general research fields: on the one hand, science still doesn't understand the true nature and role of emotions in human cognition, and therefore, man cannot reproduce them exactly; on the other hand, and despite the last two decades of empirical neurological evidence towards the active involvement of emotions into cognitive tasks, emotions are still considered by hundreds of experts as neither necessary nor primordial. Consequently, emotions are secondary aspects in the main design of any kind of an action regulation system.

Consequently, a change is necessary. Emotions cannot be something that should be embedded into a pre-existing artificial device, but they must be embodied within them. Emotions are at the same time part of the physical body and the informational process of the body sensors. Human bodily structure allows man to feel the world under a specific meaning route, the emotional one. Embodying emotions is the real task, future, and goal of the whole research field. At the end, the field needs to create feeling machines. Yes, machine learning, integration of perceptive data, data categorization, action, and goal selection or communication among agents, among others, are important and unsolved problems of the contemporary research on cognitive AI. Because of the impossibility of solving the whole problem of human cognition, researchers have fragmented it into smaller, more tractable pieces, trying to achieve easier solutions to them. And this is the current state of the research, necessary but unsatisfactory. The convergence of all these fields led to the artificial conscious existence, something for which will be absolutely necessary in creating synthetic emotions.

IJSE'S ROLE AND CURRENT STATE

The International Journal of Synthetic Emotions is the first and leading journal in the world devoted specifically to the artificial or synthetic emotions researches. As it states on the website, the mission of IJSE is to provide a forum for the advancement of knowledge and methods necessary for the creation of artificial devices with emotions. IJSE approaches the field of synthetic emotions, offering a unique interdisciplinary platform for all international researchers on this topic. The journal presents a new common space of the richest and best ideas about synthetic emotions. Also discussed is a conceptual framework that enables a synergy and symbiosis among computer scientists, cognitive scientists, robot and synthetic agent designers, as well as psychologists, neuroscientists, and philosophers.

After two years of the journal, it can be affirmed that this editorial project is a solid reality and that IJSE accomplishes a new role as the conceptual meeting point between the several types of experts of this interdisciplinary research area. Every published work contains rich and different approaches to artificial emotions. Somebody could think that this diversity could lead to a lack of agreement or that this is the example of the dominant confusion in this field. On the contrary, each contribution sheds light upon the multiple faces of the studies on synthetic emotions; all the authors, although not connected directly, contribute to the improvement of the understanding and implementation of synthetic emotions. This is a collective creation of knowledge in which all the involved researchers are designing the basis of a shared future independently.

The journal's first year had great contributions that the author of this preface comments on briefly below.

a. **Modelling the Experience of Emotion** (pages 1-17) was written by Joost Broekens (Man-Machine Interaction Group, Delft University of Technology, The Netherlands). Accepting the challenge of thinking about a new paradigm for synthetic emotions, Prof. Broekens made a critic review of the basic prevailing ideas on the field and suggested how emotions could be modelled. This is a brave attempt to face the pending problems of the field as well to clarify conceptual problems that could otherwise add confusion. Finally, he reinforced the idea of considering emotion as an experience, and consequently, presented ideas on how computational modelling of emotion cold help to better understand the experience of emotion, providing evidence that several computational models of emotion already addressed the issue.
b. **Review of Kansei Research in Japan** (pages 18-29) was written by Seiji Inokuchi (Takarazuka University of Arts and Design, Japan). This paper gave light to a forgotten and key aspect of the engineering implementation of emotional aspects: Japanese Kansei research. Despite the continuous and excellent relationships between Western and Japanese AI & Robotics researchers (for example I've enjoyed recently from a JSPS fellowship), the general literature on synthetic emotions neglects any direct reference to Kansei Engineering. This paper was a first step towards a true connection between Eastern and Western specialists.
c. **Simplifying the Design of Human-Like Behaviour: Emotions as Durative Dynamic State for Action Selection** (pages 30-50) was written by Joanna J. Bryson (University of Bath, UK) and Emmanuel Tanguy (University of Bath, UK). The authors created a new model, the Dynamic Emotion Representation (DER), which integrates emotional responses and keeps track of emotional intensities changing over time. Besides demonstrating their system with a virtual actor, they also demonstrate how even a simplified version of this representation can improve goal arbitration in autonomous agents; i.e., more simple, more reliable.

d. **Emotion as a Significant Change in Neural Activity** (pages 51-67) was written by Karla Parussel (University of Stirling, Scotland). Working on neural nets, specifically feed-forward networks of leaky integrate-and-fire neurons, Prof. Parussel tested a hypothesis according to which neuromodulators act as signals to actions than can be labelled as driving or satisfying emotions (two classes of emotions). This paper is a good example of how theoretical literature can be experimentally checked by computational means.

e. **Automatic, Dimensional, and Continuous Emotion Recognition** (pages 68-99) was written by Hatice Gunes (Imperial College London, UK) and Maja Pantic (Imperial College London, UK and University of Twente, EEMCS, The Netherlands). One of the most important aspects of the interest of human emotions is the emotion recognition process, which makes possible a true HRI. This paper shows how natural emotions (and not a simplistic and short idealized model of them) can be detected and processed, from the help of several techniques they analyze: dimensional and continuous affect modelling, sensing, and automatic recognition from visual, audio, tactile, and brain-wave modalities.

f. **Emotion in the Pursuit of Understanding** (pages 1-11) was written by Daniel S. Levine (University of Texas at Arlington, USA) and Leonid I. Perlovsky (Harvard University, USA). From the knowledge of their neural and cognitive modelling expertise, the authors suggest a neural network model in which emotional and rational processes are intertwined. At the same time, they suggest from the existing literature, a beautiful, powerful, and simple hypothesis: humans have a *knowledge instinct* that drives them to make sense of their environments, that is, a genetic aesthetic driving force behind cognitive processes.

g. **Chatterbox Challenge as a Test-Bed for Synthetic Emotions** (pages 12-37) was written by Jordi Vallverdú (Universitat Autònoma de Barcelona, Spain), Huma Shah (Universitat Autònoma de Barcelona, Spain), and David Casacuberta (Universitat Autònoma de Barcelona, Spain). The Turing test involves a semantic knowledge of the world, but the common mistake of all researchers who try to win the Turing test with their chatbots is to consider semantics as a linguistic property of things, instead of the emotional interaction between words and feelings (from specific bodies). This paper showed the unsatisfactory results of checking the performances of several chatbots and how the emotional drive of these artificial entities must be emotionally designed in order achieve any human-like appearance.

h. **Effects of Polite Behaviors Expressed by Robots: A Psychological Experiment in Japan** (pages 38-52), by Tatsuya Nomura (Ryukoku University, Japan), and Kazuma Saeki (Ryukoku University, Japan). Going one step beyond the habitual difficulties involved into robotics research, humanoid robotics is faced with several problems, most of them the result of the complexity of human social interactions. This experiment analyzes how a robot can express polite behaviours and which is the human answer to this action.

All these excellent pieces of research are a perfect example of the latest and most innovative approaches to the multidimensionality of artificial emotions, and in some cases are very brave and critical with their own fields. The authors are always looking for a better research future, always creating new roads for knowledge.

OBJECTIVES

The objectives of IJSE Editorial Board for the future will be to maintain this journal as an open intellectual platform for all researchers who think on how natural or artificial entities make decisions and act. As this author wrote in the preface of the first issue "In a world of super-specialised experts, this journal aims to be a bridge and meeting space for the different researchers who work in the field of synthetic emotions: neurologists, computer scientists, robotic engineers, philosophers, artists, and so forth. The advancement of science comes from those who are brave, who look for new thinking spaces, who create new ideas. We are at the frontier of true knowledge and inspired work. The suggested diversity of approaches will not imply a lack of depth of analysis, nor a simplification of the ideas or concepts involved. We wish to build a complex editorial project, which facilitates such a meeting point between different kinds of experts."

The author of this preface further posits is possible to observe repeatedly a general behaviour when making talks to several audiences (graduate, undergraduate, postdocs) from several backgrounds (engineering, humanities, social sciences, cognitive,..):

1. At the beginning the same faces of agreement or boredom... "yes, I know that there is a relationship between emotions and rationality, but what the H*** can a philosopher show me?"
2. In the middle of a lecture there are plenty of interested persons following along with the ideas and bad jokes, some others who clearly are fighting themselves about the meaning of some new ideas they've heard, and finally, a few who have experienced an illumination about some weird aspect of their research for which they think they've found a new solution. Obviously, the sleeping students in the population are not counted under this analysis, as well as those skeptics who, because a feeling of disgust towards bearded philosophers like me, (and following a new fallacy (ad bearded philosopher hominem) have not followed any of the presented ideas, considering that they have all the knowledge they need to solve their academic problems.
3. At the end: some quickly abandon the room, some others discuss some of the exposed ideas, another group take the opportunity of an office visit to talk pleasantly with their colleagues about their last weekend, and a few come to me to ask for PPT slides and to establish a short discussion about some part of the talk (surely, they think that they need to offer some words to justify getting the full files for the lecture). Some hours later, emails will be received asking for some details about my talk. And then, back again to the silence of one's desk.

The students are all following specific and traceable emotional dispositions that are translated into different kinds of attitudes and cognitive tendencies. It is difficult to see when talking about emotions that students and the professor are feeling them all throughout the process. There is no distance between the world, the words we use to express it, and the self. Emotions are the force that bridges these domains of reality. People are faced with the embodied nature of emotions, as the end point of understanding, to the fulfilment of knowledge necessities.

For all the previous aspects, it is necessary to maintain a true interdisciplinary journal in which experts from several domains of expertise can share, learn, discuss, or imagine new ways of creating artificial emotions. This is a complex project; perhaps researchers in this field swim against the contemporary tide of overspecialization, but it is necessary to be open to different ideas to solve the complexities of the emotional design.

FUTURE TRENDS

The future of IJSE is in the hand of the massive community of researchers who are more or less involved into the analysis of emotions, especially those who are trying to design more humanoid and/or intelligent devices. Nevertheless, as Editor-in-Chief, the author of this preface has some bureaucratic duties as well as research goals. Among these, the editor in chief must encourage two different kinds of issues, published alternatively: a) normal issues with invited or open calls collected papers; b) specialized numbers about one topic with a guest editor.

It is very important to be open to new ideas, new debates, or new points of view from young, senior, acclaimed, or unknown researchers in pursuit of the highest quality and the most innovative approaches, because synthetic emotions are a very complex problem. The truth is that complexity, although present, it is not the most important aspect of synthetic emotions: there is the pervasiveness of emotions as a qualitative and subjective experience, and there also is the difficulty of creating the main architectural design of an emotional device. *Qualia* and emergence are perhaps the two keystones of the future research of emotions, because in order to create emotions, it is not enough to talk about simulating some facial expressions, but about how to create a machine that feels the world according to its own structure. This is the real meaning of embodiment. In the process of creating such a machine, it is vital to start from the scratch reproducing basic cognitive systems (plants, insects…) and increase the complexity progressively, looking for the emergence of more complex emotions, and consequently, of better cognitive systems and consciousness itself. To be is to feel, in any kind of reality that your brain wishes to offer to you. Nervous system cognition and emotions are several faces of the same phenomena: conscious existence. Even in the case of the lack of self-consciousness, emotions drive all throughout the cognitive and social processes. They are the frame from which humans understand the world. And their understanding is not a mental activity, but also a physical one: man knows the laws of the universe through his body. To conceptualize them is a different step.

Meanwhile, and coming back to the real research, the journal devotes specialized issues of different aspects of the research: computational neuroscience and emotions, robot musicians and emotional performance, anthropology of emotions, human-robot interaction, emotions' physical measurement, electronic art and new ways to think about bodies and emotions, emotional architectures design….there are plenty of topics that must be analyzed in order to make an advance into the field. The journal must also pay attention to any specific technology or technological advance that can improve the understanding of emotions as well as their simulation.

As a final and concluding remark, this author wants to thank to this community of experts for devoting their researches to such a difficult, fascinating, and beautiful topic. Emotions create the meaning of the world, and by working in the future of artificial emotions researchers are at the same time looking for new meanings of reality. The author hopes for a long future for IJSE.

Chapter 1
Modeling the Experience of Emotion

Joost Broekens
Man-Machine Interaction Group, Delft University of Technology, The Netherlands

ABSTRACT

Affective computing has proven to be a viable field of research comprised of a large number of multidisciplinary researchers, resulting in work that is widely published. The majority of this work consists of emotion recognition technology, computational modeling of causal factors of emotion and emotion expression in virtual characters and robots. A smaller part is concerned with modeling the effects of emotion on cognition and behavior, formal modeling of cognitive appraisal theory and models of emergent emotions. Part of the motivation for affective computing as a field is to better understand emotion through computational modeling. In psychology, a critical and neglected aspect of having emotions is the experience of emotion: what does the content of an emotional episode look like, how does this content change over time and when do we call the episode emotional. Few modeling efforts in affective computing have these topics as a primary focus. The launch of a journal on synthetic emotions should motivate research initiatives in this direction, and this research should have a measurable impact on emotion research in psychology. In this paper, I show that a good way to do so is to investigate the psychological core of what an emotion is: an experience. I present ideas on how computational modeling of emotion can help to better understand the experience of emotion, and provide evidence that several computational models of emotion already address the issue.

INTRODUCTION

In this position paper I argue that efforts in computational modeling of emotion should focus more on returning results to psychology, and I propose a research direction that can achieve this.

DOI: 10.4018/978-1-4666-1595-3.ch001

Computational models of natural phenomena are useful for two main reasons. First, the model itself can be used to simulate and predict the phenomenon that is modeled. Consider for example the weather. A detailed computational model of clouds, temperature fronts, pressure systems and geological factors predicts the weather for the next couple of days. This is obviously useful, and it is a quality of the model related to its usefulness when applied in a particular context (predicting the weather). Second, any model is the instantiation of a theory or set of hypotheses, whether these hypotheses are simple or complex, widely validated or new. For a model to be computational, it needs to be executable by a computer (the model must be a computer program that can *run*). Regardless of the particular peculiarities of the computer system that is used to run the program, a fairly detailed description of the model is always needed. The computer needs detailed step-by-step instructions that match the model. Therefore, a *computational model* is a detailed instantiation of a theory or set of hypotheses. The predictions produced by a running computational model are predictions of the theory that a model is based on. Obviously, the usefulness of these predictions critically depends on two factors: the credibility of the theory used as basis for the model, and the credibility of the extra assumptions that were needed to build the computational instantiation of that model (the correctness of the implementation). This means that a computational model also has an intrinsic quality: it can be used to evaluate a theory. For example, predictions produced by a computational model of the weather can be used to evaluate the theory of the weather that underlies the computational model. Incorrect predictions motivate changes to the theory.

This view of computational models is not different in the area of affective computing. Affective computing is a research field that is concerned with the development and use of computational models of emotion. Typically, such models are used in the domains of emotion recognition, emotion elicitation (production), and emotion effects (e.g., on cognition, behavior). In following sections I will discuss emotion and affective computing in more detail, but first I will give a more concrete example of a computational model of emotion elicitation that has both qualities, the applied quality any model has that produces useful output, and the intrinsic quality a model has provided that it is grounded in theory. Consider the work by (Gratch & Marsella, 2001). They propose a model of emotion elicitation, implemented in a pedagogical software agent. The role of the software agent is to guide a trainee through a virtual-reality based training session. The software agent can—partly as a result of the model of emotion—deliver a more believable training simulation (more believable than training without emotional agents). This hopefully results in a training session that better matches reality, giving participants in the training a better preparation for real life situations. This is an applied quality of the computational model of emotion. If the modelers did a faithful job of transforming the theory they used as basis for their model into a computational instantiation then the behaviors of the agent are in essence predictions of the theory underlying the computational model. This is the intrinsic quality of the computational model of emotion. Predictions of this kind can be used as a motivation for changes to the emotion theory underlying the model (Broekens, DeGroot, & Kosters, 2008).

The applied quality of a computational model is solely based on its potential for generating useful output. Useful means that the model serves some goal. In virtual training systems (Gratch & Marsella, 2004; Henninger, Jones, & Chown, 2003), the goal is to enhance believability of the agent in order to increase the effect of the training on the trainees. In tutor and support systems (Bickmore & Picard, 2005; Graesser, Chipman, Haynes, & Olney, 2005; Heylen, Nijholt, Akker, & Vissers, 2003), the goal is to enhance the relation between the user and the system such that the system is used more often, longer and/or more effectively. In entertainment computing (Nakatsu, Rauterberg, & Vorderer, 2005), the goal is to increase enjoyment by increasing active experience (sufficient motor behavior of the user while playing for example a game) and presence (the feeling of being "in the game"). Affective computing techniques can be used to develop affectively interesting gaming characters (Broekens & DeGroot, 2004) but also to sense the user's affective state to adapt gameplay (Hudlicka, 2008a). In autonomous agent research (Coddington & Luck, 2003; Gmytrasiewicz & Lisetti, 2000; Steunebrink, Dastani, & Meyer, 2008), the goal is to enhance (and reason about) the artificial agent's decision making process. It is obvious that if the reason for developing a computational model of emotion is different depending on the domain, then the usefulness of the model depends on the domain.

The intrinsic quality of the computational model (i.e., its potential to evaluate the underlying theory) however does not depend on the domain. As mentioned above, this quality depends on the plausibility of the theory on which the model is based and the plausibility of the assumptions used to develop the computational instantiation of that theory. As a result, any model of emotion that fulfills these two criteria has intrinsic quality, and can be used to evaluate the theory on which it was based.

Figure 1 depicts the two senses of usefulness just discussed. I explain the figure in detail. In psychology there are several types of theories of emotion that are suitable as basis for computational models of emotions (e.g., cognitive appraisal theory, factor-based theories of emotion, and motivation/drive/needs theories of emotion). These theories are widely cited and actively used as basis for current computational models of emotion. The computational models are developed for different domains (as explained above). The results of the studies are therefore domain-specific results. In affective computing, mostly the domain-specific results are reported upon. Such results include *our virtual character is more believable*, *our agent can reason more efficiently*, and *our tutor agent helps users to better learn*. These are good results, and a proportion of these results is fed back to the domain itself; the results are generalized. Such generalizations could include *emotional game agent (NPCs) are more enjoyable than non-emotional agents and we can explain that because they increase the feeling of presence*. And, *affective virtual characters increase the training effect of virtual reality training and we can explain that because the model of emotion increases believability of the agent and therefore the training is more effective*. Notice, however, that these generalizations are still domain specific and do not feed back to the emotion theory that was used as basis for the computational model of emotion. There is surprisingly little feedback (thin arrow

Figure 1. Current state of the flow of results in affective computing research. Arrows denote the size of the impact of the results.

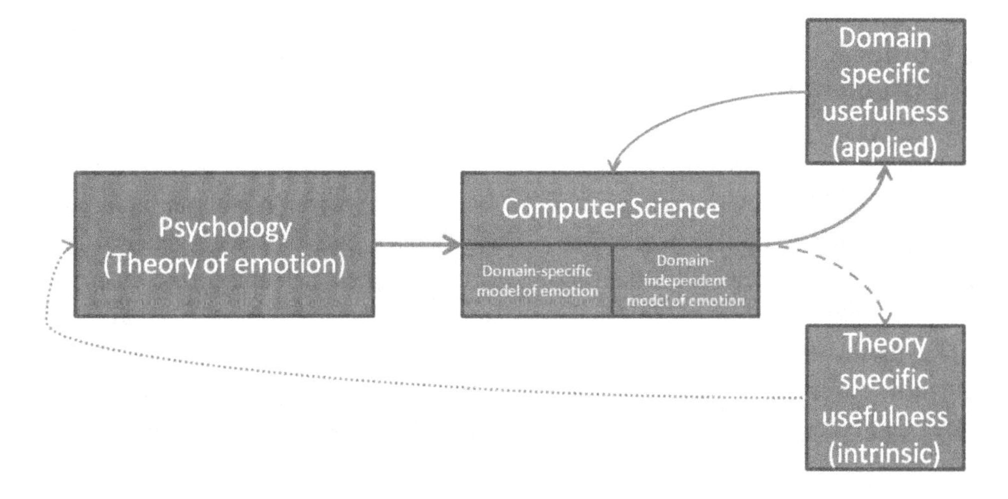

from *Theory specific usefulness* to *Psychology*) to the psychology community on the predictions of their own theories generated by computational modeling (and I will substantiate this claim later). I call these results *predictions* on purpose, they are as much predictions of a particular emotion theory as a weather simulation is a prediction of a theory of the weather and a simulation of a super-nova explosion is a prediction of a theory of star formation and death. This lack of feedback to psychology is striking, given the fact that there definitely are affective computing researchers (e.g., Breazeal & Scassellati, 2000; Broekens, 2007; Canamero, 2000; Gratch & Marsella, 2004; Hudlicka, 2008b; Lahnstein, 2005; Sloman, 2001), that try to faithfully model emotion according to the psychological theories and report the results relevant to the theory (denoted by the significantly thicker arrow from *Computer Science* to *Theory specific usefulness*).

In this paper I argue that computational modeling of emotion should focus more on returning results to psychology, and I propose a research direction that can achieve this. First I discuss affective computing and emotion. Then I show that there currently is a lack of impact on psychology. Finally I present ideas on how computational modeling of emotion can help to better understand the experience of emotion, and provide evidence that several computational models of emotion are already addressing the issue.

Affective Computing Background and Future Challenge

In the past decade, affective computing has proven to be a viable field of research comprised of a large number of multidisciplinary researchers resulting in work that is widely published and used. Although this is not a review article, I feel it is appropriate to discuss the vast terrain affective computing by now covers. The reason for doing so is (a) to give an overview to those readers not familiar with the large amount of work that has been done, and (b) to show there really is a gap in the research focus.

First, a large body of research studies automatic emotion recognition in a wide variety of domains (Cowie et al., 2001; Hanjalic & Li-Qun, 2005; Pantic & Rothkrantz, 2000; Picard, 1997). These models typically try to affectively label facial expressions, sounds, and gestures but also Web sites and other forms of written texts. The main idea is to extract affectively relevant features from the signal, where the signal can be images, movies, sounds, and so forth. Combinations of features together correlate with particular affective labels such as happy or sad (often as indicated by human subjects analyzing the same signals). Newer research tries to not only extract static features (such as the mouth having a certain angle) but also dynamic features, that is, movement. These more detailed analyses are needed to differentiate between fake and genuine emotions. This branch of research is strongly related to signal processing, pattern recognition and machine learning: try to identify relevant features, build a predictive model based on those features and use the model to label the signal.

Second, a large part of the affective computing research community is involved in computational modeling of causal factors of emotion in order to use these models in human-computer and human-robot interaction (see Bickmore & Picard, 2005; Breazeal, 2003; Fong, Nourbakhsh, & Dautenhahn, 2003; Hudlicka, 2003; Paiva, 2000). Two aspects play a key role: modeling the emotion elicitation and modeling the emotion expression. One often does not go without the other (how to express an emotion without having a model that generates one, and why generating one if you don't express it). Important examples of these approaches are Kismet the social robot (Breazeal & Scassellati, 2000), companion robots such as the Aibo, the iCat, the Huggable and Paro (see Broekens, Heerink, & Rosendal, in press; Fong et al., 2003), and a large number of emotional agents used for tutoring systems (e.g., Graesser et al., 2005; Rickel & Johnson, 1997) and virtual reality training (e.g., Elliott, Rickel, & Lester, 1999). Early research was primarily aimed at exploring the possibility of creating such affective agents (with the underlying assumption that affective agents are more believable than non-affective agents), while later research is more focused on measuring the effects on users of embedding such agents in particular domains (gaming, training, tutoring) and the effects on users of social and companion robots.

Third, a smaller part of the affective computing community is explicitly concerned with modeling the effects of emotion, such as affective influences on cognition (Broekens, Kosters, & Verbeek, 2007; Canamero, 2000; Gadanho, 2003; Hudlicka, 2008b; Marinier Iii, Laird, & Lewis, 2009; Velasquez, 1998), formal modeling of cognitive appraisal theory (Broekens et al., 2008; Gmytrasiewicz & Lisetti, 2000; Marsella & Gratch, 2009; Meyer, 2006), integrating emotional states in agent reasoning (Coddington & Luck, 2003; Meyer, 2006; Steunebrink, Dastani, & Meyer, 2008) and models of emergent emotions, such as emerging from the interaction between a simple adaptive agent and its environment (Canamero, 2000; Lahnstein, 2005; Scheutz, 2004; Velasquez, 1998). Later in this article, I will come back to these modeling efforts, as some of these are surprisingly close to the research efforts that, according to emotion psychologists, are needed to study the experience of emotion (Barrett, Mesquita, Ochsner, & Gross, 2007).

Two recent developments related to affective computing are social robotics (for a review see Fong et al., 2003) and long-term human-computer relationships (Bickmore & Picard, 2005). Key to these areas of research is the realization that, although computational modeling of emotion is needed for social robots and interfaces, it is not sufficient. Issues such as attachment and friendship, mutual dependency and shared understanding are essential too. Interestingly, Breazeal & Scassellati (2000) already started to study these issues with Kismet and Dautenhahn (1995) already argued these to be important for social intelligence in artifacts.

A general pattern in the affective computing research just reviewed is a strong focus on practical outcome. For example, a tutor agent, a virtual character, an affective interface, an emotion recognition mechanism, enhanced human computer interaction. As a consequence, many reported results relate to the applied quality of the computational model of emotion: its ability to produce useful output in the domain for which it was developed. This obviously skews the number of results towards the "applied" box instead of the "intrinsic" box (Figure 1).

However, part of the motivation for affective computing as a field is the promise to better understand emotion through computational modeling. The question is what it means to "better understand emotion"? Or, more appropriately for the current discussion, when is a "better understanding" happening? I think that this must involve feeding back the results from computational studies of emotion to psychology. Considering the lack of citations *to* affective computing *from* leading publications on emotion, such as Barrett et al. (2007), Frijda, Manstead, and Bem, (2000), Scherer, Schorr, & Johnstone, (2001), and more importantly *The Handbook of Emotions* (Lewis, Haviland-Jones, & Barrett, 2008) the affective computing community did not add a lot to the understanding of emotion, at least not to the extent that psychologists cite the work.

This is rather counterintuitive as in psychology there is a strong need to better understand the structure of, and mechanisms that underlie emotion. Sometimes mathematical and computational principles are even used to do this (Lewis, 2005; Reisenzein, 2009; Wehrle & Scherer, 2001). Also approaches that are less mathematically inclined do express a need for a better understanding of the underlying mechanisms of emotion (Barrett et al., 2007). These needs are expressed in terms of understanding how neural workings are related to higher-level psychological constructs. Nevertheless, computer models are very useful to better understand neural workings. The point is that to understand structure and mechanism, simulation is a very powerful research method. A simulation of a phenomenon not only shows a relation between constructs but also posits a possible explanation for why that relation exists.

In her seminal book and in later papers Picard (1997, 2003) and others state that one of the four major topics in affective computing is computers that *have* emotions (the others are recognizing, expressing and understanding emotions). Obviously it is currently unclear what it means for a computer to have emotion (is it alive, does it need consciousness, etc.). I think this, although somewhat sci-fi-like, goal is a valid long-term research goal, but it is less useful for the current discussion. We can interpret *having* a little less strict by adding *models that simulate* in front of it. Now the short-term goal would be *models that simulate having*, or, *models that help us understand what having is for humans*. In psychology, a critical and neglected aspect of having emotions—of emotion in general—is the *experience* of emotion (Barrett et al., 2007). The experience of emotion can be summarized as the answer to the following four questions: what does the phenomenological content of an emotional episode look like, how does this content change over time, when do we call the episode emotional, and how do neurobiological processes instantiate the experience? Little computational modeling research in the affective computing community has these topics as a primary focus. I think that a focus on these topics helps to restore the impact balance because it directly contributes to answering questions relevant to emotion psychology.

The launch of a journal on synthetic emotions should spark research initiatives in *theoretical affective computing* (or *computational affective science* if you like that term better). This research should be cited in the psychology literature. Currently, this does not happen often, while the inverse citation relation is abundant: all affective computing researchers know it is practically impossible to get a paper published without referring to the standard emotion works.

In this article I argue that a good way to restore the impact balance is to investigate the psychological core of what an emotion is: *an emotional experience*. I present ideas on how the experience of emotion can be investigated using computational models. More importantly, I provide evidence that—from a psychological point of view—some computational models of emotion are already addressing the issue. I therefore propose a challenge: to have one chapter on computational modeling of emotion in the fourth edition of *The Handbook of Emotions*.

Not a Definition of Emotion

Emotion is a complex topic, and agreement on one solid definition does not really exist. I will not attempt to define emotion here, as many excellent works have been published from different perspectives that together do much more credit to the diverse and multimodal nature of emotion (Frijda et al., 2000; LeDoux, 1996; Lewis et al., 2008; Ortony, Clore, & Collins, 1988; Panksepp, 1998; Picard, 1997; Rolls, 2000; Scherer et al., 2001). In this section I explain what the different emotion-related terms usually refer to, and the above-mentioned references are a collective source for this explanation.

Typically, affect refers to the underlying core of emotion, mood and affective attitude towards persons and things. Emotion, mood and affective attitude are different but strongly related and influence each other. In general, emotion is related to facial expression, feeling, cognitive processing, physiological change and action readiness. Furthermore, emotion refers to a short but intense episode that, in addition to the previously mentioned aspects such as facial expressions, is characterized by "attributed affect to a causal factor." An emotion is a noticeable if not powerful experience. For example, I feel (and notice I am) happy about seeing an old friend. In contrast, mood refers to a silent presence of moderate levels of affect, not necessarily related to the preparation of action. Mood is not (consciously) attributed to a causal factor. I can feel frustrated for half a day without knowing why. Affective attitude refers to how one generally feels about something or someone, not specifically because of that thing or person. For example, I *like* popular science books, and I feel *enthusiastic* about theme parks. To complicate matters a little, affect is also used as commonplace term for everything that has to do with the above.

There are several theoretical views on how to think about emotion. These views can be categorized in multiple ways, but I find the following categorization that uses two axes particularly useful. The first axis defines the level of abstraction at which emotion is studied: social, psychological, biological, and physiological. The second axis defines the way emotion is represented: categories of emotion, components that form an emotion, and principal factors. For example, the well-known six basic emotions as proposed by Paul Ekman are categorical (fear, anger, happiness, etc.). Cognitive appraisal theories are componential, as these describe emotion as a combination of the activation of different sub processes (evaluation of an event in terms of novelty, goal conduciveness, etc.). On the other hand, (Russell, 2003) proposes a description of emotion using two continuous factors (Pleasure, Arousal).

Emotion is a multimodal phenomenon and studying it benefits from a multidisciplinary standpoint. Across disciplines, there exist commonalities. For example, many (if not all) emotion researchers believe that there are two common affective factors that are useful to describe a mood, emotion or attitude: valence and arousal. Within a discipline, these factors can be studied in different ways: are these factors the psychological core of emotion, which areas or mechanisms in the brain are involved, are these always independent (orthogonal), are they artifacts of statistical analysis of many factors, and so forth. Other common views exist, for example, with regards to theories that explain emotion elicitation (where does the emotion come from). Most agree that an emotion is the result of an evaluation of the situation in terms of personal relevance. It depends on the discipline which aspect of this evaluation is highlighted. Is it a cognitive evaluation, is it conscious, holistic, component-based, automatic, biologically hard-wired, social, and so forth? For a recent overview and reflection upon emotion elicitation, see Gratch, Marsella, and Petta (2009). For a quick and broad introduction to the different emotion theories and the history of these see chapter 5 in Eysenck (2004) or chapter 3 in LeDoux (1996).

The Citation Asymmetry and the Experience of Emotion

I first substantiate the claim that there is an impact asymmetry between affective computing and the psychology of emotion, and I will do this in a very simple way. If the latest edition of the standard psychological reference manual for emotion research scholars (Lewis et al., 2008) does not contain even a single reference to the most important results in affective computing, while all affective computing literature contains many references to emotion theories, then there is a serious asymmetry. I would claim there is no such thing as affective computing for beginning scholars in emotion research (and this is an easy claim to investigate as it involves polling a representative group of psychology students on their awareness of affective computing).

Why is the impact of affective computing on psychology so small? I argue there are three main causes that might explain this asymmetry in citation. The first one is that the affective computing community has a strong focus on applied model quality, that is, the ability to use the model in a particular domain is seen as the end result of a study (thick arrow going to the "applied" box in Figure 1). This is clear from the literature overview just presented: many approaches use emotions for a particular purpose in a system, and when that has been done successfully the study is done. Computer scientists doing such studies do not relate their results to the theory of emotion they used. This is not needed. If the goal of your research is to, for example, develop an affective interface, the results are evaluated in terms of the effectiveness of the interface, not in terms of the predictions of the theory used as basis for the interface.

The second cause has to do with how results are communicated to emotion psychologists, assuming there are any (how are the results depicted by the thin arrow to the "psychology" box in Figure 1 communicated). Research results are not communicated in an effective way to the psychological research community. Computer scientists have a different language and have different publication outlets. A related issue is that in computer science it is common to publish results on conferences, and many of these conferences are not indexed by popular search engines used by psychologists. Even when the results are related to the emotion theory, these are often described in too technical a manner (including formalisms, program code, etc.) or use unconventional terminology. A related aspect is that emotion psychologists are used to read detailed discussions of how a particular new finding relates to findings and theories of others, while computer scientists do not discuss their results in this way. Computer science research is problem oriented, while psychology research is exploratory. As a result, when the problem is solved (e.g., I have an emotional avatar) the research is done.

Third, assuming emotion psychologists find and understand affective computing publications, they do not feel that the studies add to their understanding of emotion. I personally think this is much more serious an issue than the first two, as it means there actually isn't an "intrinsic" quality box (Figure 1). This feeling can be due to two things. The implicit assumptions needed to develop a computational model based on a theory of emotion cloud the validity of the predictions coming out of the running model. As a result it is difficult to claim that the computational model is a valid instantiation of the theory. Second, the topics addressed in affective computing are simply not relevant to the understanding of emotion. The first issue is a methodological one (Broekens et al., 2008), and although important I will not address it here. The second issue is the one I will discuss in the rest of this article.

Do affective computing researchers address the relevant topics from the point of view of emotion psychologists? I think the answer to this question is sometimes. Consider emotion recognition research. The typical problem that is addressed is "how can we extract the (real vs. fake) affective meaning of an expression"? This question is seen as the problem, and the tools used to solve this problem are signal processing and machine learning. As a result, advances in this field are mainly advances in signal processing and machine learning, not in understanding emotion expression. Obviously the computer science model builders understand more and more of emotion expression, but they use insights from the psychological literature to do so. Automatic emotion recognition is a special form of signal processing (typical publication venues are the signal processing journals and conferences). The same argument can be made for artificial emotion expression. The problem to be solved is "plausible emotional expression," and as a result, expressing emotions is a particular form of rendering (typical publication venues are the graphically oriented and robotic journals and conferences).

So, when do affective computing researchers address relevant problems for emotion psychologists? I think there are two areas that are directly relevant to emotion psychologists: computational models of emotion elicitation (production) and computational models of emotion effects on thought and behavior. These models do not address the issue of *having* emotions in the strict sense (as explained above), but they do help us better understand the experience of emotion. In the remainder of this article I argue that affective computing modeling efforts can help our understanding of the experience of emotion. I also present three different models of emotion generation of which I claim shed light on the experience of emotion, thereby providing evidence of the feasibility such models.

Modeling the Experience of Emotion

In a recent review of emotion research it has been argued (successfully in my opinion) that what is currently lacking is a focus on what an emotion *is* (Barrett et al., 2007). According to the authors, this is due to several reasons (including a focus on behaviorism, fear of phenomenologically oriented research, etc.) that I will not further discuss here. However, an important observation is that there has been a strong focus on causal (and preferably external) factors for emotion *not* on a thorough description of what the experience of emotion feels like and how such feelings arise (Barrett et al., 2007). The authors argue for efforts into investigating both content, a phenomenological description of the experience itself, and process, an explanatory description of the relation between the phenomenological experience, the psychological processes and biological and neurological underpinnings. The authors' motivation for this approach is a good one: one does not know what to explain if there is no adequate description of the explanandum, that is, the experience of emotion. Following Barrett et al. (2007), a phenomenological description of emotion is a description that includes "affect, perceptions of meaning in the world, and conceptual knowledge about emotion bound together at a moment in time, producing an intentional state where affect is experienced as having been caused by some object or situation." Such a description contains the following key factors (loosely ordered from emotion generation to emotion effects).

- **Situational content:** the appraisal (in the cognitive appraisal theory sense) content including causal events, goal conduciveness, novelty, and norm compatibility.
- **Relational content:** the dominance relation between people, or more generically, the social context of an emotion.
- **Appraisal detail:** the commonalities and subtle differences between different forms of anger, sadness, and so forth (Barrett et al., 2007) call this part "beyond appraisal dimensions." An important distinction made is the difference between felt and reported experiences. Currently many of the appraisal theories address the latter not the first. Both are important, but a good description of the felt experience is important from a phenomenological point of view (and more useful when searching for neural correlates).
- **Affective associations:** such as past feelings, hypothetical feelings, and online experiences.
- **Core affect:** a description of the pleasure and arousal intensities during the emotive period.
- **Arousal content:** a feeling of being active versus passive, including the difference between actual and felt arousal, relation to attention processes, and so forth.

An important related issue is the relation between time and the experience of emotion. What is the dynamic interplay between the above mentioned aspects, and how do they vary over the onset and decay of an emotional episode?

As mentioned above, there are three ways via which the experience of emotion could be unraveled (Barrett et al., 2007). First we should have a good description of the phenomenological content of emotion experience, second we should investigate the psychological processes involved, and third we should investigate the neural correlates of this content and processes (what the authors call a neural reference space).

There are three ways in which computational modeling can help. First, to investigate the neural correlates of emotion experience, computational models can be used to simulate biologically plausible neural networks involved in emotion, as is commonly being done in computational cognitive neuroscience. This type of model is strongly grounded in biological and physiological accounts of emotion but the findings generated are difficult to link to the phenomenological content of the experience of emotion. The conceptual gap between physiological and neurological theories of emotion that are suitable for computational modeling on the one hand, and a phenomenological description of emotion on the other, currently is too big.

Second, we can use formal modeling techniques to describe the emotion experience itself. The model is a formal representation of what is known about the content and flow of the experience of emotion, but cannot be used to generate new predictions, because the mechanisms responsible for the content and flow are not modeled. For example, one could model the phenomenological content of emotion using a network of nodes probabilistically connected to each other with edges. Each node contains a content description, and the edges define possible transitions. As a result, this network specifies the flow of emotion experience. The network can be executed to simulate possible flows of phenomenological experience, but it can never generate new findings.

Third, computational modeling can help to find plausible mechanisms that explain and predict the phenomenological content of emotion, as well as the effects of emotion on behavior and cognition. In this case, the model is mechanism-based specified at the psychological level aimed at bridging the gap between neuronal processes and phenomenology. In this article I focus on this type of computational model. The simulation results produced by these models are interpretable in terms of the experience of emotion, while at the same time the model proposes mechanisms that could be responsible for the generation of the experience and its effects. There obviously is a huge diversity with regards to where the mechanisms in such models reside in the neural-psychological-phenomenological space. Some are oriented towards explaining the link between neural workings and mental mechanisms, others towards the link between mental mechanisms and phenomenology.

Affective computing can help emotion psychology by developing such "generative phenomenological models" (for want of a better term). I present three examples of existing models. The models I describe focus on modeling emotion elicitation, but models that focus on emotion effects exist too (e.g., Hudlicka, 2008b). Two key characteristics of the models I discuss are (a) that the model is based on a theory that explains emotion elicitation and (b) the results of the predictions are interpreted in terms of a phenomenological description of emotion experience. The advantages of such an approach are that the model can be executed, can be used to generate new experiences, and these experiences can then be verified in (or compared to) psychological experiments. The three different approaches discussed are a logic, formal approach (Steunebrink et al., 2007), an agent-based approach (Marsella & Gratch, 2009), both of which are cognitive appraisal based, and a behavioral, biological approach (Lahnstein, 2005) that is compatible with an emotion theory such as the one proposed by Rolls (2000). Each study sheds light on one or several of the six previously mentioned aspects of the experience of emotion as proposed by Barrett et al. (2007).

Lahnstein (2005) proposes a model of the onset and decay of an emotive episode as a result of an anticipatory and subsequent reactive evaluation phase. In this model she uses a simple robot that is able to learn behavior based on reward, and control its behavior based on the prediction of future reward. The model uses a form of reinforcement learning. In the discussion, we assume the model has had several learning experiences, that is, the model is partly trained. She proposes that the valence part of the emotive episode can be modeled as a combination of the expected reward—the reward that is anticipated given a certain action—and the experienced reward—the reward received when the action is executed. According to Lahnstein (2005), the positive valence signal has four typical dynamics, three of which I think are particularly insightful (see Figure 2). Importantly, she proposes phenomenological qualities for these different dynamics. In the first case, the prediction of positive reward would correlate with feelings of hope, optimism and positive expectancy (phase 1) and the evaluation of the received reward that is smaller than expected would correlate with disappointment (phase 2). In the second case, the experience of phase one is the same, while the experience of phase two would correlate with happiness, contentment and satisfaction. In the third case, the first phase is again the same, but the second phase is correlated with happiness (and I would add positive surprise as the reward is larger than expected). I think we can easily add to her proposal plausible phenomenological accounts of these three dynamics if the valence signal is negative (e.g., fear in the first phase, and in the second phase panic when the punishment is even worse, relief when the punishment is less, and despair when the punishment is confirmed). In a series of small simulation experiments she shows that these positive valence dynamics actually occur in a simple learning robot. By doing so, she predicts, using a generative model, how the content of the emotion experience would look like for an adaptive organism with regards to *core affect*. Further, she also predicts what the online *affective associations* could be (happiness, disappointment, etc.).

The results just presented are compatible with the theory of emotion proposed by Rolls (2000), who states that emotion is the result of a combination of six reinforcement-related factors including whether reward or punishment is given or withheld, the intensity of the reinforcement and the occurrence of both a reward and a punishment at the same time. Rolls behavioral account of emotion is a significant (although debated) addition to our understanding of emotion in the context of adaptive behavior. I would claim that the modeling work by Lahnstein (2005) is a significant contribution to our understanding of the possible dynamics of emotion in relation to adaptive behavior.

A very different branch of study in affective computing is how to formalize appraisal theories. As an example, I will discuss a recent attempt by (Steunebrink et al., 2007). In their study they formalize the OCC appraisal model (Ortony et al., 1988) by extending an already existing BDI (Belief, Desire, Intention) based agent program-

Figure 2. Three different situations of the predicted and received reward, taken from Lahnstein (2005)

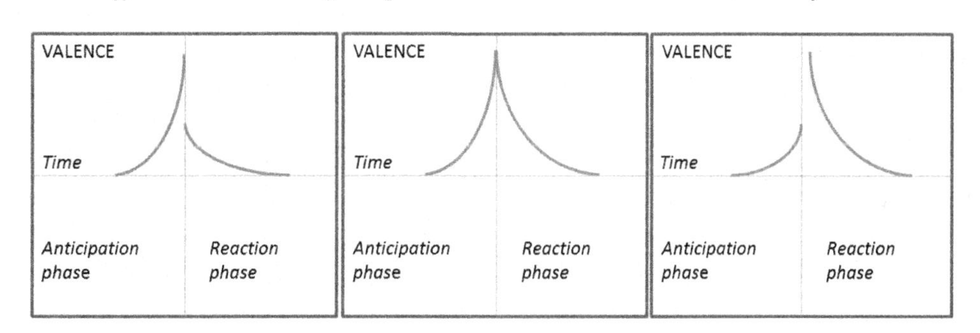

ming logic. The details of this logic are out of scope in this article, but I will have to explain a little about the underlying ideas. First, they have a system that is capable of formally representing beliefs, goals, agents, plans, abilities, commitment and the execution of plans as well as the relations between these elements. Second, they define the different emotions that can be found in the OCC model, for example, they define *hope*(p, g) as the emotion of hope of an agent, that a particular plan p will end up satisfying goal g. In an analogue fashion they define *fear*(p, $-g$) and all other emotions in the OCC model. Third, they formalize what hope would be for an agent according to the OCC model given that the agent has a formal structure around events, goals, and so forth as they defined it. So for hope this would be *hope*(p, g) $\leftrightarrow$ (I(p, g), *Commitment*(p)), which means that an agent hopes for plan p to fulfill goal g if and only if it has the intention to fulfill goal g with plan p and it has a commitment to executing plan p. This, in their view, maps to what is describe in the OCC model about hope; hope is being pleased about the prospect of a desirable event. Prospect is thus interpreted as "having a plan for," and desirable is interpreted as "being a goal." Fear on the other hand is formalized as follows: *fear*(p, $-g$) $\leftrightarrow$ (*hope*(p, g) & *Belief*(*execute*(p) $\rightarrow$ $-g$), which in their formal system means that fear about not fulfilling a goal g due to a plan p, occurs if and only if there is a hope for that plan fulfilling the goal, and the agent beliefs there is a possibility that execution of that plan might end up in not fulfilling the goal. In other words, fear involves uncertainty about successfully executing a plan aimed at a particular goal.

Regardless of what one thinks of the different assumptions that are the basis of this formalization (e.g., it might be argued that a prospect does not necessarily imply having a plan), the formal notation does serve emotion research, and in particular the *situational content*. First it makes very explicit what the consequences are of particular assumptions and theory translations. For example, fear in their case can only be derived from hope, meaning that the experience of fear would always be accompanied by a feeling of hope. This is a testable prediction, first to be evaluated on face value by emotion psychologists, then by experimentation. Second, one can derive things about the situation that elicits the emotion. A striking one is the following derivation. If an agent does not believe in the existence of a plan to accomplish a goal, it will neither hope for that goal nor fear the consequences (Steunebrink et al., 2007). This can be logically derived in a very easy way, as having a plan is a precondition for having hope and having hope is precondition for having fear. Third, formalization might learn us new things or confirm things we knew but never made explicit. For example, fear and hope differ by the fact that fear involves uncertainty about the plan. This can be derived from the following: (a) the intention for a particular plan is a prerequisite for having hope, (b) this intention exists if and only if the agent believes it can execute the plan, believes it wants the goal and believes that executing the plan actually results in the goal (Steunebrink et al., 2007), and (c) fear exists if and only if there is hope and the agent believes that the execution of the plan might *not* result in the goal. As a consequence, the agent believes that the execution of the plan could result in both the goal and not the goal. This is the essence of uncertainty. Again, this is a prediction entirely derived from a formal structure based on a theory of emotion (OCC). I claim that these kinds of models and their predictions are an important contribution to the phenomenological description of appraisal: the model describes how the *situational content* influences the resulting emotion. Unfortunately, the way the results are reported prevents the average emotion psychologist to pick up on these results, apart from perhaps those with a particular interest in formalisms (Reisenzein, 2009).

Finally, I will discuss an example of how affective computing can result in theory refinement useful for understanding the experience of emotion. (Marsella & Gratch, 2009) propose a computational model of appraisal, called EMA (EMotion and Adaption), that can be executed and used to explain the dynamics of an emotional episode. This is an important aspect of the experience of emotion: how does the emotion unfold over time, and what are the detailed specifics of the emotion. I will summarize the approach taken by Marsella and Gratch as well as their own example, to demonstrate that their model can indeed shed new light on emotion dynamics. An important assumption in their model is that appraisal processes (the processes that affectively evaluate the relation between an agent and its environment) are always quick and shallow. Now, how can such quick and shallow processes result in complex emotions such as blame and guild, classically associated with effortful cognitive processing? The mechanism they propose is cyclic re-appraisal. Appraisal processes continuously evaluate external and internal events, and in parallel cognitive processes infer meaning and predict longer term consequences. New information generated by both types of processes as well as new events occurring in the world are evaluated continuously, and therefore the appraisal processes continuously reevaluate the agent-environment state. Because the appraisal processes are always shallow, but the state can become more complex (e.g., a remembered or a cognitively inferred future state), complex emotions occur later as a result of the quick and shallow evaluation of this more complex state (relief occurs after a couple of cycles, while fear for a nearing object can result immediately). So in essence, the authors claim that the complexity of appraisal is not in the appraisal processes but in the state generation mechanisms, and that the "apparent complexity" of certain appraisal processes (such as blame, guild, etc.) is an emergent property of the cyclic re-appraisal process. As such, they propose a clear separation between inference processes and appraisal processes. This all would be limited to very interesting philosophical contemplation, if it were not for the fact that EMA is not only a theory but also a computational model that can be used to verify these hypotheses. They show how the case of a bird that unexpectedly flies into the window during a lab experiment involving actors can be accurately described by their computational model. I will only summarize their main findings, by explaining the two key phases in the re-appraisal process of the bird scenario. In the first phase, the actor hears the sound of the bird flying into the window. This event triggers the appraisal processes, of which one responds (*expectedness*). It signals that this event is not expected, resulting in the emotion of surprise. As a result of the actions associated with surprise (attention-focusing, action-readiness) the actor sees a bird close by. This event (see_bird) triggers *expectedness* again, again resulting in surprise. The state of readiness and the nearing object cause the agent to infer that there might be injury of the actor involved. This fact (injury_possible) triggers the *desirability* appraisal process. The process evaluates the situation low desirable, and, to summarize a couple of steps here, the actor prepares to strike the bird and moves back to protect her head. The resulting emotion is anger. The second phase now kicks in. As a result of moving back the perspective towards the bird changes. New information is available (the bird is no longer approaching, it is a small bird). The potential for injury is reevaluated, and the situation is re-appraised as positive. As a result of the positive evaluation and the by now predictable situation, the emotion of relief is triggered. However, at the same time, the situation of the bird is now more clear and appraised as low desirable for the bird resulting in concern.

This new version of the EMA model is an interesting case for this article. It does exactly what would be expected from a computational model aimed at investigating the experience of emotion. It is thoroughly based on assumptions from the psychological literature. It proposes an executable mechanism that is used to explain observed emotional behavior of the actor as consequences of these assumptions. It focuses on *appraisal detail* and *situation content*, and proposes a detailed description of the content as well as the time course of the appraisal and correlated emotional experience. (Marsella & Gratch, 2009) clearly show that if the assumptions of a computational model are made explicit, the model can be seen as an executable instantiation of a theory. In this particular case, the authors opted for validating their own theory, but their approach can equally well be used for evaluating theories of others. As a matter of fact, it would be interesting to see predictions (in addition to explanations) of observable human behavior generated by EMA.

These three examples show that appraisal detail, situation content and core affect can be computationally modeled to better understand the dynamics of the experience of emotion. All three models are based on emotion theory, and when executed generate testable predictions. Furthermore, the three models are insightful with respect to the mechanisms that could be responsible for the flow of emotion experience.

CONCLUSION

In this article I show that affective computing is not picked up in standard psychological emotion literature. I propose three main reasons for this. First, affective computing researchers often focus on the end result of a model of emotion (the models *applied quality*), such as the ability to correctly recognize human emotion expression and the ability to produce plausible artificial emotions. The validity of the model they use to generate these results is not their primary concern. As a result this validity is not evaluated nor reported upon and the computational model cannot be judged on its *intrinsic quality*, the ability to evaluate the theory it was based on. Second, the way affective computing researchers report their research is often not compatible with the way emotion psychologist are accustomed to read research results. Affective computing researchers could invest a little more effort in trying to discuss their results in relation to existing theories and findings in the emotion literature, something that is done, for example, in the work by (Marsella & Gratch, 2009), but not in the work by (Steunebrink et al., 2007). Both studies contain findings relevant for psychology, as I have argued in this article, however, the latter fails to elaborate on these findings in a for psychologists understandable way. Third, affective computing researchers typically attack problems that reside in the "technical" domain: emotion recognition, emotion expression rendering, virtual reality, gaming, and so forth, while emotion psychologists want to better understand emotion per se. I have shown that affective computing is able to help address what has been identified as the core of emotion research (Barrett et al., 2007), namely the experience of emotion. I also show how this can be done, and explain in detail three different approaches that do so. I think that these three examples show that affective computing is ready for a split. A long-standing promise is that affective computing can shed light on feelings and what it means to have emotions. I believe it can, but for that we need to be conscious about why a particular model of emotion is developed: is it outcome oriented or theoretical. This is the split; applied affective computing next to theoretical affective computing. If one does not like such an applied / theoretical distinction, then please note that these are just labels to emphasize the rational for doing the research and these approaches are by no means mutually exclusive. Alternatively, we could simply adopt the term computational affective science (with an eyewink to computational cognitive science).

ACKNOWLEDGMENT

I would like to thank Eva Hudlicka for the helpful discussions we had as well as her suggestions on an earlier draft.

REFERENCES

Barrett, L. F., Mesquita, B., Ochsner, K. N., & Gross, J. J. (2007). The experience of emotion. *Annual Review of Psychology*, *58*(1), 373–403. doi:10.1146/annurev.psych.58.110405.085709

Bickmore, T. W., & Picard, R. W. (2005). Establishing and maintaining long-term human-computer relationships. *ACM Transactions on Computer-Human Interaction*, *12*(2), 293–327. doi:10.1145/1067860.1067867

Breazeal, C. (2003). Emotion and sociable humanoid robots. *International Journal of Human-Computer Studies*, *59*(1-2), 119–155. doi:10.1016/S1071-5819(03)00018-1

Breazeal, C., & Scassellati, B. (2000). Infant-like social interactions between a robot and a human caregiver. *Adaptive Behavior*, *8*(1), 49–74. doi:10.1177/105971230000800104

Broekens, J. (2007). *Affect and learning: A computational analysis*. Unpublished PhD thesis, Leiden University.

Broekens, J., & DeGroot, D. (2004, November). Scalable and flexibel appraisal models for virtual agents. In Q. Mehdi & N. Gough (Eds.), *Proceedings of the International Conference on Computer Games: Artificial Intelligence, Design and Education (CGAIDE 2004)*, Reading, UK (pp. 208-215).

Broekens, J., DeGroot, D., & Kosters, W. A. (2008). Formal models of appraisal: Theory, specification, and computational model. *Cognitive Systems Research*, *9*(3), 173–197. doi:10.1016/j.cogsys.2007.06.007

Broekens, J., Heerink, M., & Rosendal, H. (in press). Effects of assistive social robots in elderly care: A review. *Gerontechnology (Valkenswaard)*.

Broekens, J., Kosters, W. A., & Verbeek, F. J. (2007). Affect, anticipation, and adaptation: Affect-controlled selection of anticipatory simulation in artificial adaptive agents. *Adaptive Behavior*, *15*(4), 397–422. doi:10.1177/1059712307084686

Canamero, D. (2000). *Designing emotions for activity selection* (No. DAIMI PB 545). Aarhus, Denmark: University of Aarhus.

Coddington, A. M., & Luck, M. (2003, May). Towards motivation-based plan evaluation. In I. Russel & S. Haller (Eds.), *Proceedings of the 16th International FLAIRS Conference*, St. Augustine, FL (pp. 298-302). AAAI Press.

Cowie, R., Douglas-Cowie, E., Tsapatsoulis, N., Votsis, G., Kollias, S., & Fellenz, W. (2001). Emotion recognition in human-computer interaction. *Signal Processing Magazine, IEEE*, *18*(1), 32–80. doi:10.1109/79.911197

Dautenhahn, K. (1995). Getting to know each other—artificial social intelligence for autonomous robots. *Robotics and Autonomous Systems*, *16*, 333–356. doi:10.1016/0921-8890(95)00054-2

Elliott, C., Rickel, J., & Lester, J. (1999). Lifelike pedagogical agents and affective computing: An exploratory synthesis. In M. Woolridge & M. Veloso (Eds.), *Artificial intelligence today* (Vol. 1600, pp. 195-212). Berlin, Germany: Springer.

Eysenck, M. W. (2004). *Psychology: An international perspective*. East Sussex, UK: Psychology Press.

Fong, T., Nourbakhsh, I., & Dautenhahn, K. (2003). A survey of socially interactive robots. *Robotics and Autonomous Systems*, *42*(3-4), 143–166. doi:10.1016/S0921-8890(02)00372-X

Frijda, N. H., Manstead, A. S. R., & Bem, S. (Eds.). (2000). *Emotions and beliefs: How feelings influence thoughts*. Cambridge, UK: Cambridge University Press.

Gadanho, S. C. (2003). Learning behavior-selection by emotions and cognition in a multi-goal robot task. *Journal of Machine Learning Research, 4*, 385–412. doi:10.1162/jmlr.2003.4.3.385

Gmytrasiewicz, P. J., & Lisetti, C. L. (2000, July). Using decision theory to formalize emotions in multi-agent systems. In *Proceedings of the 4th International IEEE Conference on MultiAgent Systems,* Boston (pp. 391-392). Washington, DC: IEEE Computer Society.

Graesser, A. C., Chipman, P., Haynes, B. C., & Olney, A. (2005). AutoTutor: An intelligent tutoring system with mixed-initiative dialogue. *IEEE Transactions on Education, 48*(4), 612–618. doi:10.1109/TE.2005.856149

Gratch, J., & Marsella, S. (2001, May). Tears and fears: Modeling emotions and emotional behaviors in synthetic agents. In *Proceedings of the 5th International Conference on Autonomous Agents,* Montreal, Quebec, Canada (pp. 278-285). ACM Publishing.

Gratch, J., & Marsella, S. (2004). A domain-independent framework for modeling emotion. *Cognitive Systems Research, 5*(4), 269–306. doi:10.1016/j.cogsys.2004.02.002

Gratch, J., Marsella, S., & Petta, P. (2009). Modeling the cognitive antecedents and consequences of emotion. *Cognitive Systems Research, 10*(1), 1–5. doi:10.1016/j.cogsys.2008.06.001

Hanjalic, A., & Li-Qun, X. (2005). Affective video content representation and modeling. *IEEE Transactions on Multimedia, 7*(1), 143–154. doi:10.1109/TMM.2004.840618

Henninger, A. E., Jones, R. M., & Chown, E. (2003, July). Behaviors that emerge from emotion and cognition: Implementation and evaluation of a symbolic-connectionist architecture. In *Proceedings of the 2nd International Joint Conference on Autonomous Agents and Multiagent Systems,* Melbourne, Australia (pp. 321-328). ACM Publishing.

Heylen, D., Nijholt, A., Akker, R. d., & Vissers, M. (2003, September). Socially intelligent tutor agents. In R. Aylett, D. Ballin, & T. Rist (Eds.), *Proceedings of the 4th International Workshop on Intelligent Virtual Agents (IVA 2003),* Kloster Irsee, Germany (pp. 341-347). Berlin, Germany: Springer.

Hudlicka, E. (2003). To feel or not to feel: The role of affect in human-computer interaction. *International Journal of Human-Computer Studies, 59*(1-2), 1–32. doi:10.1016/S1071-5819(03)00047-8

Hudlicka, E. (2008a, August). Affective computing for game design. In *Proceedings of the 4th International North American Conference on Intelligent Games and Simulation,* Montreal, Quebec, Canada (pp. 5-12).

Hudlicka, E. (2008b, November). Modeling the mechanisms of emotion effects on cognition. In *Proceedings of the AAAI Fall Symposium on Biologically Inspired Cognitive Architectures,* Arlington, VA (pp. 82-86). AAAI Press.

Lahnstein, M. (2005, April). The emotive episode is a composition of anticipatory and reactive evaluations. In L. Cañamero (Ed.), *Agents that want and like: Motivational and emotional roots of cognition and action. Papers from the AISB '05 Symposium,* Hatfield, UK (pp. 62-69). AISB Press.

LeDoux, J. (1996). *The emotional brain*. New York: Simon and Shuster.

Lewis, M., Haviland-Jones, J. M., & Barrett, L. F. (Eds.). (2008). *Handbook of emotions* (3rd ed.). New York: Guilford Press.

Lewis, M. D. (2005). Bridging emotion theory and neurobiology through dynamic systems modeling. *The Behavioral and Brain Sciences, 28*(2), 169–194.

Marinier Iii, R. P., Laird, J. E., & Lewis, R. L. (2009). A computational unification of cognitive behavior and emotion. *Cognitive Systems Research, 10*(1), 48–69. doi:10.1016/j.cogsys.2008.03.004

Marsella, S. C., & Gratch, J. (2009). EMA: A process model of appraisal dynamics. *Cognitive Systems Research, 10*(1), 70–90. doi:10.1016/j.cogsys.2008.03.005

Meyer, J.-J. C. (2006). Reasoning about emotional agents. *International Journal of Intelligent Systems, 21*(6), 601–619. doi:10.1002/int.20150

Nakatsu, R., Rauterberg, M., & Vorderer, P. (2005, September). A new framework for entertainment computing: From passive to active experience. In *Proceedings of the 4th International Conference on Entertainment Computing (ICEC 2005),* Sanda, Japan (pp. 1-12). New York: Springer.

Ortony, A., Clore, G. L., & Collins, A. (1988). *The cognitive structure of emotions*. Cambridge, UK: Cambridge University Press.

Paiva, A. (2000). *Affective interactions: Toward a new generation of computer interfaces?* New York: Springer.

Panksepp, J. (1998). *Affective neuroscience: The foundations of human and animal emotions*. New York: Oxford University Press.

Pantic, M., & Rothkrantz, L. J. M. (2000). Automatic analysis of facial expressions: The state of the art. *IEEE Transactions on Pattern Analysis and Machine Intelligence, 22*(12), 1424–1445. doi:10.1109/34.895976

Picard, R. W. (1997). *Affective computing*. Cambridge, MA: MIT Press.

Picard, R. W. (2003). Affective computing: Challenges. *International Journal of Human-Computer Studies, 59*(1-2), 55–64. doi:10.1016/S1071-5819(03)00052-1

Reisenzein, R. (2009). Emotions as metarepresentational states of mind: Naturalizing the belief-desire theory of emotion. *Cognitive Systems Research, 10*(1), 6–20. doi:10.1016/j.cogsys.2008.03.001

Rickel, J., & Johnson, W. L. (1997, February). Integrating pedagogical capabilities in a virtual environment agent. In *Proceedings of the 1st International Conference on Autonomous Agents*, Marina del Rey, CA (pp. 30-38). ACM Publishing.

Rolls, E. T. (2000). Precis of the brain and emotion. *The Behavioral and Brain Sciences, 20*, 177–234. doi:10.1017/S0140525X00002429

Russell, J. (2003). Core affect and the psychological construction of emotion. *Psychological Review, 110*(1), 145–172. doi:10.1037/0033-295X.110.1.145

Scherer, K. R., Schorr, A., & Johnstone, T. (Eds.). (2001). *Appraisal processes in emotion: Theory, methods, research*. New York: Oxford University Press.

Scheutz, M. (2004, July). Useful roles of emotions in artificial agents: A case study from artificial life. In *Proceedings of the 19th National Conference on Artificial Intelligence,* San Jose, CA (pp. 42-47). AAAI Press.

Sloman, A. (2001). Beyond shallow models of emotion. *Cognitive Processing, 2*(1), 177–198.

Steunebrink, B. R., Dastani, M., & Meyer, J.-J. C. (2007, July). A logic of emotions for intelligent agents. In *Proceedings of the 22nd National Conference on Artificial Intelligence (AAAI 2007),* Vancouver, British Columbia, Canada (pp. 142-147). AAAI Press.

Steunebrink, B. R., Dastani, M., & Meyer, J.-J. C. (2008, July). A formal model of emotions: Integrating qualitative and quantitative aspects. In *Proceedings of the European Conference on Artificial Intelligence (ECAI '08),* Patras, Greece (pp. 256-260). IOS Press.

Velasquez, J. (1998, October). Modeling emotion-based decision making. In *Proceedings of the AAAI Fall Symposium on Emotional and Intelligent: The Tangled Knot of Cognition,* Orlandon, FL (pp. 148-149). AAAI Press.

Wehrle, T., & Scherer, K. R. (2001). Towards computational modeling of appraisal theories. In K. R. Scherer, A. Schorr, & T. Johnstone (Eds.), *Appraisal processes in emotion: Theory, methods, research* (pp. 350-365). Oxford, UK: Oxford University Press.

This work was previously published in International Journal of Synthetic Emotions, Volume 1, Issue 1, edited by Jordi Vallverdu, pp. 1-17, copyright 2010 by IGI Publishing (an imprint of IGI Global).

Chapter 2
Review of Kansei Research in Japan

Seiji Inokuchi
Takarazuka University of Arts and Design, Japan

ABSTRACT

This paper gives a historical review of Kansei-based media technologies in Japan. Kansei is a Japanese word, the meaning of which covers sensibility, sentiment, emotion, and feeling. Kansei research started in the field of music, because music is the most acceptable of the arts to computer science. In the 1990s, the applications of Kansei machine vision became widespread in many industrial fields, including electronic production, automobile manufacture, steel-making, the chemical industry, the food industry, and office appliances, among others. Kansei technologies are also applied to human interface systems, including the field of brain science, for human communication.

INTRODUCTION

In the 1980s, pattern recognition and artificial intelligence, which yielded very fruitful successes in the application of computer science, brought us close to computer systems. However, in practical applications, the information to be manipulated by computer systems was logical, symbolic, and verbal. The delicate nuances of input patterns were filtered out during preprocessing. Kansei information processing began in this epoch. This paper describes the survey of the dawn and the development of Kansei research in Japan.

Kansei comes from a Japanese word, the meaning of which covers sensibility, sentiment, susceptibility, the senses, emotion, and/or feeling. It is a subjective concept in contrast to the objective concept of knowledge processing. We can find a similar concept in pathos, which is contrasted with logos. Figure 1 shows that knowledge information processing realizes "how to understand" and Kansei information processing simulates "how to feel" (Inokuchi, 1995). In Kansei information processing research, considerable effort has been directed toward human communication, especially non-verbal communication.

DOI: 10.4018/978-1-4666-1595-3.ch002

In 1993, the research project "Kansei information processing," supported by the Ministry of Education, Culture and Science of the Japanese government, began exploring a new field in the form of a collaboration of psychologists and computer engineers (Tsuji, 1992). This project aimed to organize scientists in computer science and psychology into an interdisciplinary research group with the following five research interests:

1. Basic research on Kansei information processing and its modeling
2. Extraction and representation of Kansei information in the media
3. Kansei information in behavioral space
4. Kansei information processing in communication
5. Kansei design and Kansei databases

Because Kansei indicates rather ambiguous meanings, this project limited the range further to a domain called shallow Kansei. That is, it focused on areas in which sensible information is yielded in the human mind from presentations in a variety of media, such as painting, illustrations, facial expression, sound, and music, and how such media representations can be generated from internal sensible information.

Figure 2 shows the social trends progressing in unison toward the formation of a Kansei society in Japan (Inokuchi, 1994). Since the 1960s, industrial production systems changed from fixed automation for mass production to flexible automation for low-volume, high-variety production. In a Kansei society, customized production had high value, and the value of individuality and personality increased.

Figure 1.

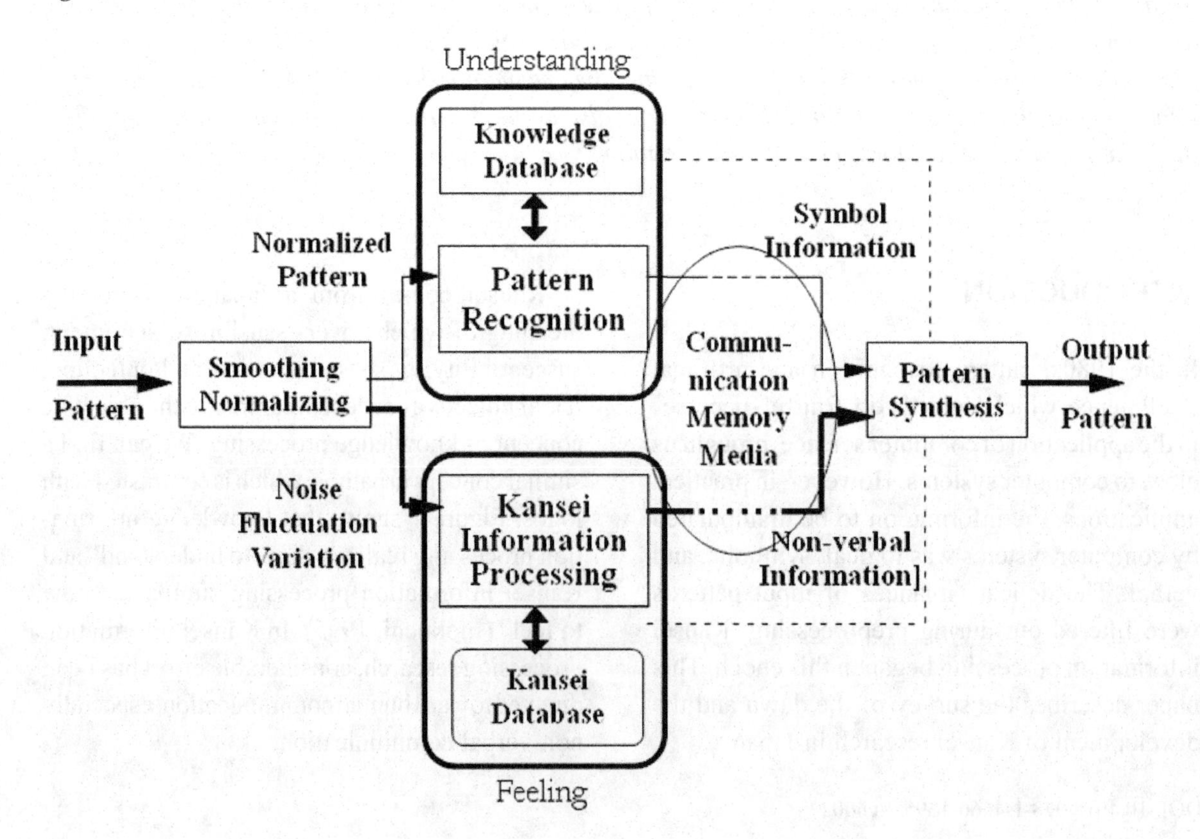

Figure 2.

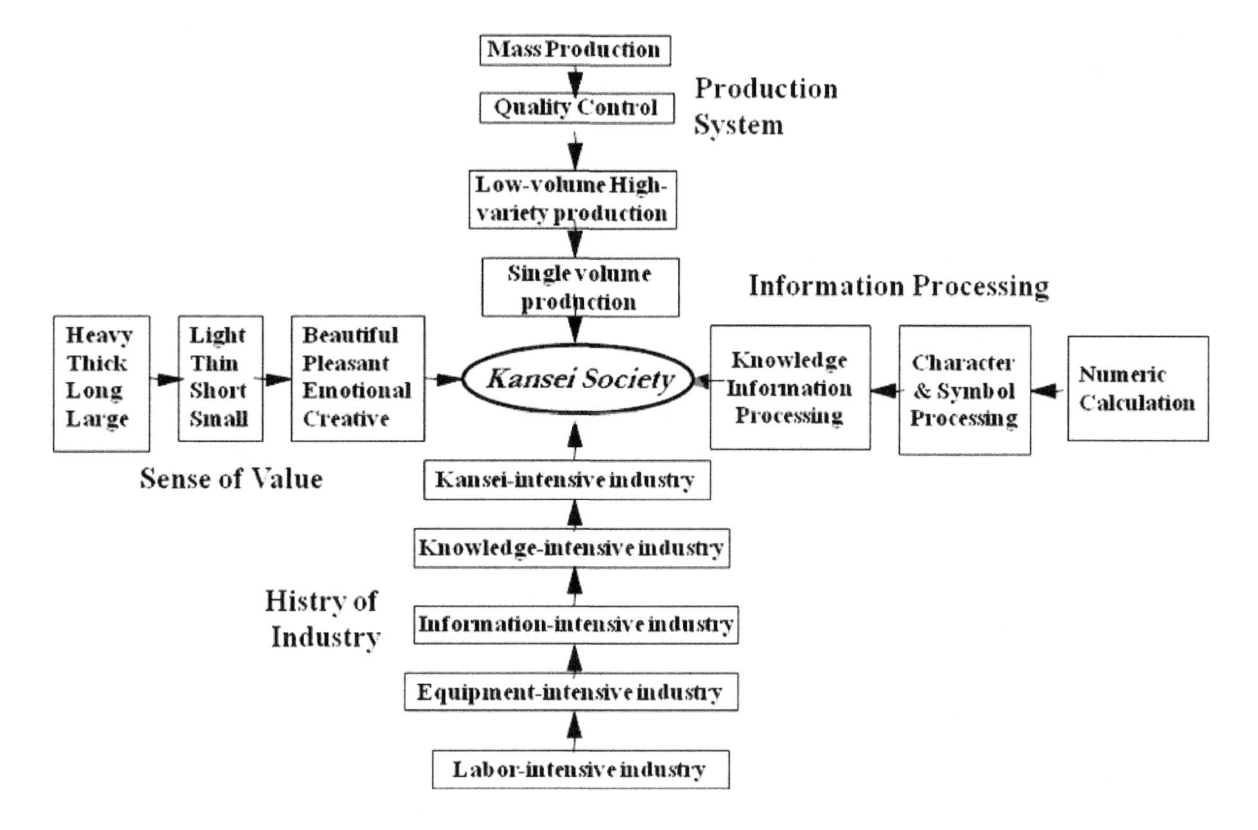

The application field of digital computers, originally limited to numeric calculation, has been extended to knowledge engineering and Kansei information processing. Concurrently, the sense of cultural values changed, corresponding to a value shift in the industry. In the 1960s and the early 1970s, when heavy industry was leading Japan, values could be summarized by "The bigger the better." Adjectives such as "heavy," "thick," "long," and "large" expressed the aims of the Japanese economy. With the prosperity of the semiconductor industry in the 1970s-1980s, the sense of value shifted to "The smaller the better." In recent years, comfort and pleasure are prized as the sense of value. Adjectives such as "beautiful," "emotional," "pleasant," and "creative" have high value. These trends have been progressing in unison toward the formation of a Kansei society.

MUSIC AND KANSEI

The study of music and emotional sensibilities started with the following problem. When a computer listens to music, it may say, "This music is in A minor and three-quarter time." However, a human being will say, "This music is deeply depressing." Then we wonder if a computer cannot also say how it feels.

Authors realized a system, which outputs the impression that a computer receives from music, using a Kansei database that contained the relationships between adjectives expressing impressions and musical primitives. The musical primitives consisted of chord progressions and rhythm. This study was presented at the International Conference on Pattern Recognition (ICPR) held in Rome in November, 1988 (Katayose, Imai, & Inokuchi, 1988). It was discussed in the session on speech recognition, because there was no music session in those days. At first, this session had few participants, but when the time for this presentation approached, many participants gathered, filling the meeting place. Many participants were vision researchers or friends of other participants, and not speech recognition people. This presentation entitled "Sentiment Extraction in Music," made a good impression on many of the attendants. The presenter showed an overhead projector sheet containing sentences expressing sentiments on the screen, while giving the recorded music.

Sentiment extraction is not based on MIDI signals but on the analysis of acoustic sound. Transcription, which extracts musical primitives as symbols from a polyphonic acoustic signal, is a very important means of data input. Polyphonic transcription requires a sound model of the instruments (envelope, tone color). To extract sentiment, it is necessary to enumerate heuristic rules of the relationships between extracted musical primitives and sentiments. The rules used in this system are generated by interviewing experienced musicians. The sentiments extracted from the music "Light and shadow of the youth" are shown in Figure 3.

Next, Kansei research on music examined synthesis of virtuoso performance. Musical nuance in great performances is measured by the transcription system described above. In our system, the information in the score is used as a guide to extract the fine velocity and the timing of key-on and key-off events. Authors constructed a rule-based system that read printed music and automatically generated a sophisticated performance. This system used two major rule categories; that is, expression rules and grouping strategies. Expression rules are used to generate concrete MIDI data from dynamic marks and motives. Grouping strategies are used to extract motives. These rules are learned from a given acoustic performance. Figure 4 shows the interpretation and performance system. This study was also presented at ICPR in 1990 (Katayose, Fukuoka, Takami, & Inokuchi, 1990).

This study led to the Rencon Workshop. Rencon (Performance Rendering Contest) is a research project that organizes contests for computer systems that generate expressive musical performances. In the field of computer science, systems evaluations are required. Because sensuousness and beauty are important for music, a subjective evaluation of generated performances is important for research on performance generation systems. Evaluation by contests in which various systems gather and compete against one another will stimulate scientific efforts. Rencon was started in 2002 from this perspective and has been held every two years.

Professional performers estimate a composer's intention behind the work, form their own performance plan, and generate performances with their excellent skills. Although the ability of computer software to play chess surpasses that of human professionals, the ability to play musical instruments has not reached the level of professional human performers. We have many issues to resolve, including how to deal with intention and affection.

Recent research developments, however, gradually begin to clarify the thought process regarding performance generation; some recent systems generate performances that are hardly distinguishable from human ones. In the 2008 Rencon, a competition was planned where systems have to generate performances of a newly created musical piece on site. The goal is to improve performance rendering techniques through such contests. At the same time, we would like to deal with performance interfaces for expression by humans.

The music and the dance, which are suitable for a computer because their description is established, were taken a lot up by Kansei study (Camurri, Hashimoto, Ricchetti, Suzuki, Trocca, & Volpe, 1999).

Figure 3.

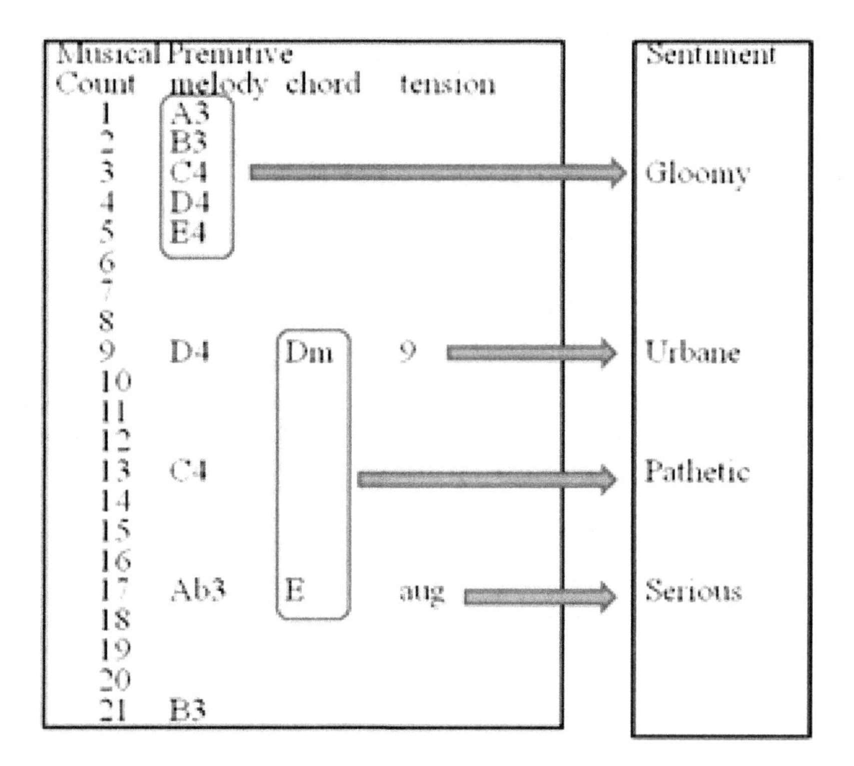

Slow and leisurely caused by speed time – 0 to 0
Sorrowful caused by key time -0 to 0
Hopeful in release time -75 to 75
Urbane in release time -75 to 75
Smart and serious in release time -75 to 75

Whole atmosphere of this music is
slow and leisurely
sorrowful
smart and serious. Level is 18.
urbane. Level is 7.
rural. Level is 6.

There is pathetic mood on chord from 5 to 33.
There is pathetic mood on chord from 37 to 65.
There is pathetic mood on chord from 69 to 97.
There is melancholy mood on chord from 105 to 115.
There is pathetic mood on chord from 133 to 153.

On release at 75, there is hopeful, urbane smart, serious.

Figure 4.

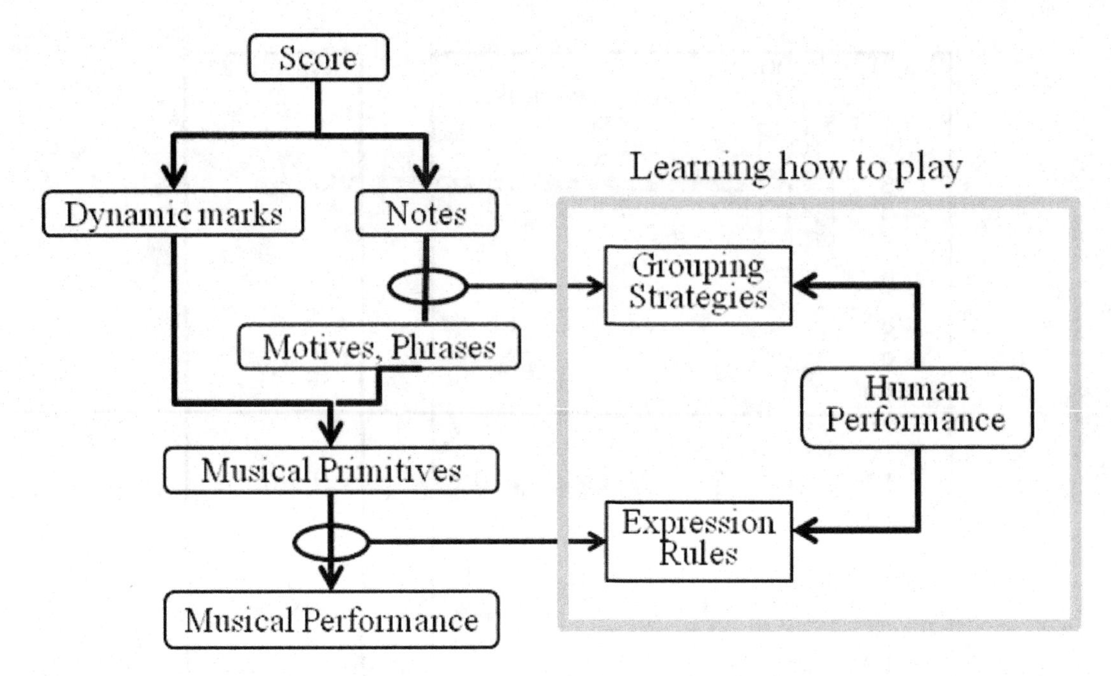

KANSEI MACHINE VISION

The applications of Kansei machine vision are widespread in various industrial fields such as electronic production, automobile manufacture, steel-making, the chemical industry, the food industry, office appliances, and so forth. These applications can be broadly divided into three types.

The first application of Kansei machine vision is in simulation of human vision. Various Kansei approaches have been tried in sensory tests, even in conventional industrial fields, for a long time. For example, various sensory evaluations have become compulsory for the inspection of paint quality in the machine and automobile industries. The technology has been introduced with great success in steel- and metal-making industries for the evaluation of flaws and surface properties, in chemical and textile industries for inspection of chemicals (Matsumoto, 1993) and fabrics, and in electrical and electronics industries for display panel inspections and LED emission display tests (Nakagawa, 1989). Inspection of printed materials has long been a subject of research for sensory tests, and the demands for quality evaluation regarding delicate color tones have become more and more severe. Sensory tests conducted on production lines are required to measure specifications such as luster, quality, and texture, which are not easy to define. Therefore, duplicating the high-resolution and multi-dimensional visual function of human experts is still a problem.

In addition, machine vision technology has made its way into fields beyond factories (Edamatsu, 1987, Fukuda, 1993); for example, the inspection of cosmetics and jewelry (Nagata, Kamei, Akane, & Nakajima, 1992), where the technology is required to make evaluations from the point of view of the consumer instead of the maker. Understanding users' tastes has therefore become important.

The second application field of Kansei machine vision is human-machine interfaces. Machine vision in human/machine information transmission, represented by keywords such as computer assistance, human-machine interface, communication, and media, is a new trend. The ability to process and incorporate physiological and visual characteristics is required in human support systems such as image retrieval using Kansei information in image databases and correcting age differences and visual characteristics. Surgical simulation using computer graphic image in medicine has great future prospects. Further, the transmission of Kansei through facial expressions is attracting attention to "face engineering," which has gained popularity in recent years. Study of portrait making is also an interesting approach in view of the overall research in face engineering; in such research, making a machine with a Kansei-like sense is a problem.

The third Kansei machine vision application is in monitoring human beings. There has been an increasing need to check the actions and expressions of human beings, such as detecting intruders in surveillance systems (Iso, Watanabe, & Sonehara, 1997) or detecting dozing drivers (Takahashi & Shimomura, 1997). Further, for individual authentication in security systems, advanced machine vision technology is required to allow the maximum possible recognition performance, corresponding to human vision, for face and fingerprint recognition. Modeling humans has therefore become an important problem.

A practical application of Kansei vision combining the first and the second fields is in pearl-quality evaluation systems. The unique color and glamorous luster of jewelry such as pearls, together with the taste of an individual, give jewelry its high value. The technical terms used to appraise pearls are extremely sensuous and can be very subjective. Attempts are under way to systematize Kansei pearl expertise (Nagata et al., 1992). The terms used to describe pearls, such as "teri" (gloss) and "iromi" (hue), have been clarified, using a psychological approach; the approach consists of a sense of depth and of grain. In addition, sensitivity analysis using neural networks is used to pick out the wavelength bands related to color appraisal, improving the discrimination correspondence ratio of experts.

Another practical application combining the second and the third fields is in facial caricature systems. Research on machine vision for faces and emotional expression goes back to the 1970s and is currently very popular with a number of diversified systems being targets of development. Among these, research in portrait making is attracting attention because of its comprehensive study of the general problems in the science of face. Recent digital cameras have many functions, including face finding, emotion extraction, and face color improvement, among others.

Facial caricatures are generated by a machine vision system called PICASSO, who was one of the great painters (Koshimizu & Murakami, 1993). It can extract individual features of a face by comparing the given face with a "mean face" introduced in advance to extract facial characteristics. In the generated caricatures, we can conclude that Kansei information regarding the individuality of the face was successfully formulated by this method of comparison to a mean face.

SYNTHESIS—RENDERING OF PEARL AND WOVEN CLOTH

The applications of Kansei technology described in the previous section are based on analysis of the real world. Kansei engineering has been more widely applied to the synthesis of computer graphics, in particular, high-quality images of jewelry and highly natural movements in the real world. The first example to appeal to the sensitivity of the person is a synthesized image of pearl, where an "analysis-by-synthesis" approach, involving a physical model with multi-layer thin film interference specific to pearls (Nagata, Dobashi, Manabe, Usami, & Inokuchi, 1997). In normal thin-film interference, the color change of the interference light largely depends on the direction of the light source. But the color change on pearl surface does not depend on the incident angle of the light. In order to simulate this phenomenon, we propose a physical model of multilayer thin-film interference called an "illuminant model" which pays careful attention to the multiple reflection of light inside a pearl as shown in Figure 5. Some of the light reaching the pearl surface goes inside the pearl, is repeatedly reflected and transmitted and is propagated to the rear of the nucleus before being distributed over the whole nacreous layer. As a result, it appears as if each point in the layer had a point light source transmitting rays in all directions. In other words, the light waves reflected on the boundary surfaces of each layer interfere with each other within the extremely short coherence distance of natural light. Here, as the phase difference of the reflected wave is determined by the angle between the reflected wave and the nacreous layer, the power spectrum of the interference light depends only on the refractive angle. As the interference takes place everywhere in the nacreous layer, each interference ray is propagated in all directions outside the pearl. Taking account of only the interference light waves propagated in the direction of viewpoints (a) and (b) in Figure 5, the light from each point on the concentric circle is the interference light propagated with the same angle of refraction, so that the phase difference, that is, the spectrum distribution must be equivalent. It follows from this that the independence of the interference light color from the direction of the light source and its change in concentric form can thus be explained. To allow a comparison of our result with real pearls, the superimposition of the synthesized image on a photo of real pearls is shown in Figure 6, a synthesized pearl (left) and a real pearl (right). It follows, therefore, that this method can effectively represent the optical phenomena of pearls. This photograph displayed a cover of *IEEE Transactions on Visualization and Computer Graphics* in 1997.

The next example is the computer graphics of naturalness of appearance and movement in the real world. The need for rendering woven fabrics arises frequently in computer graphics (Uno, Mizushima, Nagata, & Sakaguchi, 2008). Woven fabrics have a specific appearance, luster, and transparency. A BRDF model is well known as the basic technology employed for expressing the appearance of a woven fabric. To represent the transparency of a woven fabric, a bidirectional transmittance distribution function (BTDF) model is required in addition to the BRDF model. This paper proposes two rendering methods for woven fabrics, particularly transparent fabrics such as lace, based on a BTDF model.

The BTDF of two woven fabrics was measured using a BRDF instrument, consisting of a fixed digital camera, a movable light source (metal halide), and a movable sample plate. Two thousand four hundred points per cloth were measured by repositioning the lamp and the plate. Then the following observations were obtained: (1) a woven fabric has the property of bidirectional transmittance and scattering and (2) transmitted light consists of two components: diffusional and directional transmission.

To express various types of woven fabrics, it is essential to use a standardized BTDF model with an ability to compress measurement data. We propose a standardized model consisting of two components, diffusional and directional transmission.

A method for automatic estimation of parameters is required in order to apply the proposed model to measurement data. The parameters were estimated using optimization algorithms. The results of rendering based on the measured BTDF and the modeled BTDF are presented in Figure 7. Both rendering algorithms are implemented as shader plug-ins for Maya. In both images, it can be observed that the transmission factor differs according to the position of the curtains, and the resulting shadows feature uneven shading. These results demonstrate that the modeled BTDF is as effective in depicting the transmission properties as the measured BTDF.

Figure 5.

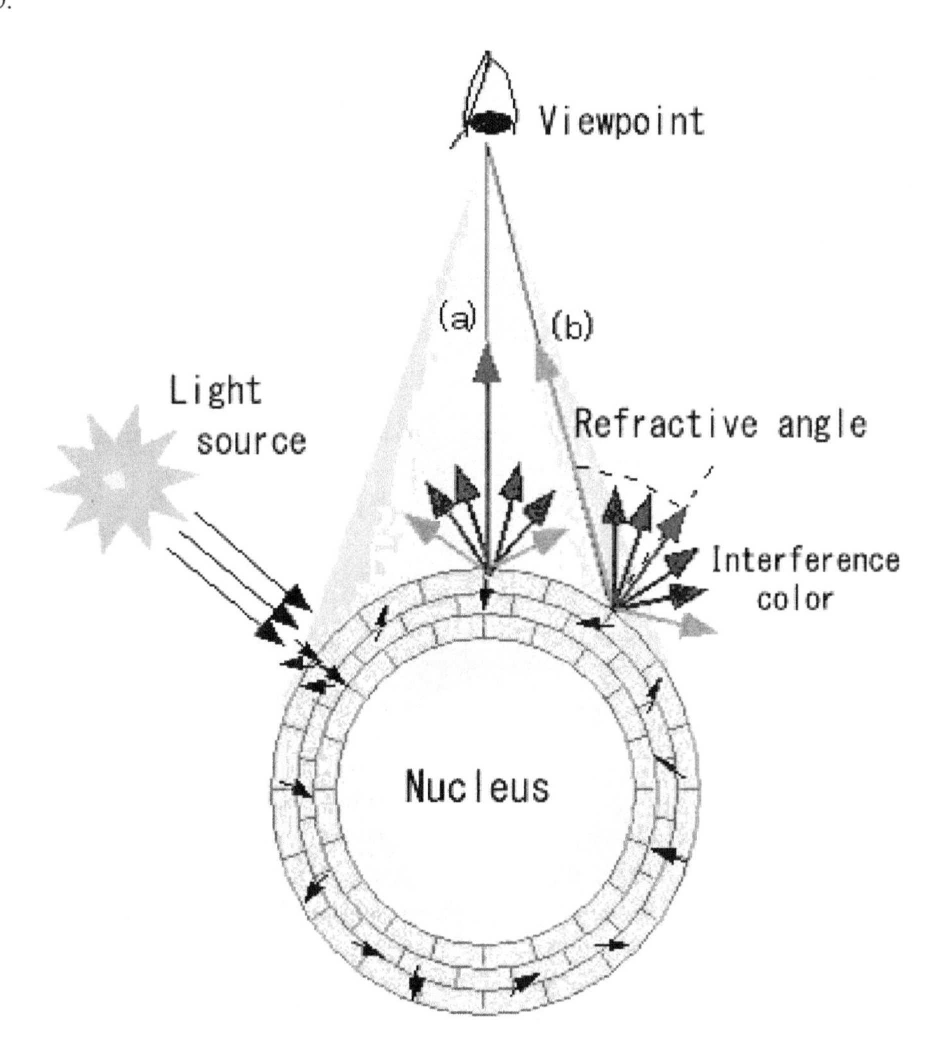

Figure 6.

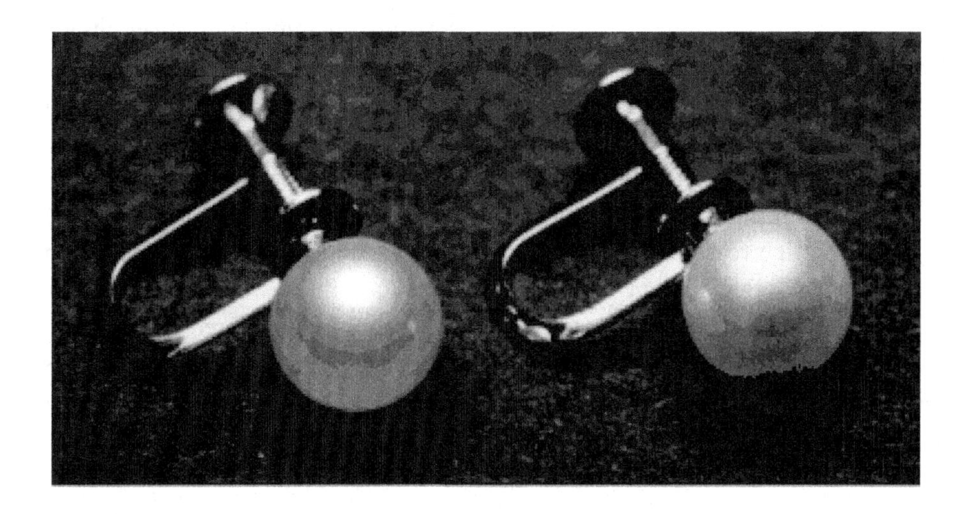

Figure 7.

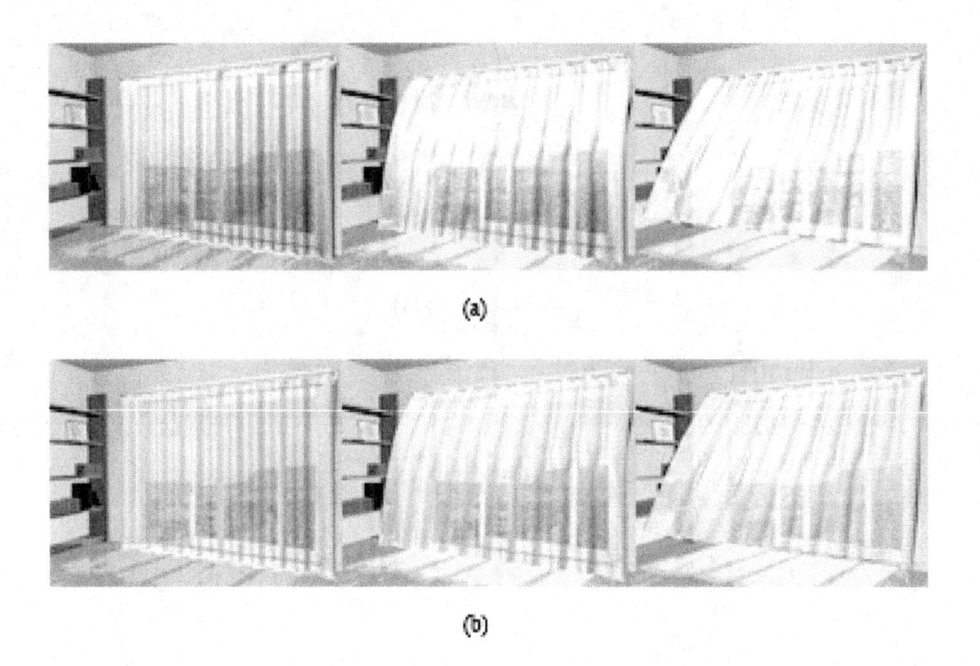

A real-time rendering algorithm of this BTDF model was implemented using a combination of OpenGL and Nvidia Cg. The algorithm was programmed using texture sampling by means of an LUT, which was constructed as a two-dimensional bitmap image translated from the four-dimensional BTDF data. The transmitted and reflected light obtained from the LUT, the background light defined by cube mapping, and a texture element were added during rendering.

SYNESTHESIA—KANSEI AND BRAIN SCIENCE

In the early stage of Kansei research, processes of the psychology including introspection method were mainly used from the reason why Kansei research was subjective activity. From the end in 1990s to the beginning of the 2000s, many physiology indices such as a change measurement of a R-R of a heartbeat, eyes measurement, nasal skin temperature, breathing, and so forth, became very important to increase the objectivity of subjective data in Kansei research. There are a lot of practical examples which help us in our real life. A trial to prevent the sleepiness of the driver by measuring awakening degree through nasal skin temperature is a good example in response to modern social needs.

More recently, brain science became the mainstream and gave much knowledge for Kansei study (Watanabe, 2009; Yamanaka, 2009). Synesthesia is a condition in which the stimulation of one sensory modality involuntarily elicits a perception in another modality. It is said that one in every 2,000 people has synesthesia, and it is about six times more common in women than in men.

Brain activity in music-color synesthetes was measured by using fMRI for two colored-hearing subjects and 11 controls when listening to music (Nagata & Fujisawa, 2009). Authors observed the brain activity in colored-music (color-key correspondence) synesthetes and non-synesthetes while listening to tonal music by using fMRI. The results showed that the fusiform gyrus, cerebellum, lateral inferior parietal lobule and superior frontal gyrus were activated only in the synesthetes, shown in Figure 8. They also found that the area of activity in the cerebellum and the color V4/V8 in the fusiform gyrus which are next to each other were activated simultaneously. This provides evidence for the synesthesia cross-wiring hypothesis that there is a neurological connection between the V4 complex and the cerebellum, and that the activity in the V4 complex occurs as a result of the activity in the cerebellum caused by listening to music.

They also observed activity in the left V4 complex selectively in synesthetes. There can be considered two types of mechanism involved in color perception. One is actual color perception evoked by visual stimuli from the external, real world. The other is imaginative color perception by color imagination.

As their results with synesthetes involved activity in the left lateral fusiform gyrus, the experience of colored-hearing synesthetes can be considered as actual color perception, that is to say, they experienced a dual representation. This also supports the idea that synesthesia appears to be an involuntary experience, instead of a voluntary one like color imagination

Figure 8.

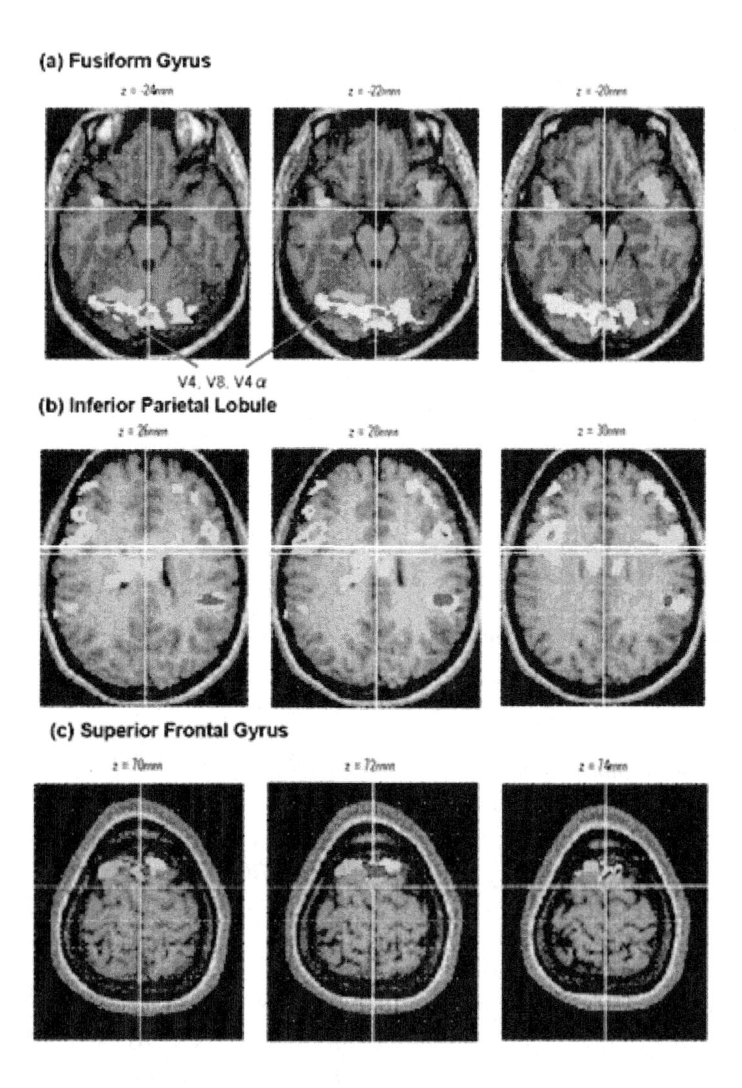

CONCLUSION

This article gave a historical review of Kansei research in Japan. Kansei research which started in the fields of audio and visual contents has been spread into the fields of physiology and brain science.

Japan developed many leading-edge robots. Recently Osaka University group created a robot actor, which can speak his bit and move around the stage alongside human actors. The 1 meter tall humanoid robot is made to be a home-sitter and a caring robot for the physically weak. His new role is what excites us, but it also sends us wondering about the human machine relationship. He seems to have emotions. Gizmo Watch, an online technology news source, says "It's time to switch from emotional robots to some fun and theater" (2008).

REFERENCES

Camurri, A., Hashimoto, S., Ricchetti, M., Suzuki, K., Trocca, R., & Volpe, G. (1999, October). *KANSEI analysis of movement in dance/music interactive systems*. Paper presented at the 2nd International Symposium on HUmanoid and RObotics (HURO99), Tokyo.

Edamatsu, K. (1987). Machine vision of medical goods. *Proc. ITV, 41*(10).

Fukuda, K. (1993). Machine vision systems for agricultural and marine products. *Factory Automation, 11*(11).

Gizmo Watch. (2008). *Wakamaru robot, robo-actor in the making hits stage*. Retrieved from, http://www.gizmowatch.com/entry/wakamaru-robot-robo-actor-in-the-making-hits-stage

Inokuchi, S. (1994). The aims of Kansei information processing. *Journal of Information Processing Society of Japan, 35*(9), 792–798.

Inokuchi, S. (1995, July). From knowledge engineering to Kansei engineering - a study on music performance. In *Proceedings of the 4th IEEE International Workshop on Robot and Human Communication,* Tokyo (pp. 7-14). Washington, DC: IEEE Computer Society.

Iso, T., Watanabe, Y., & Sonehara, N. (1997, June). Automatic detection of a masked person for security system. In *Proceedings of the 2nd Symposium on Sensing via Image Information,* (pp. 167-172).

Katayose, H., & Inokuchi, S. (1989). The Kansei music system. *Computer Music Journal, 13*(4), 72–77. doi:10.2307/3679555doi:10.2307/3679555

Katayose, H., Fukuoka, T., Takami, K., & Inokuchi, S. (1990, June). Expression extraction in virtuoso music performances. In *Proceedings of the 10th International Conference on Pattern Recognition,* Atlantic City, NJ (pp. 780-784). Washington, DC: IEEE Computer Society.

Katayose, H., Hirai, S., Horii, C., Kimura, A., & Sato, K. (2001). Kansei interaction in art and technology. In M. J. Smith, G. Salvendy, R. J. Koubek, & D. Harris (Eds.), *Usability evaluation and interface design: Cognitive engineering, intelligent agents and virtual reality* (pp. 509-513). Mahwah, NJ: Lawrence Erlbaum Associates.

Katayose, H., Imai, M., & Inokuchi, S. (1988, November). Sentiment extraction in music. In *Proceedings of the 9th International Conference on Pattern Recognition,* Rome (pp. 1083-1087). Washington, DC: IEEE Computer Society.

Katayose, H., Kanamori, T., Kamei, K., Nagashima, K., Sato, K., Inokuchi, S., et al. (1993). Virtual performer. In *Proceedings of the 1993 International Computer Music Conference,* Tokyo (pp. 241-248). ICMA.

Kato, H., Wake, S., & Inokuchi, S. (1993). Cooperative musical partner system: JASPER (Jam Session Partner). In *Proceedings of the Conference on Human Computer Interaction* (pp. 509-513).

Koshimizu, H., & Murakami, K. (1993). Facial caricaturing based on visual illusion - a mechanism to evaluate caricature in PICASSO system. *Transactions of the IEICE. E (Norwalk, Conn.), 76-D*(4), 470–478.

Matsumoto, S. (1993). *Image processing applications to chemical industry* (Tech Rep. IEE).

Mcgregor, R., Mershon, D. H., & Pastore, C. M. (1994). Perception, detection, and Diagnosis of appearance defects in fabrics. *Textile Research Journal, 64*(10), 584–591. doi:10.1177/004051759406401006doi:10.1177/004051759406401006

Nagata, N., & Fujisawa, X. T. (2009). Functional neuroimaging of synesthesia. *Journal Systems. Control and Information, 53*(4), 149–154.

Nagata, N., Dobashi, T., Manabe, Y., Usami, T., & Inokuchi, S. (1997). Modeling and visualization for a pearl-quality evaluation simulator. *IEEE Transactions on Visualization and Computer Graphics, 3*(4), 307–315. doi:10.1109/2945.646234doi:10.1109/2945.646234

Nagata, N., Kamei, M., Akane, M., & Nakajima, H. (1992). Development of a pearl quality evaluation system based on an instrumentation of "Kansei". *Trans. IEE Japan, 112-C*(2).

Nakagawa, Y. (1989). Visual inspection of electronic devices. *Trans. IEE Japan, 109-D*(7).

Takahashi, H., & Shimomura, R. (1997). Image processing technologies for driving assist. *Journal of ITE, 51*(6), 746–750.

Takashima, A., Nishimoto, M., Takahashi, R., Fujisawa, T. X., & Nagata, N. (2008, March). *Colored-hearing synesthesia: The relationship between color and music tonality*. Paper presented at the 4th Annual Meeting of the UK Synaesthesia Association, Edinburgh, UK.

Tsuji, S. (1992). *Kansei information projects - what is Kansei information*.

Uno, H., Mizushima, Y., Nagata, N., & Sakaguchi, Y. (2008, August). Lace curtain: Measurement of BTDF and rendering of woven cloth - production of a catalog of curtain animations. In *Proceedings of the International Conference on Computer Graphics and Interactive Techniques (ACM SIGGRAPH 2008),* Los Angeles (no. 30). ACM Publishing.

Watanabe, K. (2009). Scientific research on Kansei - laboratories versus real-life. *Journal of Japan Society of Kansei Engineering, 8*(3), 427–431.

Yamanaka, T. (2009). Kansei-design and brain-functions research. *Journal of Japan Society of Kansei Engineering, 8*(3), 445–448.

This work was previously published in International Journal of Synthetic Emotions, Volume 1, Issue 1, edited by Jordi Vallverdu, pp. 18-29, copyright 2010 by IGI Publishing (an imprint of IGI Global).

Chapter 3
Simplifying the Design of Human-Like Behaviour:
Emotions as Durative Dynamic State for Action Selection

Joanna J. Bryson
University of Bath, UK

Emmanuel Tanguy
University of Bath, UK

ABSTRACT

Human intelligence requires decades of full-time training before it can be reliably utilised in modern economies. In contrast, AI agents must be made reliable but interesting in relatively short order. Realistic emotion representations are one way to ensure that even relatively simple specifications of agent behaviour will be expressed with engaging variation, and those social and temporal contexts can be tracked and responded to appropriately. We describe a representation system for maintaining an interacting set of durative states to replicate emotional control. Our model, the Dynamic Emotion Representation (DER), integrates emotional responses and keeps track of emotion intensities changing over time. The developer can specify an interacting network of emotional states with appropriate onsets, sustains and decays. The levels of these states can be used as input for action selection, including emotional expression. We present both a general representational framework and a specific instance of a DER network constructed for a virtual character. The character's DER uses three types of emotional state as classified by duration timescales, keeping with current emotional theory. We demonstrate the system with a virtual actor. We also demonstrate how even a simplified version of this representation can improve goal arbitration in autonomous agents.

DOI: 10.4018/978-1-4666-1595-3.ch003

INTRODUCTION

Emotion is a popular topic in AI research, but most existing work focuses on the appraisal of emotions or mimicking their expression for HCI (see review below). Our research is concerned with their role in evolved action-selection mechanisms. In nature, emotions provide decision state which serves as a context for limiting the scope of search for action selection (LeDoux, 1996). This state is sustained more briefly than traditional (life-long) learning, but longer than simple reactive responses.

Improving the realism of emotion representations can allow us to not only improve the realism of intelligent virtual actors, but also to make programming them easier. Rather than needing to describe the exact details of a facial expression, a behaviour script can simply specify abstract concepts like *emphasis* or intentional, communicative expression gestures such as *smile in greeting*. In real-time, the agent can then interpolate these instructions with its current emotional state. This latter in turn reflects the agent's recent experiences. For example, a FAQ agent that has just been accessed might respond with more apparent enthusiasm than one that has been interacting with a client and receiving verbal abuse (Brahnam & De Angeli, 2008). For commercial applications this is often desirable, since companies do not want to be represented by "stupid" agents. Another place where real-time emotion tracking is useful is for home assistance agents. Instructions (e.g., to take medication or remind the user that the stove is on) need to be reliable and clear, yet they cannot be always presented identically or else even patients with severely compromised short-term memory can become habituated. Using recent interaction history as a seed to vary delivery style is one mechanism for maintaining variation in presentation style, as well as potentially increasing user engagement.

To this end, we have developed mechanisms for modelling both the temporal course of emotional state and the interactions between such states. We have an elaborate model for complex, human-like emotions for generating realistic facial expressions, the Dynamic Emotion Representation (DER) (Tanguy, Willis, & Bryson, 2003; Tanguy, 2006). For applications with less demand for emotional complexity, we also present a simplified system called Flexible Latching. This provides basic goal arbitration as a part of an action selection mechanism without requiring as much programming. Both systems track systems of emotion and/or drive intensities which change and interact over time. The actions and emotional response of agents containing such durative-state models depends on their recent history as well as their individual priorities or personality and their environment.

Our durative-state systems assume other independent mechanisms for appraising the agent's situation and expressing the emotional responses. Developers using our representations can specify and describe both the number and the attributes of fundamental emotions and express how they interact. In this respect, these emotion representation systems are similar to spreading activation action-selection systems (e.g., Maes, 1991). They are designed to be the root of an agent's action selection, determining the current goal structure. Note that in this fully modular system, additional "higher order" emotions may either be interpreted as emerging from the interactions of fundamental emotions, or they can be introduced with explicit representations—the choice is left to the developer.

We begin this article with a review of the concepts and literature. We next give a detailed description of the relatively complex mechanism, the DER, capable of producing biomimetic human-like emotions. We then describe for the more basic action-selection aspects of goal arbitration Flexible Latching. Finally, we describe full implementations of each mechanism demonstrating their roles as parts of complete systems.

BACKGROUND

Action Selection and Durative State

Action selection is one of the fundamental problems of intelligence (Prescott, Bryson, & Seth, 2007). For an agent (whether biological or artificial), *action selection* is the ongoing problem of choosing what to do next. For a developer, action selection presents two problems:

- designing the agent's action-selection process, and
- determining the level of abstraction at which the process will operate.

A physical agent must ultimately perform precise control of motors or muscles, but this is almost certainly not the level at which decision making should occur. We know animals that have lost their higher cognitive capacity (e.g., lost their forebrains) can still perform species-typical behaviours, although they may not be performed in appropriate contexts (Carlson, 2000). Also in animals, complex actions such as grasping or moving a hand to a mouth can be triggered by stimulating individual nerve cells in associative cortecies (Graziano, Taylor, Moore, & Cooke, 2002), while targeted scratching of irritants can be controlled from the spine (Bizzi, Giszter, Loeb, Mussa-Ivaldi, & Saltiel, 1995).

Artificial action selection also normally operates on a set of pre-defined primitive acts (Bryson, 2000). Even where these actions are acquired through machine learning, they still tend to be segmented into discrete actions, gestures or target postures which can then be reassembled in a desired order (Brand, 2001; Schaal, Ijspeert, & Billard, 2004; Whiteson, Taylor, & Stone, 2007; Wood & Bryson, 2006).

To date, *durative state* like emotions and drives has not been adequately incorporated in standard action-selection architectures (Bryson, 2008). We call this state "durative" in contrast to long-term learning and to the transient state associated with real-time decisions. Certainly many (if not most) current AI architectures do address emotions and/or drives in some way. However, few current best-practice techniques of action selection include fully integrated emotion systems. Some systems use emotions as relatively isolated systems, essentially social effectors for human-robot interaction (Breazeal & Scassellati, 1999; De Rosis, Pelachaud, Poggi, Carofiglio, & De Carolis, 2003; Velásquez & Maes, 1997). An outstanding exception from within this general approach is from Marcella and Gratch (2002), whose emotional system does affect action selection by changing their military-training system's basic reasoning to better simulate civilian reactions to troops.

Most AI research that does postulate agent-centric utility for affect has focussed on it as a sort of reward accumulator. Emotions serve as additional pieces of internal state to assist in learning and applying action selection policies (Broekens, Kosters, & Verbeek, 2007; Gadanho, 1999; Hiller, 1995; Zadeh, Shouraki, & Halavati, 2006). Some of this research has been inspired partly by the controversial somatic marker hypothesis (Tomb, Hauser, Deldin, & Caramazza, 2002).

Several elaborate architectures have been proposed but not yet constructed which postulate similar referential or marker roles for emotional systems, but operating at a higher self-referential level (Minsky, Singh, & Sloman, 2004; Norman, Ortony, & Russell, 2003; Sloman & Croucher, 1981). Such elaborate theories of the role of emotion in metacognition are beyond the scope of this article. We discuss basic action selection, not reflective reasoning.

We believe emotions and drives are absolutely integral to action selection, determining the current focus of behaviour attention. A similar perspective is taken by Morgado and Gaspar (2005), but these mechanisms are not incorporated into a full architecture. At the other extreme of implementation detail, Breazeal (2003) like us treats both moods and drives as essential mechanisms for maintaining homeostatic goals. She has an extremely elaborate robotic system built around her architecture. Here we will emphasise usability considerations as a general-purpose element of animal-mimetic AI systems.

Representing Emotional State

Computational emotion models should include two parts:

- mechanisms eliciting emotions from external and internal stimuli, including potentially the agent's own goals, beliefs and standards;
- emotion representations keeping track of the emotional states and their changes over time.

In the design of emotion models the distinction between mechanisms eliciting emotions and emotion representations is useful; the assessment of an emotional event can be the same but its impact on the actions and future emotional state of the virtual actor can vary according to its *current* emotional state. For instance the event of knocking over a cup of tea might make somebody already angry lose their temper, whereas if this person was happy in the first place this negative event might have little impact, just a slight reduction of happiness. An appropriate emotion representation can enable programmers to reduce the complexity of mechanisms eliciting emotional responses by allowing them to assess an identical event in the same way, regardless of context.

Most existing emotion theories are concerned with mechanisms eliciting emotions (Frijda, 1986; Izard, 1993; Lazarus, 1991; Plutchik, 1980; Sloman, 2003). In contrast, the duration of emotions and the way different emotions interact are not the focus of much research. The same imbalance is found in computational models of emotions—the focus is on the mechanisms eliciting emotions and on their expression, but their representation is typically trivial.

But if we want to use emotions and other durative state in a biomimetic way—as a key part of action selection—we need something more. Thus we recommend a modular and temporal approach to representing durative state.

- Since emotions and drives are integral to an agent's motivation system, their number should be flexible and correlated to the tasks the agent needs to perform. This includes social goals such as achieving agreement with a user. Thus a good durative state system should be able to represent any number of persisting states, such as moods, emotions and drives;
- A single event may have multiple different consequences for different goals and therefore different emotions. Thus an appraised emotional impulse should be able to affect more than one state, and do so positively or negatively depending on their interactions.
- Similarly, the state of some goals may have ramifications on others, so they should also be able to have impact on others. At the same time, we do not necessarily want to fully connect all durative state, since that could lead to an impossibly complex system to develop. Rather, connections between durative state modules should be optional and configurable.
- Finally, a complex agent requires not only AI, but also the easy expression of developer intelligence (Bryson & Stein, 2001). Thus our approaches always focus on usability. For example the DER (described in the next section) is configured by using an XML file.

The Dynamic Emotion Representation

We describe here an elaborate and powerful system for creating realistic emotions for real-time, human-like agents such as robots or VR avatars. This is the Dynamic Emotion Representation (DER). Each emotion in the DER is described with characteristic intervals of onset, sustain and decay, and each emotion may either excite or inhibit any other.

Besides simplifying the emotion elicitation process, the DER makes it easier to generate variety in the behaviour of real-time interactive character-based AI systems, since the same stimuli can result in significantly different (but locally coherent) responses, depending on the agent's emotional state. The DER also greatly simplifies scripting for virtual actors by decomposing the problems of specifying the emotionally salient events from describing the agent's individual reaction to or expression of characteristic emotional states. For instance, a script could specify the general action of grabbing an object. Detailed characteristics of this action, such as the location and effort of the grasp (Badler, Allbeck, Zhao, & Byun, 2002; Blumberg, 1996), could be modified per the current DER state, producing different animations and implying different interpretations. The DER presents a powerful mechanism for specifying virtual agent personalities, by allowing developers to (for example) specify characteristic moods or other emotion-related attributes such as tension level.

The DER was inspired by a variety of appraisal theories (Izard, 1993; Frijda, 1986; Lazarus, 1991; Ortony, Clore, & Collins, 1990; Plutchik, 1980), and the pioneering work of several influential researchers (Picard, 1997; Sloman, 2003). Many other AI systems use appraisal to influence the decision processes and behaviours of virtual actors (André, Klesen, Gebhard, Allen, & Rist, 1999; Cañamero, 2003; Delgado-Mata & Aylett, 2004; Gratch & Marsella, 2004). Relatively few systems provide dynamic emotion representations on multiple time scales like the DER, and none of these are as configurable as our system. We present a more thorough review of the most closely related systems below, but first we present the DER.

Three Responses to one Series of Events

Before explaining the details of the DER we will first clarify its utility with a concrete example of its use. This example involves a specific instance of a DER system (described below) where there are representations corresponding to three different time courses:

- **behaviour activations:** action-selection impulses corresponding to states such as "happy" or "angry." These are elicited by events (either internal or perceived) and result in basic emotion-related behaviours such as smiling. Behaviour activations *trigger* pre-organised behaviours, which follow their own time course after their activations. Activations can be associated with intensity levels.
- **emotions:** such as happiness or anger. This is durative state, which varies gradually in response to events and the passage of time. Emotions provide a context influencing the current actions. The interaction between emotions and behaviour activations is complex—the emotional impulses that elicit behaviour activations can also increase compatible emotion levels and decrease incompatible ones, while the state of the emotions can influence the appraisal which elicits the activations.
- **moods:** longer-term durative state. Moods are similar to emotions, but change much more slowly. In the demonstration, we use

tension and energy as interacting mood components. During the short period of the demonstration described next, they are essentially fixed environments that differentiate the various conditions. However, moods too alter as a consequence of events, though slowly, doing so in response to emotion or other internal stimuli.

We illustrate this system embedded in a facial avatar system called EE-FAS (described further below) (Tanguy, Willis, & Bryson, 2006). EE-FAS provides the actual behaviour primitives or gestures, such as the capacity for smiling; the DER determines when and how much to express smiling.

Figure 1 shows a DER in three different mood contexts responding to the same series of six elicited emotional impulses coming from an appaisal mechanism: three happiness-elicited impulses followed by three anger-elicited impulses. Graph *d* shows these impulses, while graph *a* shows the response in a negative mood (high tension, low energy), *b* a neutral mood, and *c* a positive mood (high energy, low tension). The Happy and Angry graphs have + symbols on them when they result in a behaviour activation—a signal being sent to the EE-FAS system to generate a facial expression (see Figure 2). The EE-FAS contains a muscle model which results in realistic transitions between target expressions.

Figure 2 shows the EE-FAS output. The intensities of the behaviour activations determine the strength of the displayed facial expressions. However the durations of facial expressions are innate characteristics and are not limited to the duration of behaviour activations. Between each screen shot shown in Figure 2, expressions decay slowly to return to its neutral position or to be replaced by a new expression. Typically a happy expression is shown by raising the lip corners and low-eyelids; and an angry expression is represented by eyebrow frowns and tight lips.

In this example, the elicited emotional impulses could be due to the appraisal of six declarations from the employer of the character: "You are our best employee (first happiness stimulus), you have helped us tremendously (second stimulus) and I should increase your salary (third). However, I can't do this (first anger stimulus)—the company is not doing well (second anger), so we will all need to work harder (third)." This sequence of events produces various reactions (such as a smile) depending on the agent's mood, but they also change the emotional state of the character. This in turn influences the character's next action.

In row 1, the first screen shot shows some response to the happiness impulse. However this activation is reduced due to the influence of negative mood. The next two impulses show no response because the happiness impulse intensities are too low to achieve behaviour activation in this mood. In the neutral mood context, row 2, the first happiness impulse produces a stronger activation than in the context of negative mood. Here the second impulse also produces an activation but the intensity of the third impulse is still too low to generate a response. The positive mood, row 3, amplifies the happiness impulses, therefore they all produce facial expressions, and these expressions have stronger intensities than in the previous contexts.

The effects of anger impulses are influenced by mood states but in addition, they are also influenced by the level of the emotion *happy* generated by the previous happiness impulses. In row 1, all three anger impulses produce behaviour activations, showing an expression of anger represented by an eyebrow frown and tight lips. The different impulse intensities, 100%, 50% and 50%, produce different strengths of expression, but the differences are not marked since the effect of negative mood and the building anger amplifies the lower intensity impulses.

In row 2, the neutral mood, the response of the first anger impulse is stronger than the responses

Figure 1. Changes of DER states due to six emotion impulses in three contexts. Graphs a, b and c show state changes in the contexts of a Negative Mood, a Neutral Mood and a Positive Mood, respectively. Graph d shows the emotion impulses initially sent to the DER in all three contexts.

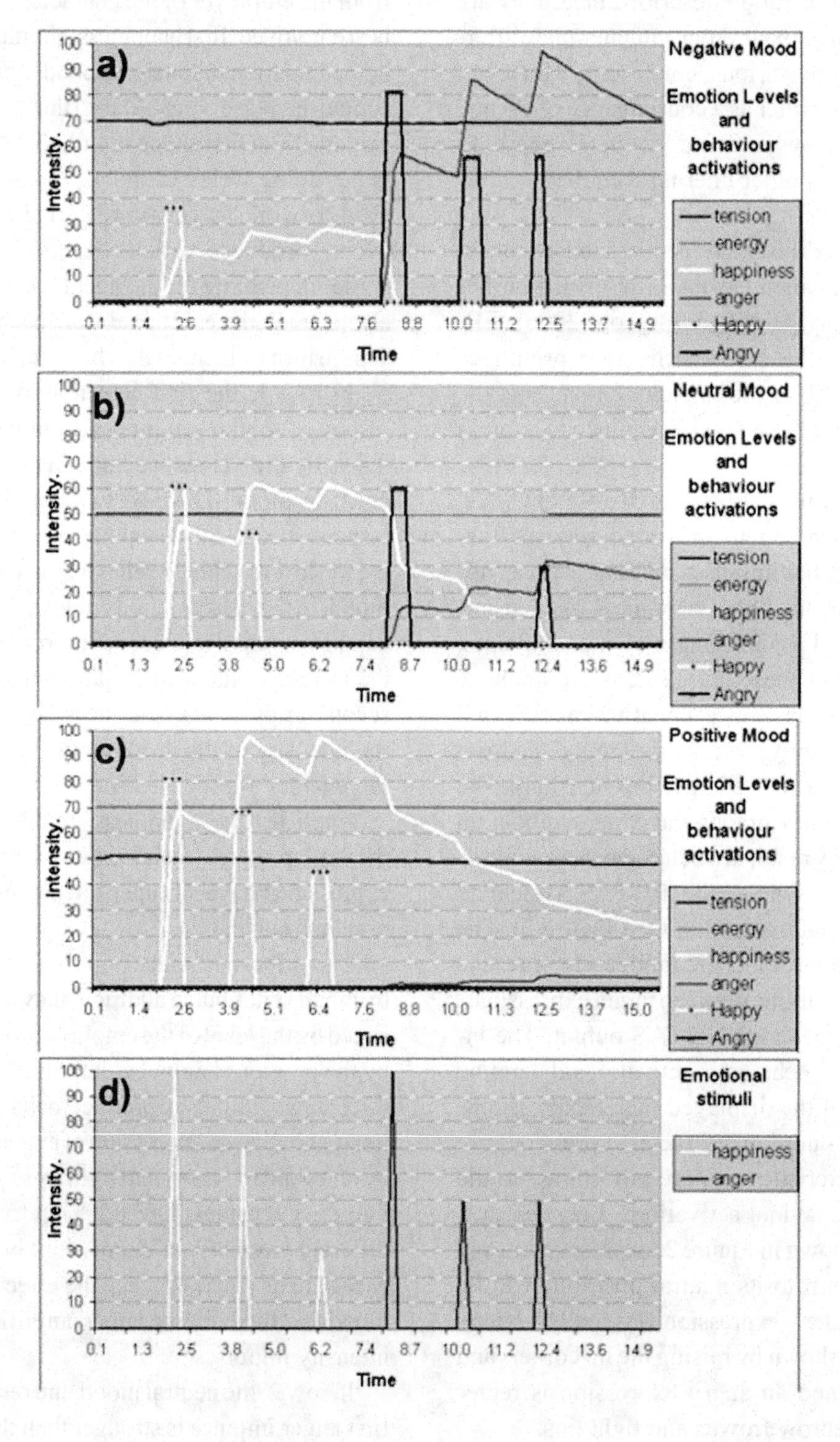

Figure 2. The top through bottom rows show EE-FAS screenshots of the Negative, Neutral and Positive Mood, corresponding to charts a, b and c of Figure 1. Columns correspond to the time when a impulses are sent to the DER, as per d of that figure.

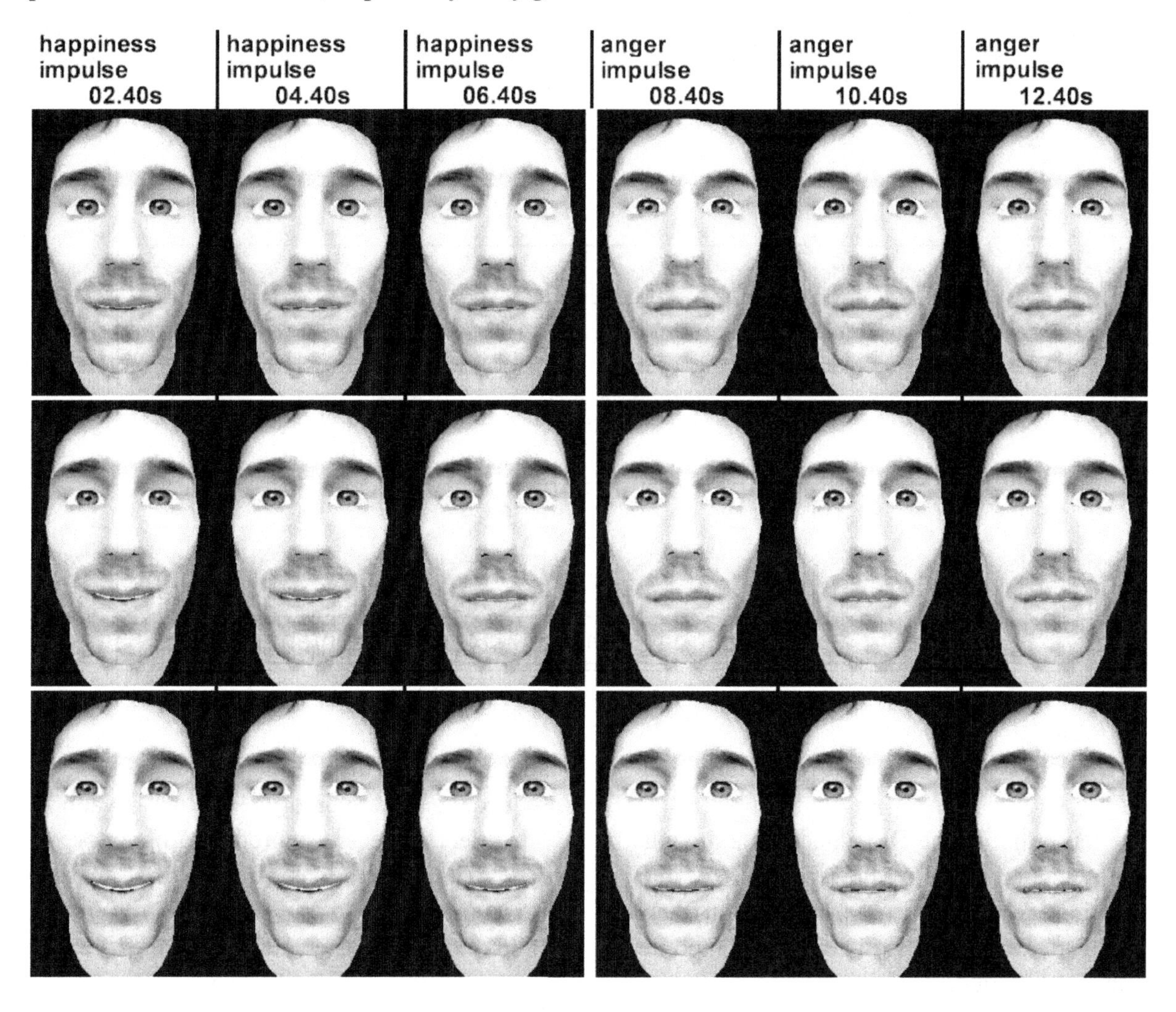

of the two other anger impulses. In fact, Figure 1 shows that no behaviour activation has been triggered by the second anger activation, therefore no new facial expression is displayed. The expression shown at the time of the second anger impulse is due to the visual momentum of the expression produced by the first anger activation which is still fading. The third anger impulse does produce an emotional expression, since happiness has decreased. The difference between these is the emotional momentum produced by the previous happiness impulses. Happiness impulses increase the level of happiness, which takes time to disappear and inhibits the effects of anger impulses. In contrast, the negative agent (row 1) never became very happy in the first place. While for the positive agent, (row 3) no anger impulses produce any behavioural response. This is due to two reasons. First, the positive mood reduces the effects of anger impulses. Second, the happiness momentum produced by the previous happiness impulses also reduces the effects of anger impulses. The largest impact of the bad news is the reduction of happiness which had previously soared.

Figure 3. Emotional stimuli are summed to compute the intensity of an emotion

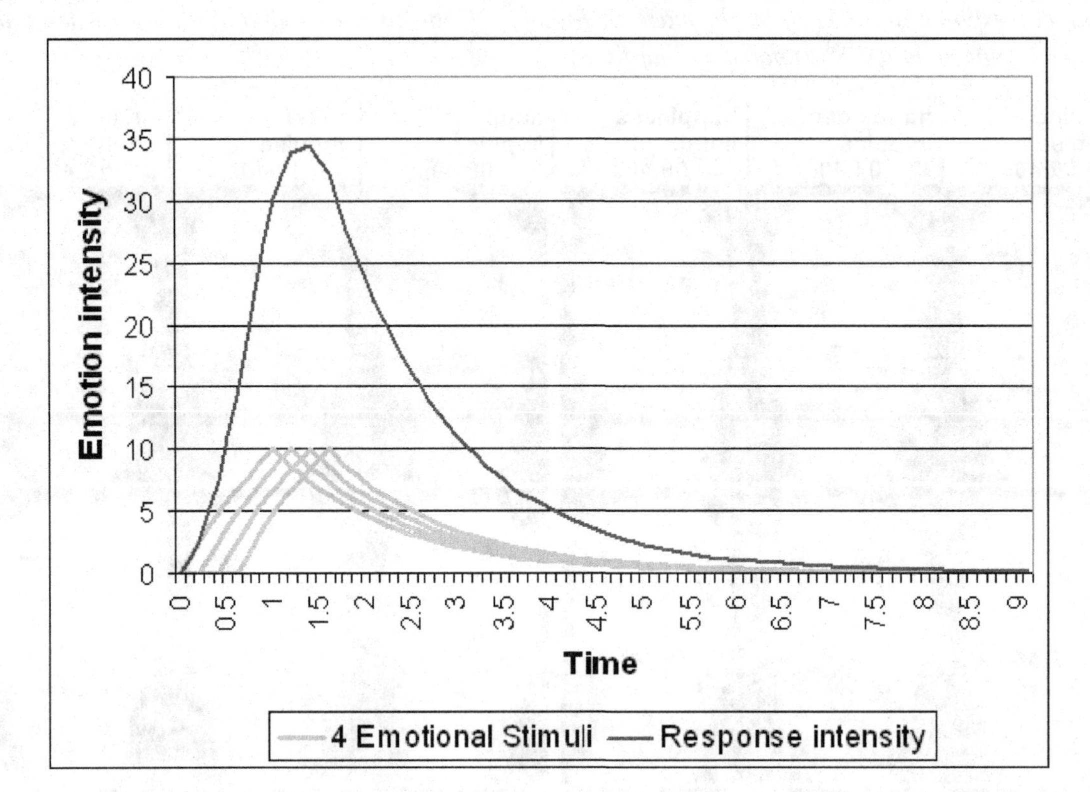

The DER Basic Representation

The basic unit of the DER model is a modular representation based on the (Picard, 1997) description of emotion intensity and emotion filters. A DER network consists of a system of modules connected by filters.

We assume an emotion appraisal mechanism, such as those based on the OCC model (Ortony et al., 1990), classifies events, actions and objects, outputting emotion types and intensities. We call this output an *emotional impulse*. Emotional impulses are defined by:

- the name of an emotion,
- an intensity value and
- a valence, which can be 1, 0 or -1.

The valence specifies whether a behaviour activation is positive, neutral or negative. Fast and slow mechanisms eliciting emotions can produce the same type of behaviour activations with different intensity or produce different types of behaviour activations affecting the same or different emotions.

Emotional impulses are transformed by the DER into emotion stimuli. The stimuli include timing information typical of an emotion type and represent intensity changes over time. The activation curve representing emotional stimuli, shown at the bottom of Figure 3, was chosen to represent the slow decay of emotion intensity (Picard, 1997). The effects of small emotional events are cumulative. Therefore emotional stimuli are summed to compute the intensity of an emotion, as shown by the top curve in Figure 3.

As shown in the example above (Figure 1), the effect of an emotional event depends on an agent's current emotional state. This is implemented in the DER by connecting modules through

Figure 4. Sigmoid functions are used as dynamic filters by changing their parameters

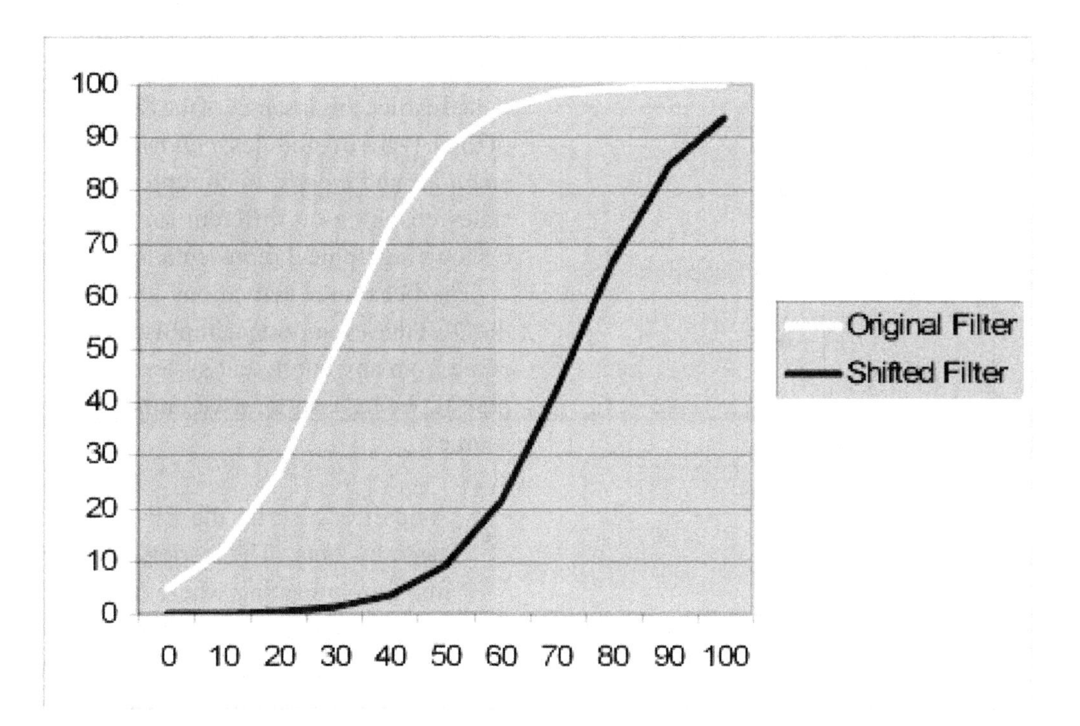

a system of *dynamic filters*. Sigmoid functions have been chosen for this role because they describe "a large variety of natural phenomena" (Picard, 1997). The sigmoid function parameters can be modified depending on the DER model's state, resulting, for example, in a shifted sigmoid curve as show in Figure 4. This effect simulates the change of sensitivity, for example, emotion threshold activation, to particular emotional stimulus in relation to the current emotional state of a person. In the DER model, we refer to each module as a *dimension*. A dimension may represent for instance a particular emotion or a particular behaviour activation. Dimensions consist of a list of dynamic filters. One dynamic filter modifies one parameter of a particular type of emotional stimulus, for example its peak intensity. Some characteristics, such as the decay duration, can be modified. In Figure 4, the horizontal axis represents the input value, such as the peak intensity of an emotional stimulus, and the vertical axis represents the output value, such as a new peak intensity value.

Modules influence each other by passing their output to a bus which modifies the parameters of other module's dynamic filters. This bus is the same one conducting the emotional stimuli; the influence on other modules occurs through their "input" filter. Figure 5 shows states affected by two types of emotional stimulus, *Anger* and *Happiness*, and whether the influence is positive or negative for each type of emotional stimuli. For instance, happy stimuli affect positively the emotional state of *Happiness* and negatively the state of *Anger*. This figure also shows that the emotional state Happiness amplifies the effects of happy stimuli and reduces the effects of angry stimuli. In practise, the higher the level of the emotional state *Happiness*, the more the sigmoid functions controlling the effects of emotional stimuli anger are shifted to the right. This mechanism decreases the positive effect of anger

Figure 5. Example of a network of influences between emotional states and emotional impulses in the DER model. D.F. stands for Dynamic Filters

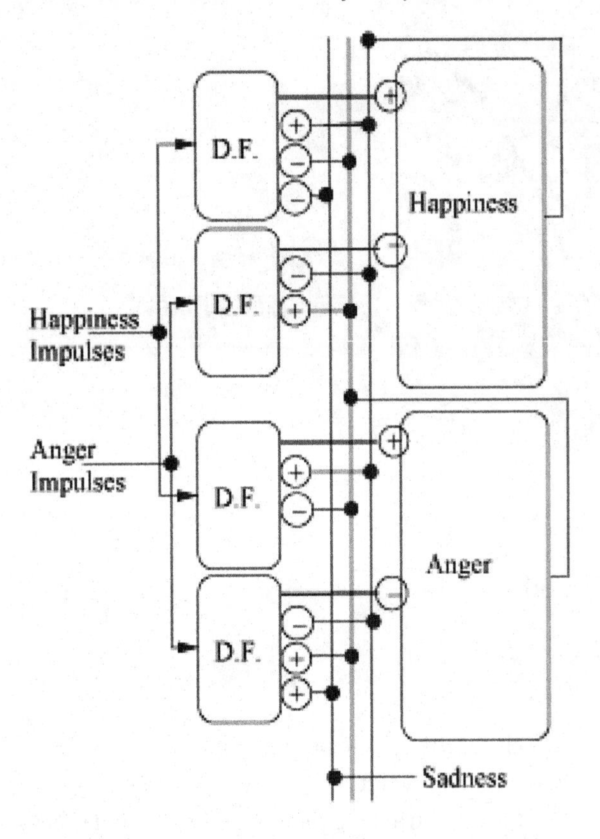

stimuli on the emotional state anger. This simulates the effects of good and bad news on different moods as demonstrated above.

The system can be configured such that any type of behaviour activation can affect any emotional state and any emotional state can influence the effects of emotional impulses on any emotional state. For the instance of the DER model integrated in the EE-FAS (described below), the tuning has been carried out using heuristic values and visualisation software plotting the resulting sigmoid functions as well as the modified emotional stimuli.

An Embedded Instance of a DER

Using the representations just described, we created an instance of a DER and integrated it into the Emotionally Expressive Facial Animation System (EE-FAS), which is a custom-built virtual reality system for producing 3D facial avatars. As mentioned earlier, this instance of the DER is composed of three types of modules: *behaviour activations*, *emotions* and *moods*. Each represents persisting states changing on different timescales. Figure 6 shows a graphical representation of this DER.

The behaviour activations are generated by the DER due to emotional impulses. Impulses can come from any intelligent system capable of appraisal. We have so-far used impulses from three sources:

- As part of a script the EE-FAS avatar essentially acts. The scripts include XML mark up indicating where impulses should be inserted. The exact nature of the agent's acting is dependent on the state of the DER (the agent's mood) and can thus be extremely varied. Example videos of this can be found on our Web page.
- By the real-time appraisal of textual interactions with users. The appraisal of text for emotional content was provided for us by the Bristol company Elzware as a Web service.
- Through button presses on a GUI interface. This interface allows for the real-time influencing of the DER which can be used in concert with the script-reading for demos.

Any behaviour activation is displayed by the EE-FAS as one of the Ekman's emotional facial expressions. However, the duration of an emotional facial expression is different from the duration of the corresponding behaviour activation, as expressions have their own innate time courses representing underlying durative (probably chemical or hormonal) state. The graphs a, b and c in Figure 1 show the behaviour activations *Happy* and *Angry*. Emotions, such as *Happiness* and *Anger*, also produced by emotional impulses, last longer than behaviour activations. In the EE-

Figure 6. A DER composed of three types of state changing on different timescales: behaviour activations, emotions and moods

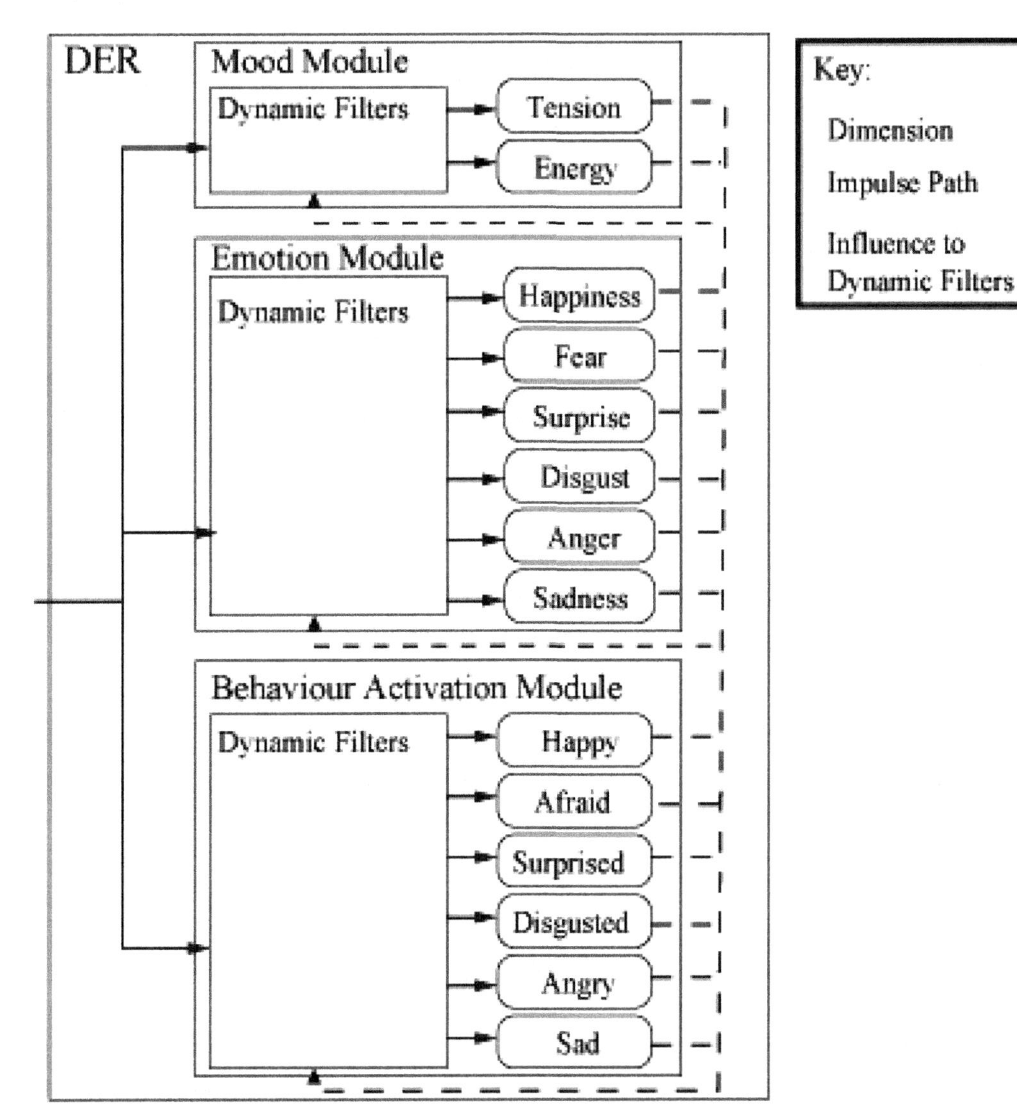

FAS, emotions are also used to select facial signals corresponding to communicative functions when these are requested, for example, by a script. For example, a semi-deliberate facial expressions can be synchronised with speech, such as emphasis or deliberate smiles. Mood changes on a slower timescale than emotions and it influences and is influenced by the effects of emotional impulses on the DER state. More detail on the design of this DER can be found elsewhere (Tanguy, 2006).

Experiments and Applications of the DER

We are evaluating both the believability and the usability of the DER through a series of applications. So far, most of these have incorporated the DER instance described above and the EE-FAS. Ellis and Bryson (2005) describe an experiment using the DER which demonstrates the importance of graphical textures to human recognition of the emotions communicated by intelligent virtual agents. There were extremely significant differences in user assessment of the emotions of the EE-FAS between three different textures: a simple, cartoon-like texture, a photo-realistic male texture, and a photo-realistic female texture. In all three cases, the textures overlay the same standard (male) facial structure. The textures themselves determined systematically what emotions viewers were likely to detect.

We have also used the system for live demonstrations both of the DER itself and of real-time chatbot technology where the natural language capabilities were provided by Elzware. We have worked on integrating the EE-FAS into an assistive home environment, making it give suggestions on typing breaks based on camera input as a prototype system. Below we describe briefly some experiments using the DER and EE-FAS to further assess the human perception of emotions.

There is an open question in psychology as to whether humans recognise emotions from facial components or from full-face configurations (Izard, 1997; Smith & Scott, 1997; Wehrle, Kaiser, Schmidt, & Scherer, 2000). Using the DER in the EE-FAS, we generated different animations from an animation script to test whether humans can recognise emotions from component-only changes—a test impossible with real human faces. By changing the state of the DER different facial signals corresponding to communicative functions are selected. We designed an experiment using videos displaying different facial component actions, such as *raise lip corners* or *eyebrow frown*. The hypothesis of this experiment was that individual facial component actions would influence subjects' perception of a virtual actor and that they communicate their own meanings.

The experiment involved 60 subjects. Each subject watched all 17 videos in randomised order and after each video the subject filled a short questionnaire about the virtual actor present in the video. We showed that emotions could be recognised with minimal cues: eyebrow frown (AU4) is interpreted as a sign of anger and displeased state; lip corner raise (AU12) is interpreted as a sign of happiness and pleased state; eyebrow oblique (AU1) is interpreted as a sign of sadness and displeased state. We thus find that facial component actions are sufficient for interpreting emotions without the presence of full-face configuration changes. The experiment also shows that eyebrow oblique is interpreted as a sign of sincerity where the combination of lip corner raise and eyebrow frown is interpreted as a sign of insincerity. The combination of these two facial component actions was in our system as an emergent property due to the presence of two emotions. All these results are highly significant with a p value under 0.001. Further details of the experimental procedure and results are reported by (Tanguy, 2006).

Comparison to Related Systems

A fundamental concept of the DER model is the division of emotion models into mechanisms eliciting emotions and emotion representations. This greatly simplifies scripting or direction for characters, since once the DER is set and an initial mood described, the script or direction can describe communicative actions abstractly rather than describing precise facial expressions. For agents situated in long-term real-time domains such as Web pages or interactive environments, this also provides a mechanism for greater variety of behaviour per scripted response, since the mood can depend on the recent interaction history.

Emotion models are heavily researched now; of these a number of researchers have made systems to which the DER is more or less similar. The main advantage of the DER is its modularity, flexibility, ease of configuration and relative autonomy (lack of required direction) once completed. Its main disadvantage is that it takes some time "out of the box" to configure, although we also distribute through our Web page a pre-configured version with the EE-FAS instance described earlier. The DER can:

- represent any number of emotions,
- represent emotions or other forms of durative state with different time scale,
- define interactions between emotions, and
- customise the influences of emotional impulses on each emotion.

Paiva et al. (2004) present an emotion model which assigns a decay function to each emotion elicited with a value higher than a personality threshold. In contrast to the DER, Paiva et al.'s work does not implement any interaction between emotions in its emotion representation. Egges, Kshirsagar, and Magnenat-Thalmann (2004) describe a generic emotion and personality representation composed of two types of affective states, moods and emotions. Any number of moods and emotions can be represented. In the implementation of their model the only influences between states is the influence of mood on emotions. Egges et al. compute the intensity of affective states by linear functions through the use of matrix operations. In the DER, sigmoid functions are used to control and change the influences of emotional stimuli on emotions and the influences between emotions. This mechanism produce non-linear behaviours closer to natural phenomena.

Bui (2004) does use a decay function to represent the durations of emotions, but the effects of new emotional impulses on an emotion are influenced by the intensity of the other emotions. Their decay functions are also influenced by personality parameters. Velásquez and Maes (1997) present another representation. The computation of the intensity changes of an emotion takes into consideration the intensity of other emotions, the decay in intensity and the previous intensity of the emotion itself. The influences of emotions on others are of the types inhibitory or excitatory. The DER model is rather like these two systems. However it differs in being highly customisable. Any durative state, such as mood, and any number of emotions can be represented, and influences of emotional stimuli on emotions can also be defined by the researcher. The main advantage of the DER model is that its representation can be adapted to different emotion theories and to different mechanisms eliciting emotions from the agent's environment. It is a tool that can help the community to model different emotion theories.

Compared to some systems though we have simplified the system slightly to make it more generic. Our definition of emotional impulses carries less information than the emotional structures described by Reilly (1996), which also contain the cause or referent of the emotions. Reilly and colleagues' interest was primarily in creating *believable* agents, like classic animated cartoon characters which exist to entertain and communicate. We have focussed instead on *realistic* models, which are more useful for experiments and long-term plotless semi-autonomous applications. The DER model focuses on the duration and interaction of emotions, cognitive referents can be tracked in other parts of an agent's intelligence, or the definition of impulse can be expanded. In our system, every emotions decays over time. An emotion such as hope might be thought to persist as long as the situation is the same. We take the position that hope will decay even if the situation stays the same. However, new appraisal of the same situation produces new emotional stimuli increasing the level of hope. Similarly, the DER could be used to represent drives like hunger. The only requirement is inverting the levels and decay function. A drive slowly increases over time, but then consummatory actions (rather than emotional impulses) such as eating can abruptly reduce its level.

Durative State for Goal Arbitration: Flexible Latching

Drives, like emotions, represent essential goals an animal needs to pursue. The hormone and endocrine systems underlying drives and emotions are an evolved system for providing smooth regulation of behaviour (Carlson, 2000). The problem of behaviour regulation includes allocating appropriate amounts of time to a variety of sometimes conflicting goals (Dunbar, 1993; Korstjens, Verhoeckx, & Dunbar, 2006). Through our experience building the DER for the EE-FAS, we realized that realistic, evolved emotions can have extremely complex interactions. If we are trying to build more expediently reliable real-time systems that self-regulate, we need a simpler and clearer system for describing the interaction of drives and emotions.

Drives as Simple Latches

The simplest way to represent drives is as a prioritised set of goals. The highest priority goal that is currently active or *released* directs the actions of the agent. For example, the goal of eating is only active when the agent is hungry, the goal of evading predators is only active when the agent is being chased. If the agent is both hungry *and* being chased, the fleeing should take priority.

The problem with this simple approach is in satiating multiple goals that gradually increase and decrease, for example the desire for food, water and sleep. When is the agent hungry enough to act on eating? If a single arbitrary threshold is chosen, then the agent will oscillate back and forth fairly rapidly between eating and not eating as eating takes its hunger just under the threshold, but then a little bit of time raises it over the threshold again.

A solution to this dithering is common in basic control theory, it is called the *latch*. Essentially, a goal is activated when a relatively high threshold value (e.g., of hunger) is achieved, but not *de*activated until a second, significantly lower threshold value occurs. Building one of these requires a simple module containing the following:

- **level:** This is the only thing that the DER refers to as *dimensions* present in our simplified representation. For drives, the level increases gradually with time, while consummatory actions can reduce it. Emotions are the inverse --- the passage of time gradually reduces the level, while perceptual events can increase it dramatically.
- **latch:** A latch consists of two thresholds and a single bit (true-false) of information. The first threshold determines when the level of a drive has reached a level such that, if the agent had not been currently influenced by the drive, it now will be; while the second threshold represents the point at which the drive will stop influencing behaviour if it previously had been. The bit simply records whether the drive's behaviour is active when the level is between the two thresholds. In biology (as in the DER) the thresholds are influenced by external circumstances such as the cost of changing behaviours or the attractiveness of an associated stimulus (e.g., rare food or an attractive mate), but we have not yet attempted to build into the simple drive system an appraisal system for such assessment. Rather, we fix the thresholds for the agents at design time.

Flexible Latching

Although the above simple latching is adequate to begin exploring complex interacting goals such as we see in primate social behaviour (Bryson, 2003), we discovered a problem as we began making more detailed models of primate social interactions.

As mentioned earlier, once a drive has passed the threshold required for it to begin influencing behaviour, it continues to do so until either

Figure 7. Performance of three action-selection systems measured in terms of the number of time steps allocated to low-level priorities. This measure indicates the overall efficiency with which higher level goals are met while the agents' basic needs are satisfied sufficiently for it to stay "alive." Latching is always more efficient than dithering, but in the case of external interruptions strict latching is significantly less so. Flexibility in reassigning latched drives after an interruption ameliorates this problem.

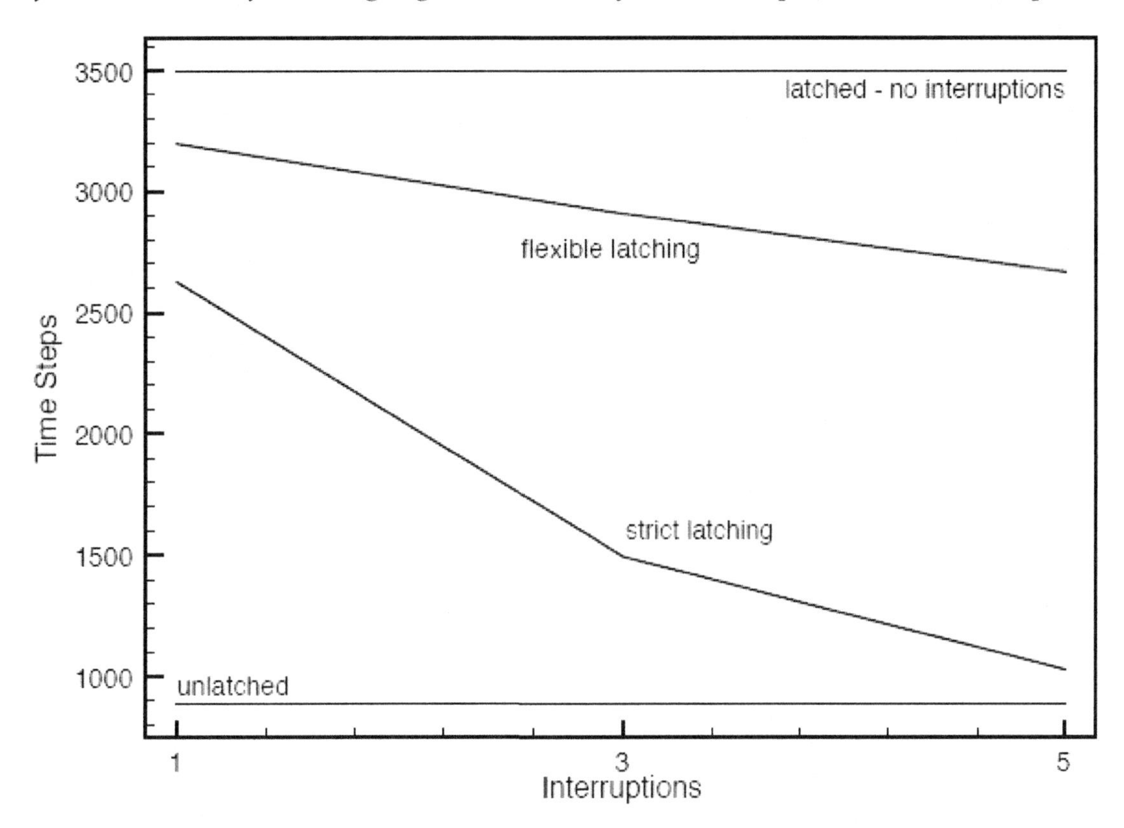

a higher-priority activity interrupts, or another threshold indicating satiation has been reached. However, sometimes a dynamic external environment intervenes in a way that causes an *external* interruption. For example, if you were eating boiled eggs until you were very nearly satiate but then ran out of eggs, would you boil some more? In our primate simulations, a monkey that had not quite satisfied itself with grooming might pursue another grooming partner for five minutes, only to then satiate after just five seconds of further grooming.

It seems that a more plausible model would be the following. When an agent is reliably engaged in an activity consummatory to its goal (or, indeed, is failing to engage in a consummatory action for some length of time) it may essentially reset its lock status and "reconsider" its current top-level drive. Such a system still escapes dithering, but also provides a more efficient pursuit of goals—a heuristic mechanism for sensing when expectations have been violated and it is sufficiently likely that a goal may no longer be worth pursuing to justify reassessment. An illustration of the efficiency brought on by flexible latching can be seen in Figure 7. The cost for this efficiency is low: really, only adding mechanisms for recognising external interruption. Reassessing priorities after interruption is the same as initial assessment which must already be implemented.

In the system evaluated in Rohlfshagen and Bryson (2008) (see Figure 7) the agents had four goals. Two high-priority goals have to do with the immediate health of the agents: eating and drinking; while two have to do with the adaptive well-being of the agents: grooming (which correlates to safety from predation, see Lehmann & Bryson, 2007) and exploring. For the grooming goal, for example, consummation is the act of grooming, while preparatory actions include selecting and approaching a partner. Eating, drinking and grooming all rely on the stability of a dynamic environment—food sources can be depleted and grooming partners can become bored and leave. Also, grooming can be interrupted by an increased urgency of the higher-priority feeding goals. The evaluation of efficiency is done in terms of how much time the agent has to devote to its lower-priority goals in a fixed-duration "lifetime." This would recognise a small class of exogenous events that might interrupt the behaviour's expression. Full details of this system, how thresholds can be set, and experimental results can be found in Rohlfshagen and Bryson (2008).

An alternative implementation of Flexible Latching would be to include a more general-purpose mechanism for recognising interruptions, rather than requiring specific modification of the consummatory actions. The system might recognise if a preparatory, non-consummatory action involved in achieving a goal has been invoked after a period of consummatory behaviour. This period could be indicated by the drive threshold being below the triggering threshold for the latch, or by a timestamp indicating a recent expression of the consummatory action. For example, one might expect a short interval between eating multiple eggs during a meal which would be required to break into the next one. However, a longer break might indicate an unexpected difficulty in finding that next egg, which indicates an interruption. The advantage of such a strategy would be that it would be robust to detecting unanticipated forms of failure. The disadvantage is that it would complicate and slightly slow the basic action-selection mechanism, since it adds an additional check to executing every action associated with a complex goal, except for the consummatory ones.

CONCLUSION AND IMPLICATIONS

This article has presented representational systems for the relatively persistent action selection state often associated with moods, emotions and drives. First, the Dynamic Emotion Representation enables a programmer to represent any number of persisting states and the interactions between them, whether excitatory or inhibitory, linear or not. The system integrates these with ordinary temporal decay. We also described working systems using these representations. Second, we described a simplification of the DER called Flexible Latching that allows an agent to arbitrate efficiently between multiple conflicting goals. Both of these systems require design to set appropriate levels for behaviour, but in fact most commercial AI systems rely more on design than on automated planning or learning. What AI requires is an iterative development approach that optimises between the intelligence the artifacts can find for themselves and what is best provided by the designer (Bryson & Stein, 2001). What we emphasise here is getting the representations and ideas right such that designers have a relatively easy job for building emotions and control. We hope our work helps roboticists and other real-time AI designers when they specify and build their agents.

Interestingly, at least two published models of consciousness are similar to our representations of durative state. Norman and Shallice (1986) describe consciousness as a higher cost attentional system which is brought on line whenever the more basic, reliable, low-cost action-sequencing mechanism is unable to proceed. This is similar to our proposals in Flexible Latching. Shanahan (2005) proposes a model of mutually-inhibiting actions in a global workspace. We do not agree that Shanahan's model can account for all of action selection, for example, see the Tyrrell (1994) critique of Maes (1991). However, his model is similar to what we propose in the DER and with Flexible Latching for arbitration between certain types of high-level tasks. It may be that spreading activation models, while not effective for modelling detailed action selection, are good models for arbitration between high-level goals. This may in turn imply that every emotion or drive an animal has a corresponding adaptive goal for the agent, and vise versa. This would indicate that in agent design, every goal set for the agent should be associated with an element of durative state. Further, every autonomous agent should have as an essential core of its action selection a mechanism for arbitrating between these goals. For life-like agents, this arbitration should be done through a system of mutual excitation and inhibition, as demonstrated in the DER.

ACKNOWLEDGMENT

This work was supported by a PhD studentship for Tanguy from the Department of Computer Science, University of Bath, and by the UK EPSRC AIBACS initiative, grant GR/S/79299/01. This paper extends a previous conference paper by TanguyIJCAI07. We would like to thank Philipp Rohlfshagen and Philip J. Willis for their contributions to the research described here. All code described here is available open-source on line and can be found from the AmonI Software page. Bryson's time on this article was supported in part by a sabbatical fellowship provided by the Konrad Lorenz Institute for Evolution and Cognition Research, in Altenberg, Austria.

REFERENCES

André, E., Klesen, M., Gebhard, P., Allen, S., & Rist, T. (1999, October). Integrating models of personality and emotions into lifelike character. In *Proceedings of the Workshop on Affect in Interaction — Towards a new Generation of Interfaces,* Siena, Italy (pp. 136-149). New York: Springer.

Badler, N., Allbeck, J., Zhao, L., & Byun, M. (2002, June). Representing and parameterizing agent behaviors. In *Proceedings of Computer Animation*, Geneva, Switzerland (pp. 133-143). Washington, DC: IEEE Computer Society.

Bizzi, E., Giszter, S. F., Loeb, E., Mussa-Ivaldi, F. A., & Saltiel, P. (1995). Modular organization of motor behavior in the frog's spinal cord. *Trends in Neurosciences*, *18*, 442–446. doi:10.1016/0166-2236(95)94494-P

Blumberg, B. M. (1996). *Old tricks, new dogs: Ethology and interactive creatures*. Unpublished PhD thesis, MIT Media Laboratory, Learning and Common Sense Section.

Brahnam, S., & De Angeli, A. (2008). Special issue on the abuse and misuse of social agents. *Interacting with Computers*, *20*(3), 287–291. doi:10.1016/j.intcom.2008.02.001

Brand, M. (2001, December). Morphable 3D models from video. In *Proceedings of the IEEE Conference on Computer Vision and Pattern Recognition (CVPR'01)*, Kauai, HI (Vol. 2, pp. II456-II463). Washington, DC: IEEE Computer Society.

Breazeal, C. (2003). Emotion and sociable humanoid robots. *International Journal of Human-Computer Studies*, *59*(1–2), 119–155. doi:10.1016/S1071-5819(03)00018-1

Breazeal, C., & Scassellati, B. (1999, October). How to build robots that make friends and influence people. In *Proceedings of the IEEE/RSJ International Conference on Intelligent Robots and Systems (IROS-99)*, Kyongju, Korea (pp. 858-863). Washington, DC: IEEE Computer Society.

Broekens, J., Kosters, W. A., & Verbeek, F. J. (2007). Affect, anticipation, and adaptation: Affect-controlled selection of anticipatory simulation in artificial adaptive agents. *Adaptive Behavior, 15*(4), 397–422. doi:10.1177/1059712307084686

Bryson, J. J. (2000). Cross-paradigm analysis of autonomous agent architecture. *Journal of Experimental & Theoretical Artificial Intelligence, 12*(2), 165–190. doi:10.1080/095281300409829

Bryson, J. J. (2003). Where should complexity go? Cooperation in complex agents with minimal communication. In W. Truszkowski, C. Rouff, & M. Hinchey (Eds.), *Innovative concepts for agent-based systems* (pp. 298-313). New York: Springer.

Bryson, J. J. (2008, March). The impact of durative state on action selection. In I. Horswill, E. Hudlicka, C. Lisetti, & J. Velasquez (Eds.), *Proceedings of the AAAI Spring Symposium on Emotion, Personality, and Social Behavior,* Palo Alto, CA (pp. 2-9). AAAI Press.

Bryson, J. J., & Stein, L. A. (2001, August). Modularity and design in reactive intelligence. In *Proceedings of the 17th International Joint Conference on Artificial Intelligence*, Seattle, WA (pp. 1115-1120). Morgan Kaufmann.

Bryson, J. J., & Thórisson, K. R. (2000). Dragons, bats & evil knights: A three-layer design approach to character based creative play. *Virtual Reality (Waltham Cross), 5*(2), 57–71. doi:10.1007/BF01424337

Bui, T. D. (2004). *Creating emotions and facial expressions for embodied agents.* Unpublished PhD thesis, University of Twente.

Cañamero, D. (2003). Designing emotions for activity selection in autonomous agents. In R. Trappl, P. Petta, & S. Payr (Eds.), *Emotions in humans and artifacts* (pp. 115-148). Cambridge, MA: MIT Press.

Carlson, N. R. (2000). *Physiology of behavior* (7th ed.). Boston: Allyn and Bacon.

De Rosis, F., Pelachaud, C., Poggi, I., Carofiglio, V., & De Carolis, B. (2003). From greta's mind to her face: Modelling the dynamics of affective states in a conversational agent. *International Journal of Human-Computer Studies, 59*, 8–118.

Delgado-Mata, C., & Aylett, R. S. (2004, July). Emotion and action selection: Regulating the collective behaviour of agents in virtual environments. In *AAMAS ' 04: Proceedings of the 3rd International Joint Conference on Autonomous Agents and Multiagent Systems,* New York (Vol. 3, pp. 1304-1305). Washington, DC: IEEE Computer Society.

Dunbar, R. I. M. (1993). Coevolution of neocortical size, group size and language in humans. *The Behavioral and Brain Sciences, 16*(4), 681–735.

Egges, A., Kshirsagar, S., & Magnenat-Thalmann, N. (2004). Generic personality and emotion simulation for conversational agents. *Computer Animation and Virtual Worlds, 15*, 1–13. doi:10.1002/cav.3

Ellis, P. M., & Bryson, J. J. (2005, September). The significance of textures for affective interfaces. In T. Panayiotopoulos, J. Gratch, R. Aylett, D. Ballin, P. Olivier, & T. Rist (Eds.), *Intelligent Virtual Agents: Proceedings of the Fifth International Working Conference on Intelligent Virtual Agents*, Kos, Greece (LNCS 3661, pp. 394-404).

Frijda, N. H. (1986). *The emotions*. Cambridge, UK: Cambridge University Press.

Gadanho, S. C. (1999). *Reinforcement learning in autonomous robots: An empirical investigation of the role of emotions*. Unpublished PhD thesis, University of Edinburgh.

Gratch, J., & Marsella, S. (2004, August). Evaluating the modeling and use of emotion in virtual humans. In *Proceedings of the 3rd International Joint Conference on Autonomous Agents and Multiagent Systems,* New York (Vol. 1, pp. 320-327). Washington, DC: IEEE Computer Society.

Graziano, M. S. A., Taylor, C. S. R., Moore, T., & Cooke, D. F. (2002). The cortical control of movement revisited. *Neuron, 36*, 349–362. doi:10.1016/S0896-6273(02)01003-6

Hiller, M. J. (1995). *The role of chemical mechanisms in neural computation and learning*. (Tech. Rep. AITR-1455). Cambridge, MA: MIT AI Laboratory.

Izard, C. E. (1993). Four systems for emotion activation: Cognitive and noncognitive processes. *Psychological Review, 100*(1), 68–90. doi:10.1037/0033-295X.100.1.68

Izard, C. E. (1997). Emotions and facial expression: A perspective from differential emotions theory. In J. A. Russel & J. M. Fernández-Dols (Eds.), *The psychology of facial expression* (pp. 57-77). Cambridge, UK: Cambridge University Press.

Korstjens, A. H., Verhoeckx, I. L., & Dunbar, R. I. M. (2006). Time as a constraint on group size in spider monkeys. *Behavioral Ecology and Sociobiology, 60*(5), 683–694. doi:10.1007/s00265-006-0212-2

Lazarus, R. S. (1991). *Emotion and adaptation*. New York: Oxford University Press.

LeDoux, J. (1996). *The Emotional Brain: The mysterious underpinnings of emotional life*. New York: Simon and Schuster.

Lehmann, H., & Bryson, J. J. (2007, September). Modelling primate social order: Ultimate causation of social evolution. In F. Amblard (Ed.), *Proceedings of the 4th Conference of the European Social Simuation Society (ESSA '07),* Toulouse, France (p. 765). IRIT Publications.

Maes, P. (1991). The agent network architecture (ANA). *SIGART Bulletin, 2*(4), 115–120. doi:10.1145/122344.122367

Marcella, S., & Gratch, J. (2002, July). A step toward irrationality: Using emotion to change belief. In *Proceedings of the 1st International Joint Conference on Autonomous Agents and Multiagent Systems*, Bologna, Italy (pp. 334–341). ACM Publishing.

Minsky, M., Singh, P., & Sloman, A. (2004). The St. Thomas common sense symposium: Designing architectures for human-level intelligence. *AI Magazine, 25*(2), 113–124.

Morgado, L., & Gaspar, G. (2005, July). Emotion based adaptive reasoning for resource bounded agents. In *Proceedings of the 4th International Joint Conference on Autonomous Agents and Multi Agent Systems (AAMAS '05),* Utrecht, The Netherlands (pp. 921-928). ACM Publishing.

Norman, D. A., Ortony, A., & Russell, D. M. (2003). Affect and machine design: Lessons for the development of autonomous machines. *IBM Systems Journal, 42*, 38–44.

Norman, D. A., & Shallice, T. (1986). Attention to action: Willed and automatic control of behavior. In R. Davidson, G. Schwartz, & D. Shapiro (Eds.), *Consciousness and self regulation: Advances in research and theory* (Vol. 4, pp. 1-18). New York: Plenum.

Ortony, A., Clore, G. L., & Collins, A. (1990). *The cognitive structure of emotions*. Cambridge, UK: Cambridge University Press.

Paiva, A., Dias, J., Sobral, D., Aylett, R., Sobreperez, P., Woods, S., et al. (2004, July). Caring for agents and agents that care: Building empathic relations with synthetic agents. In *AAMAS '04: Proceedings of the 3rd International Joint Conference on Autonomous Agents and Multiagent Systems,* New York (pp. 194-201). Washington, DC. IEEE Computer Society.

Picard, R. W. (1997). *Affective computing*. Cambridge, MA: MIT Press.

Plutchik, R. (1980). A general psychoevolutionary theory of emotion. In R. Plutchik & H. Kellerman (Eds.), *Emotion: Theory, research, and experience* (pp. 3-33). New York: Academic Press.

Prescott, T. J., Bryson, J. J., & Seth, A. K. (2007). Modelling natural action selection: An introduction to the theme issue. *Philosophical Transactions of the Royal Society, B— Biology, 362*(1485), 1521-1529.

Reilly, W. S. N. (1996). *Believable social and emotional agents*. Unpublished PhD thesis, School of Computer Science, Carnegie Mellon University, Pittsburgh.

Rohlfshagen, P., & Bryson, J. J. (2008, November). Improved animal-like maintenance of homeostatic goals via flexible latching. In A. V. Samsonovich (Ed.), *Proceedings of the AAAI Fall Symposium on Biologically Inspired Cognitive Architectures,* Arlington, VA (pp. 153-160). AAAI Press.

Russel, J. A., & Fernández-Dols, J. M. (1997). *The psychology of facial expression*. Cambridge, UK: Cambridge University Press.

Schaal, S., Ijspeert, A., & Billard, A. (2004). Computational approaches to motor learning by imitation. In C. D. Frith (Ed.), *The Neuroscience of Social Interaction: Decoding, Imitating, and Influencing the Actions of Others*, (pp. 199-218). New York: Oxford University Press.

Shanahan, M. P. (2005). Global access, embodiment, and the conscious subject.*Journal of Consciousness Studies, 12*(12), 46–66.

Sloman, A. (2003). How many separately evolved emotional beasties live within us? In R. Trappl, P. Petta, & S. Payr (Eds.), *Emotions in humans and artifacts* (pp. 35-114). Cambridge, MA: MIT Press.

Sloman, A., & Croucher, M. (1981, August). Why robots will have emotions. In *Proceedings of the 7th International Joint Conference on Artificial Intelligence (IJCAI '81)*, Vancouver, British Columbia, Canada (pp. 1537-1542). William Kaufmann.

Smith, C. A., & Scott, H. S. (1997). A componential approach to the meaning of facial expressions. In J. A. Russel & J. M. Fernández-Dols (Eds.), *The psychology of facial expression* (pp. 295-320). Cambridge, UK: Cambridge University Press.

Tanguy, E. A. R. (2006). *Emotions: The art of communication applied to virtual actors* (Bath CS Tech. Rep. CSBU-2006-06). Bath, UK: University of Bath.

Tanguy, E. A. R., Willis, P. J., & Bryson, J. J. (2003). A layered dynamic emotion representation for the creation of complex facial animation. In T. Rist, R. Aylett, D. Ballin, & J. Rickel (Eds.), *Intelligent virtual agents* (pp. 101-105). New York: Springer.

Tanguy, E. A. R., Willis, P. J., & Bryson, J. J. (2006). A dynamic emotion representation model within a facial animation system.*International Journal of Humanoid Robotics, 3*(3), 293–300. doi:10.1142/S0219843606000758

Tanguy, E. A. R., Willis, P. J., & Bryson, J. J. (2007, January). Emotions as durative dynamic state for action selection. In *Proceedings of the 20th International Joint Conference on Artificial Intelligence*, Hyderabad, India (pp. 1537-1542). Morgan Kaufmann.

Tomb, I., Hauser, M. D., Deldin, P., & Caramazza, A. (2002). Do somatic markers mediate decisions on the gambling task? *Nature Neuroscience*, *5*(11), 1103–1104. doi:10.1038/nn1102-1103

Tyrrell, T. (1994). An evaluation of Maes's bottom-up mechanism for behavior selection. *Adaptive Behavior*, *2*(4), 307–348. doi:10.1177/105971239400200401

Velásquez, J. D., & Maes, P. (1997, February). Cathexis: A computational model of emotions. In *Proceedings of the 1st International Conference on Autonomous Agents (Agents '97)*, Marina Del Ray, CA (pp. 518-519). ACM Publishing.

Wehrle, T., Kaiser, S., Schmidt, S., & Scherer, K. R. (2000). Studying the dynamics of emotional expression using synthesized facial muscle movements. *Journal of Personality and Social Psychology*, *78*(1), 105–119. doi:10.1037/0022-3514.78.1.105

Whiteson, S., Taylor, M. E., & Stone, P. (2007). Empirical studies in action selection for reinforcement learning. *Adaptive Behavior*, *15*(1), 33–50. doi:10.1177/1059712306076253

Wood, M. A., & Bryson, J. J. (2007). Skill acquisition through program-level imitation in a real-time domain. *IEEE Transactions on Systems, Man, and Cybernetics. Part B, Cybernetics*, *37*(2), 272–285. doi:10.1109/TSMCB.2006.886948

Zadeh, S. H., Shouraki, S. B., & Halavati, R. (2006). Emotional behaviour: A resource management approach. *Adaptive Behavior*, *14*(4), 357–380. doi:10.1177/1059712306072337

This work was previously published in International Journal of Synthetic Emotions, Volume 1, Issue 1, edited by Jordi Vallverdu, pp. 30-50, copyright 2010 by IGI Publishing (an imprint of IGI Global).

Chapter 4
Emotion as a Significant Change in Neural Activity

Karla Parussel
University of Stirling, Scotland

ABSTRACT

It is hypothesized here that two classes of emotions exist: driving and satisfying emotions. Driving emotions significantly increase the internal activity of the brain and result in the agent seeking to minimize its emotional state by performing actions that it would not otherwise do. Satisfying emotions decrease internal activity and encourage the agent to continue its current behavior to maintain its emotional state. It is theorized that neuromodulators act as simple yet high impact signals to either agitate or calm specific neural networks. This results in what we can define as either driving or satisfying emotions. The plausibility of this hypothesis is tested in this paper using feed-forward networks of leaky integrate-and-fire neurons.

INTRODUCTION

Driving and Satisfying Emotions

Emotions in a natural agent are either pleasant or unpleasant, but never neutral, (Nesse, 1990). We can understand emotions as being either positive or negative, (Zhang & Lee, 2009). This may be useful when describing emotions from a personal perspective, but this description carries connotations and an implicit judgment on their utility. We need to differentiate between the experience of an emotion and its effect. For example, it may be argued that anger is a negative emotion because it is unpleasant to experience. An equally valid argument is that anger has positive motivational benefits. Nesse gives an example of the rationality of anger. In a long term, committed social partnership where one party is tempted to defect, the threat of an irrational and spiteful retaliation because of the betrayed partner's anger decreases the likelihood of a defection continuing or even taking place at all.

We could also think of emotions as being either attractive or repulsive. This may be useful when describing emotions within the context of a dynamical system but it is less applicable when describing animal or human behavior. For example

DOI: 10.4018/978-1-4666-1595-3.ch004

sadness and fear are repulsive emotions that we normally seek to minimize but people deliberately invoke sadness by watching soap operas and other melodramas. They deliberately invoke fear when reading or watching thrillers or by participating in fun-fair rides or extreme sports. In the latter case, people engage in these activities because they are also exciting and fun. Emotions can be simultaneously attractive and repulsive.

Rolls (2005, p. 118) describes emotions in terms of rewards and punishments. An animal will work for a reward, but will work to escape or avoid a punishment.

Emotions are proposed as being states elicited by rewards and punishers and changes in reward and punishment (Rolls, 1999, p. 60). Contentment can be considered a rewarding emotional state for example, but how is this different from the emotion of joy? Rolls uses the concept of positive and negative reinforcers and punishers as determined by whether the reinforcer or punisher increases the probability of a response by the agent.

These terms may be useful when describing observations of animal behavior but they are less descriptive when referring to emotional experiences or an appreciation of why rewards and punishers have the effect that they do. Animals *experience* reward and punishment. From the perspective of the animal, reward and punishment is more than mere habituation and conditioning.

It can be seen that the utility and limitations of the descriptions that we use partially depend upon the context in which they are employed. Can we decide on terms that are unambiguous regardless of whether we are referring to the experience of emotions or observations of animal behavior? It is proposed here that emotions can be thought of as being either *driving* or *satisfying*. These terms describe both the experience and behavioral effect of being in an emotional state and are also neutral as to its utility. This is more than a mere linguistic exercise; there is a theoretical basis behind these terms.

Rolls (2005, p. 128), discusses how *taxes* orient an organism toward or away from stimuli in its environment. Phototaxis bends a plant toward a light source for example. An organism may move toward sources of nutrients or away from materials with physical properties detrimental to its health.

Animals need to maintain homeostasis. Various bodily processes need to be kept relatively constant. Critical resources must be kept replete regardless of the environment that the agent may inhabit. Examples of these resources include levels of food, water and oxygen. Internal physiological variables must also be kept within a certain range. For example, natural agents will seek warmth when it is too cold and try to cool down when it is too hot.

Panksepp (1998) describes how sensations generate pleasure or displeasure depending on the homeostatic equilibrium of the body. For example, food tastes better when we are hungry (p. 164). Panksepp also discusses the idea of emotional attractors in the brain as reflected by repetitive patterns of electrical activities that are triggered by specific environmental stimuli (p. 94).

When discussing homeostasis we can think of driving emotions occurring when the organism needs to reassert the internal equilibrium of its physiological processes. Satisfying emotions would ensue when equilibrium is reasserted or maintained. Although successful adaptation to an environment is more than a matter of maintaining homeostasis, the concepts apply equally well to neutral actions and behaviors that have no intrinsic value to the maintenance of the body. For example, animals may be driven to seek out others to breed and socially bond with, and can be satisfied and settle down when they do.

So far we have only judged emotions as being driving or satisfying. If these terms are to be non-ambiguous then we need to be able to determine their classification through quantifiable measurements rather than via interpretation.

The Hypothesis

The brain can be understood as a self-organizing system (Kelso, 1995; Von der Malsburg, 2003). The way that a normal brain functions internally is not directly determined by an external controller. Instead the brain reacts to signals from the agent's senses.

If the brain self-organizes then there must be attractors or relatively stable states that it can settle into. When other physical systems self-organize they normally do so as their own internal energy dissipates or is minimized. Patterns can emerge instantaneously in a chaotic system but also disappear again just as quickly. Patterns persist in a self-organizing system because there is insufficient energy or activity to break them apart. We can see this happen with crystallization when a liquid becomes supersaturated as it cools. If the liquid is re-heated then the activity of the molecules is increased and the patterns start to break up.

It was discussed above how Panksepp refers to emotional attractors in the brain as seen by repetitive patterns of electrical activities. The assumption made in this paper is that the brain self-organizes by settling into stable states, or attractors, as characterized by a reduction in internal activity. This assumption is consistent with how models of artificial neural networks developed by the author are understood to self-organize.

Feed-forward networks of leaky integrate-and-fire neurons can be made to self-organize by minimizing the strength of their input activity. This consequently also reduces the internal activity of the network (Parussel, 2006). The networks act as minimal disturbance systems. Incoming activation is directed to neurons in the output layer and the action that corresponds to the winning neuron is performed accordingly. If the action has desirable consequences then the appropriate input signals fed to the network are temporarily reduced in strength. Actions that reduce the strength of the input signal have a greater chance of being performed again in the future. If an action does not subsequently decrease the strength of the input signal then other actions have an equal chance of being performed.

It was shown that the networks can be biased toward exploration using inhibitory neuromodulators in the middle layer. This agitates the network out of any relatively stable state to increase the chance of it exploring other actions, (Parussel, 2006). The networks can also be biased toward exploitation using excitatory neuromodulators at the output layer, (Parussel & Cañamero, 2007). Emotions can be modulated by altering the levels of neuromodulators in a brain. Kelley (2005) and Fellous (2004) argue that emotions provide a multi-level communication of simplified but high impact information. Fellous (1999) also argues that emotion can be seen as continuous patterns of neuromodulation of certain brain structures

The hypothesis made here is that neuromodulators are used to either aid or hamper the brain in minimizing its internal activity. It is theorized that neuromodulators are used for this purpose to act as simple yet high impact signals to either agitate or calm specific neural networks. This results in what we can define as either driving or satisfying emotions. Driving emotions significantly increase the internal activity of the brain and result in the agent seeking to minimize its emotional state by performing actions that it would not otherwise do. Satisfying emotions significantly decrease the internal activity of the brain and increase the probability of the agent in continuing its current behavior to maintain its emotional state.

Noble (1997) argues that Artificial Life simulations cannot prove theories concerning the real world. The role of such models is to establish the plausibility of a theory. The theory can then be referred back to the relevant empirical science in order to be proven in the natural world. The plausibility of the above hypothesis given the stated assumptions and observations is tested in this paper.

METHOD

The System

A self-organizing biologically inspired neural network has been developed so as to explore the functionality provided by neuromodulation. The intention is to increase our understanding of emotions by researching the functionality of the mechanisms underlying them.

The artificial life animat concept has been abstracted to provide the simplest possible context for testing the effect of neuromodulation when applied to an artificial neural network. A stimulus-response agent has been created that can neither sense an environment nor be affected by one. The only thing that it interacts with is a body with two resources, labeled "Energy" and "Water" (see Figure 1).

Each change in resource level is passed to the agent controller as an input signal. Before being input, they are scaled to the largest increase and decrease that has occurred to each resource so as to be within the range [0, 1]. They are then inverted so that desirable changes, such as increases to a resource level, result in a reduced signal to the agent controller.

Figure 1. Agent as a system schematic; body, agent controller, actions

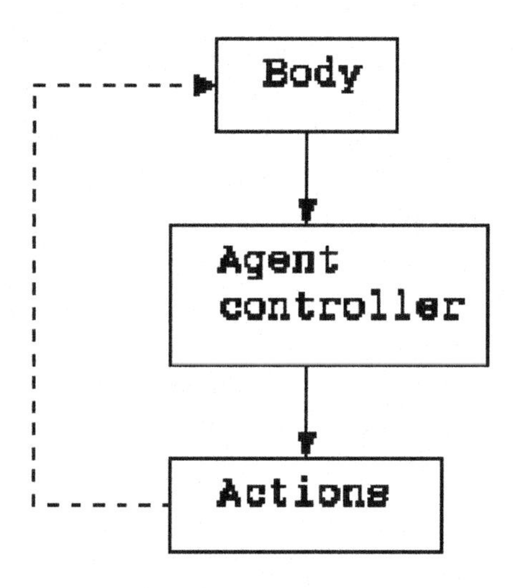

The agent can execute a set of actions that either increase or decrease by a given amount the energy or water level in the body, plus two neutral actions. Neutral actions are useful because if they are used differently to each other then it throws doubt on how well the agent is adapting. The 'Inactive' action is used by default when an agent fails to choose for itself. This can happen if no activation reaches the output neurons of its neural network. It results in each resource of the agent being reduced by the maximum cost. The effect of this is more costly to the agent than if it deliberately chose the most costly action available to it as that would only result in a reduction of one resource.

The Neural Network

The agent adapts using a feed forward neural network of spiking leaky integrate-and-fire neurons based on the model described in Koch (1999, p. 339) and Wehmeier, Dong, Koch, and Essen (1989).

The network learns which outputs should be most frequently and strongly fired to minimize the subsequent level of input signal in the next turn. Each neural network is made up of three distinct layers; input, middle and output.

For each resource, the input layer has two neurons that output to the middle layer. One neuron signals the need for the resource and the other neuron signals the satisfaction of that need. There are situations in which an effective behavior for an agent may be to decrease a need but not satisfy it. Alternatively there may be situations in which an agent needs to store more resources than it is used to doing. In these experiments the agent is tasked only with maximizing its resources.

There is one output neuron per action. The network is iterated over a fixed number of times within a single turn. The action corresponding to the output neuron with the greatest average activation is then performed. The action performed by the agent directly and immediately alters the level of a resource. This consequently determines the strength of the corresponding input signal fed to the network in the next turn. This is fed via the input neurons corresponding to the resource affected by the action. This allows the network to act as a minimal disturbance system (W¨org¨otter & Porr, 2004) as it settles upon actions that reduce its total input activation.

The Neuron

Spiking neurons were used in the neural network, each one acting as a capacitor to integrate and contain the charge delivered by synaptic input. This charge slowly leaks away over time. The neurons have a fixed voltage threshold and base leakage which are genetically determined.

The neurons also have an adaptive leakage to account for how frequently they have recently spiked. If a neuron spikes then its leakage is increased by a genetically determined amount. If the neuron does not spike then the leakage is decreased by that same amount[1]. Resistance is constrained within the range [0, 1]. This model was inspired by the adapting integrate-and-fire models described in Koch (1999, p. 339).

The spiking threshold is the same for all neurons in the network and is constant. The neurons are stochastic so that once the spiking threshold has been reached, there is a random chance that a spike will be transmitted along the output weights. Either way the cell loses its activation[2].

The neurons send out a stereotypical spike. This is implemented as having a binary output. The weights connecting the neurons are constrained within the range [0, 1].

Local Learning Rule

The learning rule employed uses spike timing-dependent plasticity (Bi & Wang, 2002). It is implemented as a two-coincidence-detector model (Karmarkar & Buonomano, 2002; Karmarkar, Najariana, & Buonomano, 2002) based on Song, Miller, and Abbott (2000) and later evolved for use in robots by Di Paolo (2003). Each neuron has its own post-synaptic recording function that is incremented when the neuron spikes and which decays over time in-between spikes. This is compared to the pre-synaptic recording function of the neuron that has transmitted the activation. Each layer of neurons has its own increment and decay rates determined prior to testing via automated parameter optimization.

Synaptic Connectivity between Layers

The multitude of connectivity between two layers is specified using a continuous value whereby the fractional part determines the chance of a connection between two neurons being made. So for example, a multitude of 1.5 would mean that every neuron in a source layer was connected to every neuron in the target layer at least once, but with a 50% chance of being made a second time. Parameter optimization most often selected multitudes of less than 1.

All connections between layers are excitatory and modifiable. Non-modifiable connections were avoided to help minimize the risk that evolution would hard-code the network topology to increase the average fitness during parameter optimization.

Modulation

A modulator is a global signal that can influence the behavior of a neuron if that neuron has receptors for it. The signal decays over time, as specified by the re-uptake rate, and can be increased by firing neurons that have secretors for it.

Neurons that are to be modulated are given a random number of receptors. These can be modulated by neurons in other layers that have secretors for those modulators. The receptors modulate either the neuron's sensitivity to input or probability of firing. The effect of this modulation is determined by the level of the associated modulator and whether the receptor is inhibitory or excitatory.

Neurons can also have secretors. These increase the level of an associated modulator. The modulator re-uptake rate, the modulation rate of the receptors and the increment rate of the secretors is determined by artificial evolution along with many other parameters of the neural network before the model is tested.

Parameter Optimization

The parameters of the networks are optimized using artificial evolution so as to make a fair comparison. Once these constrained evolutionary runs are finished the parameters are hard-coded and tested as a population of 450 agents in order to determine the average performance of the neural network. An average fitness is required because the mapping from genotype to phenotype is stochastic. This is due to the randomization of weights and the connectivity between neurons. The fitness function used during parameter optimization was Energy + Water + Age – absolute (Energy − Water).

The absolute difference between the energy and water resource is subtracted from the fitness as both resources are essential for the agent to stay alive. Age is important for the fitness function during parameter optimization when agents are more likely to die before the end of their evaluation.

Minimal Disturbance Networks

The network learns which outputs should be most frequently and strongly fired to minimize the subsequent level of input signal in the next turn.

It is easier to understand how the neural network functions if it is seen as a dynamical system (D.Beer, 1995). Understanding an agent as a self-organizing dynamical system removes the question of when to switch behaviors as the transition happens continuously over time. It also means that it is more appropriate to think of attractive and aversive external stimuli than positive or negative reinforcement. The system can therefore be self-organizing and more autonomous. Self-organization removes the question of when to teach the network and when to recall information encoded in it.

W¨org¨otter and Porr (2004) provide an overview of the field of temporal sequence learning. They discuss how the learning paradigm of disturbance minimization, as opposed to reward maximization, removes the problem of credit structuring and assignment. The two paradigms are not equivalent. Whereas maximal return is associated with a few points on a decision surface, minimal disturbance uses all of the points. In a minimal disturbance system, every input into the system drives the learning process. If there is no signal then the system is seen as being in a stable state. Rewards and maximal return are not sought, as is the case with credit assignment learning. Instead, any disturbance-free state is satisfactory.

Minimizing Free-Energy

The dynamics of a self-organizing system can be understood using the concept of an energy landscape (Heylighen, 2000; Kauffman, 1993, p. 176).

Using an analogy of a ball rolling along a peak, ridge or plateau, then given sufficient energy it will roll down a slope and minimize its own potential energy. The ball will not be able to later return unless its kinetic energy is first increased. This process will continue until the ball comes to a stop at the bottom of the landscape, or within a local depression that requires more kinetic energy than the ball currently has for it to escape. Valleys correspond to attractors in a dynamical system, the speed that the system moves into them being determined by the steepness of the slope.

This is not a new concept in neural network theory, an energy function was first used with Hopfield networks (Hertz, Krogh, & Palmer, 1991, p. 21). This allows an "energy landscape" to be imagined whereby patterns memorized, being attractors in the system, can be seen as local minima in the landscape. As with the analogy of the ball, assuming the influence of gravity, a particle placed anywhere on this imaginary surface will roll down to the nearest basin.

Adaptive Performance of the Networks

The synaptic weights between the input and the middle layer of the network can be thought of as providing "activity diffraction" to allow the input signals to filter through the system at different speeds. The synaptic weights between the middle layer and the output layer can be thought of as providing "activity integration," integrating those signals back into combinations that allow particular output neurons to fire more frequently than others.

The network is feed-forward rather than recursive. The output neurons do not connect back to the input layers but they can affect them indirectly. The action that corresponds to the output neuron that has the highest average activation over all the iterations within a turn is performed by the agent. If this increases or decreases a resource in the body then this change is reflected in the subsequent input signals fed to the neural network.

Because activity filters through the network at different speeds, some output neurons will fire earlier than others. If an action is rewarding and subsequently results in a reduction of input signal to the network, synaptic activity will be reduced for the other neurons and therefore will be less likely to fire. If an action is not rewarding, the input signal is not reduced, other neurons will eventually fire and other actions will be tried instead.

Biasing a Network for Either Exploration or Exploitation

Neuromodulators can be used to bias a neural network to function in a certain way depending on how they are used. The networks used here can be biased toward either exploration or exploitation by using inhibitory or excitatory receptors respectively (Parussel, 2006; Parussel & Cañamero, 2007).

The network can be biased toward exploration if the hunger and thirst input units secrete corresponding modulators, for which the middle layer units have a random set of inhibitory receptors (see Figure 2 a). Alternatively, the network can be biased toward exploitative behavior if the middle layer secretes a single modulator for which the output layer has excitatory receptors (see Figure 2 b). A variant of the exploitation network that can be externally influenced using modulators can be seen in Figure 2 c. This network was optimized for use without modulators but was tested with inhibitory receptors applied to its input layers.

Exploitation

With a non-modulating or exploratory network, the more rewarding an action, the stronger the activation of the corresponding output neuron. In contrast, a network biased for exploitation provides reduced activations for all of its output

Figure 2. Modulated variants of the neural network agent controller

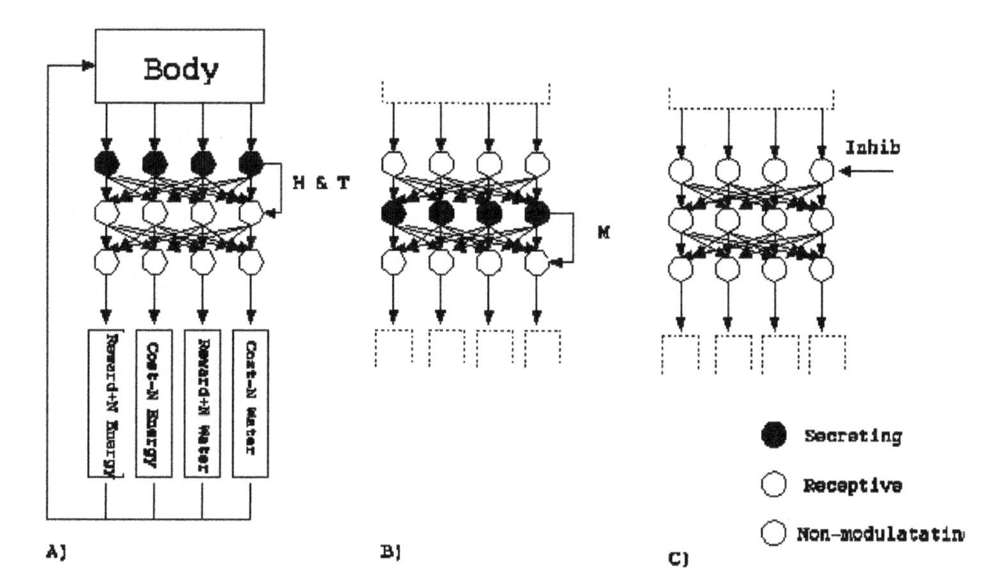

neurons by default and uses modulation to excite the output neurons which are rewarding.

The excitatory receptors at the output layer increase the activity of the network. If the network performs an action that reduces the overall input level, the winning neurons in the output layer will benefit more from excitatory modulation than the less activated neurons that are losing.

If the network performs a sub-optimal action then the input signal is reduced less than if an optimal action was chosen. This means that other middle layer neurons are more likely to fire. Each middle layer neuron will also increase the level of the modulator and each is more likely to fire different output neurons. Consequently, the modulator cannot be used to excite any particular output neuron more than all the others when a sub-optimal action is performed.(See Figure 3)

Exploration

It was discussed earlier how activity filters through the network at different speeds with some output neurons firing earlier than others. If an action is rewarding and subsequently reduces the input signal to the network, activation of the other neurons will be reduced and they will be less likely to fire. If an action is not rewarding, the input signal is not reduced, other neurons will eventually fire and other actions will be tried instead.

The hunger and thirst modulators of the exploration agent optimized for use with discrete actions inhibit the neurons in the middle layer. The strongest firing neurons have more activation to lose when being inhibited. These are also the neurons more likely to be firing the output neurons that lead to actions that reduce total input activity into the network. So by inhibiting the neurons in the middle layer the 'diffraction' of activation throughout the network is reduced and other actions have a greater chance of being performed. This increases exploratory behavior. (See Figure 4)

Relevance of Exploration and Exploitation to Emotions

Emotions can help the reasoning process (Damasio, 1994). Evans puts this idea in a game-theoretical framework in his search hypothesis

(Evans, 2002). A rational agent confronted with an open-ended and partially unknown environment, emotions constrain the range of outcomes to be considered and subjectively applies a utility to each. The search hypothesis can be seen as an example of an agent moving from exploration of possible outcomes to an exploitation of the action providing the current expected highest expected utility.

However, the best course of action does not need to be learnt through experience. Nesse (1990) defines emotions as specialized states of operation that give an evolutionary advantage to an agent in particular situations. LeDoux (1998) describes a distinguishing characteristic of cognitive processing as flexibility of response to the environment. Emotions provide a counter-balance to this by narrowing the response of an agent in ways that have a greater evolutionary fitness.

As an example, predator avoidance driven by fear is an ideal behavior to be selected for and optimized by evolution. It is a behavior that needs to be maintained until the prey reaches assured safety regardless of whether it is able to continually sense the predator or not (Avila-Garc´ıa & Can˜amero, 2005). Nor will the prey benefit from being distracted by less important sensory input while it is still in danger. Successful fleeing behavior might not require exploration of different actions when instead exploitation of known strategies for a successful escape should be given priority. On the contrary, positive emotional states are thought to promote openness to the world and exploration of new courses of actions (Blanchard & Can˜amero, 2006).

Figure 3. The structure of a typical modulating network

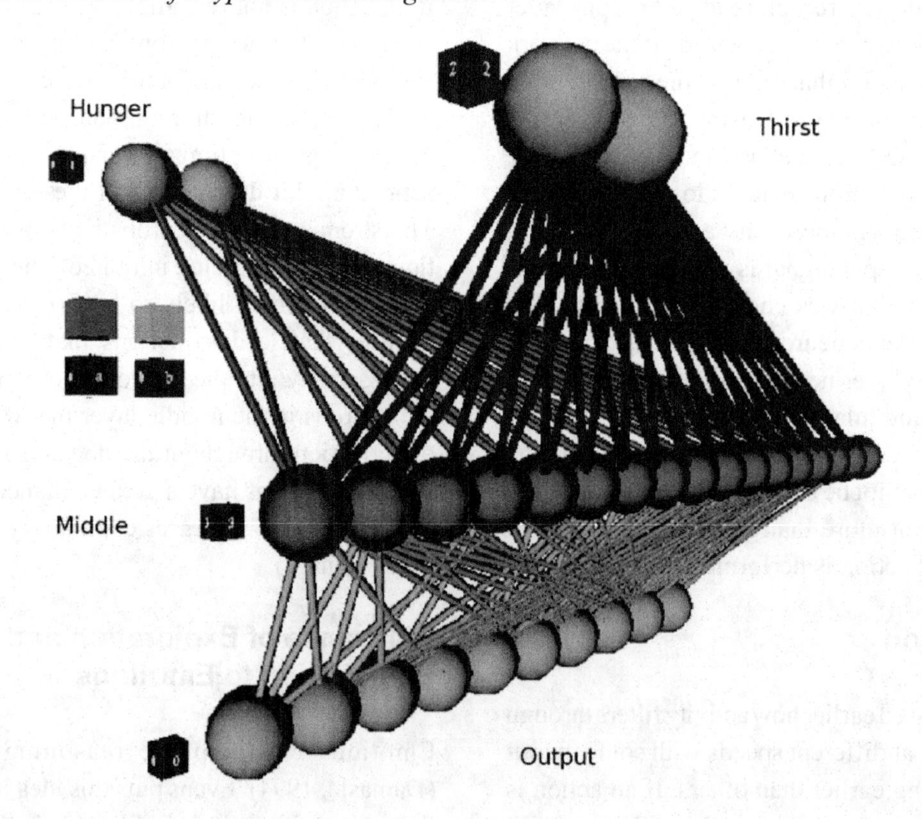

Figure 4. A modulating network in action

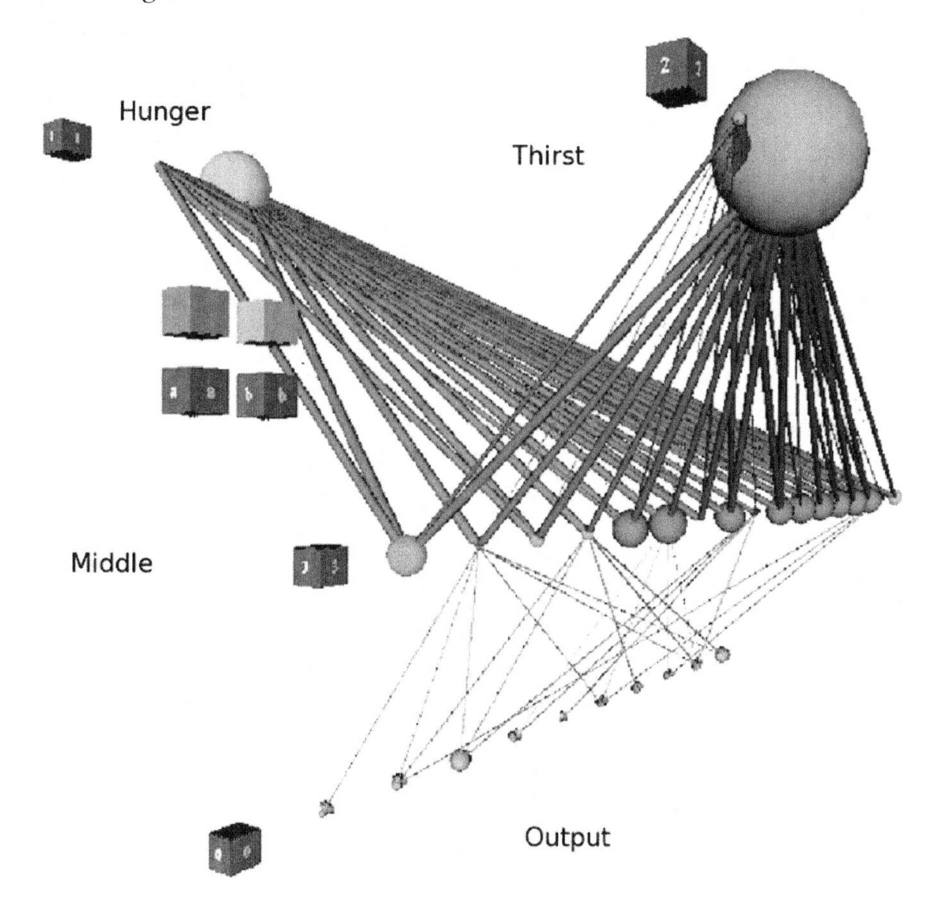

RESULTS

Changing the Level of Overall Activity

In dealing with the networks described here, it has been observed that it is not as important whether receptors have an excitatory or inhibitory effect on a neuron so much as whether release of modulator increases or decreases activity for the entire network.

The exploitation network has the middle layer excite the output layer when modulating the sensitivity to input of the neurons. Yet when modulation is decreased network activity is increased. Conversely, the exploratory network has the input layer inhibit the middle layer via modulation, yet this decreases overall activity (see Figure 5). This graph shows the average activation for all the neurons for both networks and how it either increases or decreases as the modulation rate is increased. The change in the activation of the exploitation network can be seen more clearly in Figure 6.

Biasing the network toward exploration requires that activity is increased so that other outputs have a greater chance of winning. Biasing it toward exploitation requires that the network is led to a more stable state by reducing its overall activity. The network controller can also be influenced to choose specific actions that would

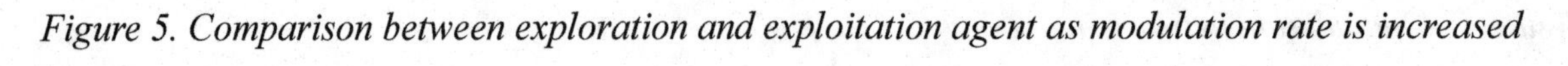

Figure 5. Comparison between exploration and exploitation agent as modulation rate is increased

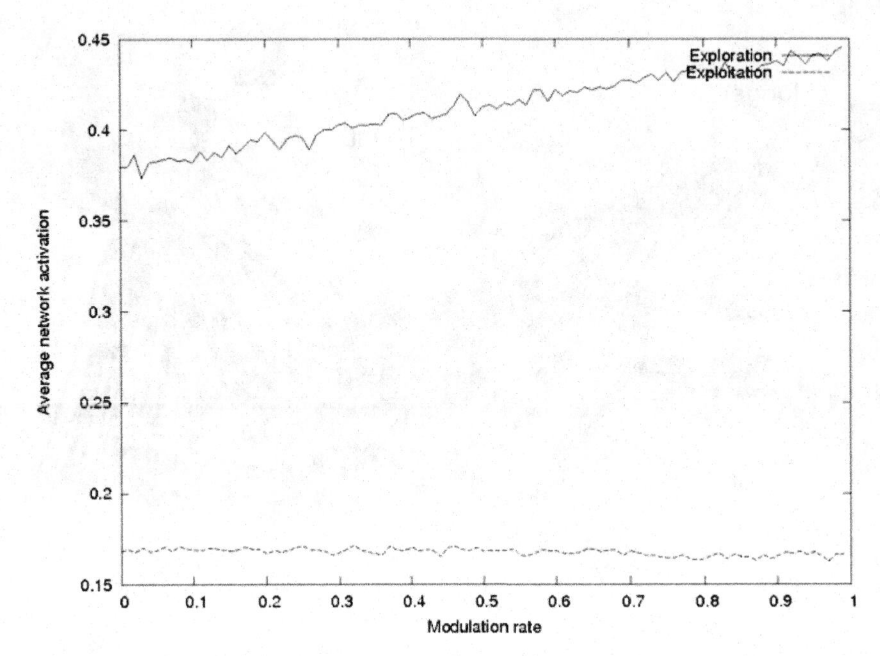

Figure 6. The exploitation agent as the modulation rate is increased

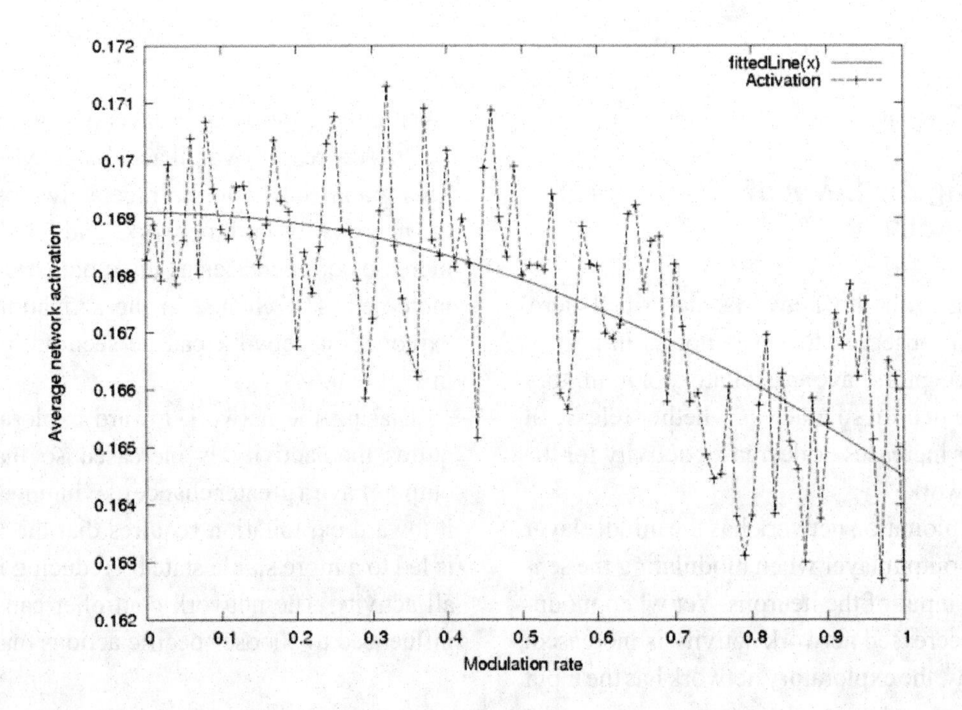

probably otherwise not be selected by an external system decreasing its overall activity.

Using the analogy of the energy landscape again, it is useful to think of a ball rolling around a local minima. Shaking the landscape via an earthquake may bounce the ball out of it and elsewhere. The stronger the earthquake the more chance there is of this happening. Stopping the earthquake all-together allows the ball to come to a rest. The network is the ball, constantly trying to come to a rest. The modulators are like a gain control for the earthquake.

Decreasing Overall Activity

Figure 6 shows the effect of increasing the modulation rate for the exploitation agent. The effect is not as dramatic as for the exploration agent as only the output layer is modulated. The output layer does not connect to any other layer and so the effect of the modulation is localized. Whereas with the exploration agent, the middle layer is modulated and this also has an effect on the output layer.

It may seem strange that the activity of the entire network can be reduced by exciting the output neurons, whether by increasing their probability of firing or by increasing their sensitivity to input. The neurons in the output layer do not connect to any other neurons and so the increase in activity does not affect any other neurons. But because excitatory modulation makes the output neurons more likely to fire, then the neurons are more likely to enter into a refractory state for a period of time. During this period, any incoming activation is immediately leaked away.

The exploitation network uses excitatory receptors at the output layer in order to reduce network activity and to bias it toward performing particular actions. A non-modulating network was also adapted to reduce network activity, but with inhibitory receptors at the input layer instead. The modulator for these receptors was released externally to the network when specific actions were performed. This was used to bias the network to perform two otherwise neutral actions (see Figure 7).

Increasing Overall Activity

Biasing a network toward exploration can also be used to stop activity dieing all-together. With a network evolved to work without modulators, a decrease in input activity eventually leads to a decrease in output activity. If an action results in the lowest possible strength of input signal and spiking-activity in the network has already declined to the minimum threshold required for hebbian learning to occur, then the network settles into a stable state. This can occur in the absence of any changes external to the system, such as the effect of an action changing or noise being added to the input signals.

If no activity reaches the neurons in the output neuron then the agent cannot choose an action for itself. In this situation the default "Inactive" action is chosen for the neural network controller by the encompassing system. This function is more costly than if the agent chose an action itself.

When testing a population of non-modulating agents for longer than 1,000 turns, spiking-activity in the network would cease over time (Parussel & Smith, 2005). This led to the weights freezing because the STDP learning rule only updated the weights when spikes occurred. The activation of the output neurons would slowly decay over time with the winning action remaining the same in the absence of any change in the effect of that action (see Figure 8). The limited use of artificial evolution for parameter optimization had settled upon a brittle strategy which depended on how long each agent was evaluated for.

A population of modulating exploration agents were then tested for the same extended period.

Figure 7. Non-modulating agent run with inhibitory receptors at the input layer

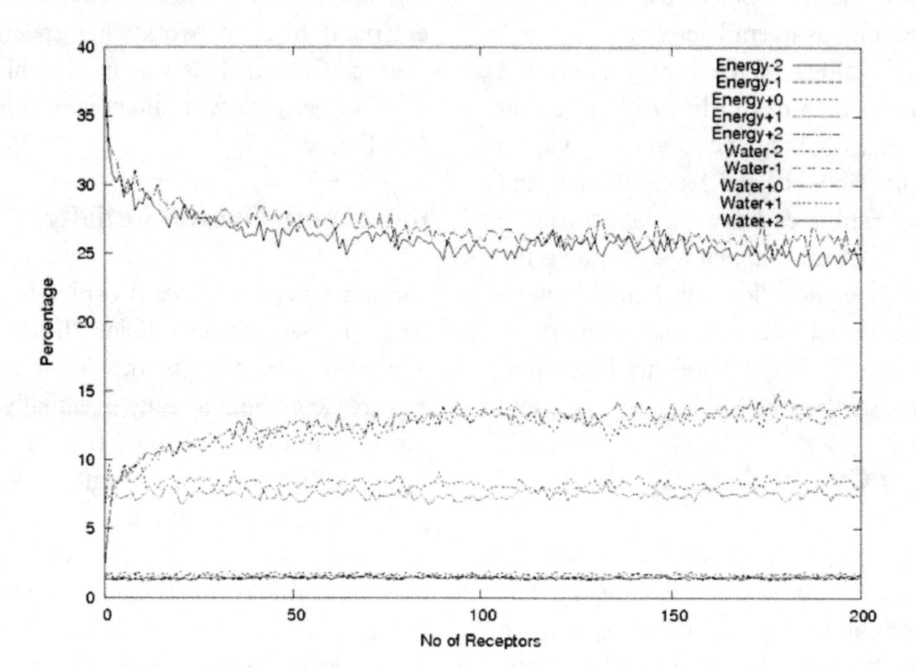

Figure 8. Non-modulating agent run over an extended period

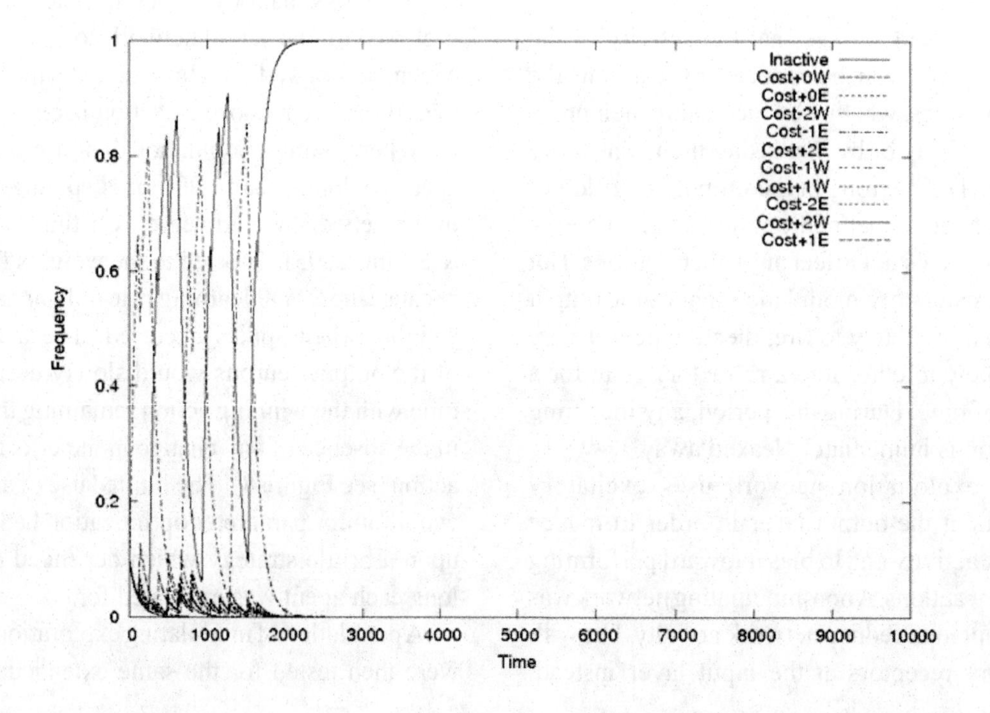

Figure 9. Exploration agent run over the same extended period of time and using the same axes as in Figure 8.

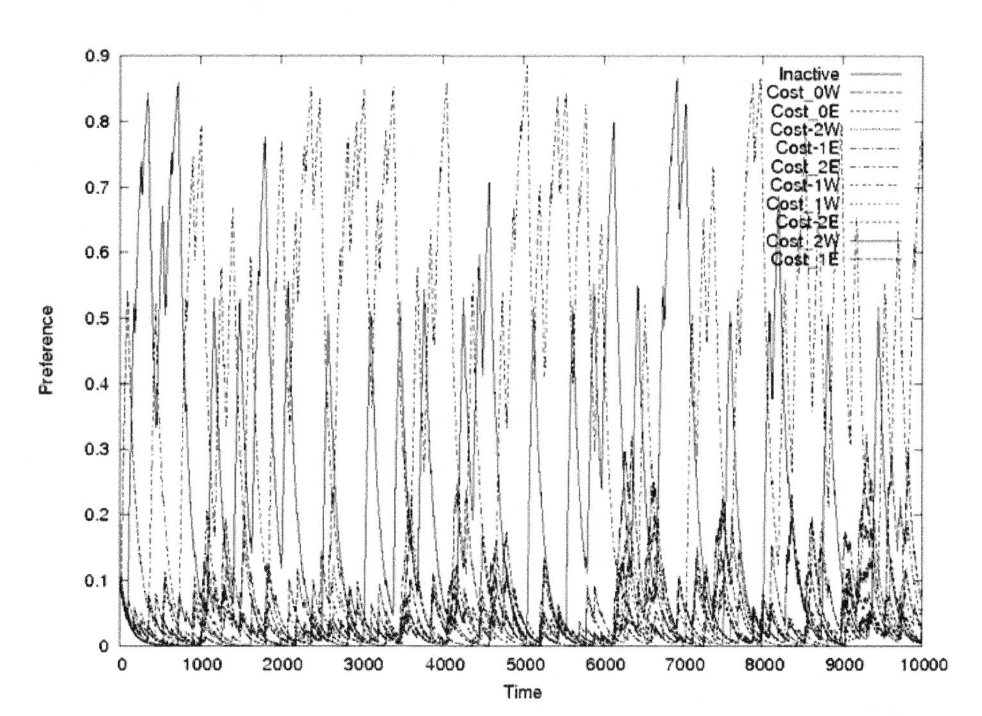

They were shown to continue transitioning between the same two winning output neurons that caused a maximum increase in energy and water, with other neurons very occasionally being chosen (see Figure 9).

When comparing the exploration agent and non-modulating agent in environments that they were not evolved for, in this case evaluated for a variable or extended length of time, then it is shown that modulation makes the agent more robust. This robustness carries with it a performance cost as the exploration agent cannot execute the actions that only reduce the overall input signal the most.

Modulation for the exploration agent, stops the system from settling into a stable state where activity declines to a point whereby the network stops alternating between actions. This agitation is achieved by increasing the global network activity of the system. This stops it reducing the strength of its inputs and settling into a stable state, even though the environment may allow for it or make this the optimal behavior.

DISCUSSION

It has been hypothesized in this paper that there exist two classes of emotions; driving and satisfying emotions. The model of emotion used here is presented as a mechanistic process within the context of a dynamical system. The brain, performing action selection by self-organizing and minimizing its internal activity, is either hampered or aided in this by neuromodulators that agitate or calm it. This has the effect of either influencing an agent to perform actions it would not otherwise do, or continuing its current behavior. Because this is a significant influence upon the behavior of the agent, we observe these effects as driving and satisfying emotions.

Applying the Hypothesis to Natural Agents

The plausibility of this hypothesis has been tested in this paper using feed forward networks of spiking integrate-and-fire neurons. The model is a simplistic one that adapts to immediate stimuli. There is no capacity for long term memory storage, adaptation to sequences of inputs or ability to associate stimuli.

But for a stimulus-response agent, the results are consistent with the hypothesis. This in itself is insufficient for us to draw conclusions about the nature of emotions in animals and humans. For that, we will need real-life observations. There is evidence though to suggest that the hypothesis may apply to natural brains. Panksepp (1998, p. 95) provides some evidence for this when discussing the localization of activity in the brain related to emotional states. Activity is decreased in the brain when happy feelings are experienced; conversely, activity is increased when sad feelings are experienced. People who have a predilection toward panic attacks exhibit overactivity in their right parahippocampal regions.

If the hypothesis is correct then it will most likely not be as simple as positive emotional states being signified by low neural activity and negative emotional states signified by high activity. Panksepp provides the example of people suffering depression exhibiting less arousal of their left frontal areas than is considered normal.

Gotlib and Hamilton (2008) provide a review of the literature concerning the neural activity of people suffering from depression. They also discuss the increased activation of the amygdala in those prone to depression. Major depressive disorder is a complex phenomenon which is essentially a psychiatric disorder of the regulation of emotion. A lack of motivation and the inability to regulate the processing of negative experiences are strong characteristics of depression. Their review discusses the idea of depression being caused by an imbalance in the activity between the limbic system and the dorsal cortical structures. Also noted is the apparent normalization of activity between the amygdala, anterior cingulate cortex and the dorsolateral prefrontal cortex following successful treatment. Minsky (1988) raises the issue of competing interests within an artificial agent giving rise to what can be observed as emotional reactions. Maybe a related point is that emotional disorders can arise from the skewed salience of competing interests, as reflected by relative levels of neural activity in the corresponding areas of the brain.

A Potential Architecture for Artificial Agents

Kelley (2005) argues that in their broadest possible sense, emotions are required for any organism or species to survive. They allow animals to satisfy needs and act more effectively within their environment. If robots are to survive as effectively then they also need equivalent systems.

Implementing these systems and seeing first-hand how they benefit artificial agents should help us appreciate the reasons why natural agents are endowed with emotions. It is envisaged that the following architecture should prove useful for the design of artificial agents. The premise behind this is the question; how can we design agents to adapt to unknown environments when we ourselves do not know what those environments will be? The approach taken here is to concern ourselves with the features and resources that are consistent between the different environments that the agent may inhabit. The state of these features shall then be signaled to a self-organizing agent controller so that it can adapt accordingly.

Separate subsystems can be hard-coded to look out for certain sensory features and to provide a signal to the neural network controller using modulators. So for example, separate subsystems may be required to recognize the difference between a clean carpet and a dirty one, or the edge of some stairs. A subsystem that recognizes a dirty carpet could send out a signal to agitate the neural network controller until the agent started to clean the carpet. Another subsystem could decrease network activity using a neuromodulator when the agent started to recharge batteries that were low. If an agent with such a controller as presented in this paper needs to replenish a critical resource or keep its physiological variables within a critical range, then it will do so by choosing actions that result in lower network activity.

For an agent to maintain homeostasis using a self-organizing system, there must be a non-linear increase in the activity of the network controller in order to signal that equilibrium of its physiological variables needs to be restored. The relative importance of repleting a resource grows as it is depleted. Taking the example of a battery level for a robotic agent, a change from 2% to 1% is absolutely critical, far more say than a change from from 15% to 14%. The increase in network activity needs to be amplified, it needs a gain control.

The signal need not carry much information, but it must be acted upon when the level of a resource becomes critical. It must increase the activity of the parts of the system that allow homeostasis to be re-asserted. Once this has been achieved, the signal is no longer required and the system can settle back into a stable state. The more significant the increase in network activity, the more the self-organizing system is driven to minimize it. As with Panksepp's example of food tasting better the more hungry we are, neuromodulators could work together to repulse and attract the agent toward specific actions or environments. If there is a significant increase in activity because the agent has a particular resource that is critically low, then a neuromodulator that decreases activity in the affected parts of the brain will have a much stronger effect.

The example of homeostasis was used because the need to maintain equilibrium of physiological processes is constant, regardless of the environment that an agent may inhabit. This mechanism need not be constrained to maintaining homeostasis though. Significant changes in network activity could be triggered because of specific external, rather than internal, sensory stimuli. An increase in network activity was used in this paper to drive an agent to re-explore the effect of actions that had previously shown to be less than optimal. But it could probably also be used to implement the role of disgust by making certain external stimuli aversive, driving the agent away from it.

Satisfying emotions could help encourage an agent to perform otherwise neutral actions. There are situations whereby an agent may need to perform an action that will indirectly minimize network activity because it leads to a more promising environment. So for example, an agent may have learnt from previous experience that being in a particular environment increases the chances of a specific resource being repleted. Learning to recognize such an environment and inducing satisfying emotions that minimized activity in the network would attract the agent toward it.

An agent may also need to perform an action that does not help in maintaining homeostasis at all. In the case of an artificial agent developed for a specific purpose, we may wish to bias it to perform actions or behaviors which are of no benefit to the robot but for example, provides us with cleaner carpets.

ACKNOWLEDGMENT

Many thanks go to Professor Leslie S. Smith for proofreading numerous drafts and providing many useful comments as to how the paper could be improved, as well as to Professor Evan H. Magill and the Computing Science department of the University of Stirling for employing me.

REFERENCES

Avila-García, O., & Cañamero, L. (2005, April). Hormonal modulation of perception in motivation-based action selection architectures. In *Proceedings of the Symposium on Agents that Want and Like: Motivational and Emotional Roots of Cognition and Action, AISB 05,* Hatfield, UK (pp. 9-16). Society for the Study of Artificial Intelligence and the Simulation of Behaviour.

Bi, G. Q., & Wang, H. X. (2002). Temporal asymmetry in spike timing-dependent synaptic plasticity. *Physiology & Behavior*, *77*(4-5), 551–555. doi:10.1016/S0031-9384(02)00933-2

Blanchard, A. & Cañamero, L. (2006, September). Developing affect-modulated behaviors: Stability, exploration, exploitation, or imitation? In F. Kaplan et al. (Eds.), *Proceedings of the 6th International Workshop on Epigenetic Robotics,* Paris (pp. 128). Lund University.

Damasio, A. (1994). *Descartes' error: Emotion, reason, and the human brain*. North Yorkshire, UK: Quill.

D.Beer, R. (1995). A dynamical systems perspective on autonomous agents. *Artificial Intelligence*, *72*, 173–215. doi:10.1016/0004-3702(94)00005-L

Di Paolo, E. (2003). Evolving spike-timing-dependent plasticity for single-trial learning in robots. *Philosophical Transactions of the Royal Society of London, Series A: Mathematical, Physical and Engineering Sciences, 361*(1811), 2299-2319.

Evans, D. (2002). The search hypothesis of emotion. *The British Journal for the Philosophy of Science, 53*(4), 497–509. doi:10.1093/bjps/53.4.497

Fellous, J.-M. (1999). The neuromodulatory basis of emotion. *The Neuroscientist*, *5*(5), 283–294. doi:10.1177/107385849900500514

Fellous, J.-M. (2004, March). From human emotions to robot emotions. In *Architectures for modeling emotions: Cross-disciplinary foundations. Papers from the 2004 AAAI Spring Symposium,* Palo Alto, CA (pp. 37-47). AAAI Press.

Gotlib, I. H., & Hamilton, J. P. (2008). Neuroimaging and depression: Current status and unresolved issues. *Current Directions in Psychological Science*, *17*(2), 159–163. doi:10.1111/j.1467-8721.2008.00567.x

Hertz, J., Krogh, A., & Palmer, R. G. (1991). *Introduction to the theory of neural computation*. Boston: Addison-Wesley.

Heylighen, F. (2000). The science of self-organization and adaptivity. In *The encyclopedia of life support systems* (pp. 253-280). Paris: UNESCO.

Karmarkar, U. R., & Buonomano, D. V. (2002). A model of spike-timing dependent plasticity: One or two coincidence detectors. *Journal of Neurophysiology*, *88*, 507–513.

Karmarkar, U. R., Najariana, M. T., & Buonomano, D. V. (2002). Mechanisms and significance of spike-timing dependent synaptic plasticity. *Biological Cybernetics*, *87*, 373–382. doi:10.1007/s00422-002-0351-0

Kauffman, S. (1993). *The origins of order: Self-organization and selection in evolution*. Oxford, UK: Oxford University Press.

Kelley, A. E. (2005). Neurochemical networks encoding emotion and motivation: An evolutionary perspective. In J-M. Fellous & M. A. Arbib (Eds.), *Who needs emotions? The brain meets the robot* (pp. 29-77). New York: Oxford University Press.

Kelso, J. A. S. (1995). *Dynamic patterns: The self-organization of brain and behavior*. Cambridge, MA: MIT Press.

Koch, C. (1999). *Biophysics of computation*. New York: Oxford University Press.

LeDoux, J. E. (1998). *The emotional brain*. New York: Simon & Schuster.

Minsky, M. (1988). *The society of mind*. New York: Simon & Schuster Inc.

Nesse, R. (1990). Evolutionary explanations of emotion. *Human Nature (Hawthorne, N.Y.)*, *1*(30), 261–289. doi:10.1007/BF02733986

Noble, J. (1997, July). *The scientific status of artificial life*. In Paper presented at the 4th European Conference on Artificial Life, Brighton, UK.

Panksepp, J. (1998). *Affective neuroscience: The foundations of human and animal emotions*. New York: Oxford University Press.

Parussel, K. M., & Cañamero, L. (2007). Biasing neural networks towards exploration or exploitation using neuromodulation. In J. M. de Sá, L. A. Alexandre, W. Duch, & D. Mandic (Eds.), *ICANN 2007: Proceedings of the 17th International Conference on Artificial Neural Networks Part II* (Vol. 4669, pp. 889-898). Springer-Verlag.

Parussel, K. M., & Smith, L. S. (2005, April). Cost minimisation and reward maximisation. A neuromodulating minimal disturbance system using anti-hebbian spike timing-dependent plasticity. In *Proceedings of the Symposium on Agents that Want and Like: Motivational and Emotional Roots of Cognition and Action, AISB 05,* Hatfield, UK (pp. 98-101). Society for the Study of Artificial Intelligence and the Simulation of Behaviour.

Parussel, K. M. (2006). *A bottom-up approach to emulating emotions using neuromodulation in agents*. Unpublished doctoral dissertation, University of Stirling.

Rolls, E. T. (1999). *The brain and emotion*. New York: Oxford University Press.

Rolls, E. T. (2005). What are emotions, why do we have emotions, and what is their computational basis in the brain? In J-M. Fellous & M. A. Arbib (Eds.), *Who needs emotions? The brain meets the robot* (pp. 117-146). Oxford University Press.

Song, S., Miller, K. D., & Abbott, L. F. (2000). Competitive hebbian learning through spike-timing-dependent plasticity. *Nature Neuroscience*, *3*, 919–926. doi:10.1038/78829

Von der Malsburg, C. (2003). Self-organization and the brain. In M. A. Arbib (Eds.), *The handbook of brain theory and neural networks* (pp. 1002-1005). Cambridge, MA: MIT Press.

Wehmeier, U., Dong, D., Koch, C., & van Essen, D. X. (1989). Modeling the mammalian visual system. In C. Koch & I. Segev (Eds.), *Methods in neuronal modeling: From synapses to networks* (pp. 335-360). Cambridge, MA: MIT Press.

W¨org¨otter, F., & Porr, B. (2004). Temporal sequence learning, prediction and control - a review of different models and their relation to biological mechanisms. *Neural Computation*, *17*, 1–75.

Zhang, Q., & Lee, M. (2009). Analysis of positive and negative emotions in natural scene using brain activity and gist. *Neurocomputing*, *72*(4-6), 1302–1306. doi:10.1016/j.neucom.2008.11.007

ENDNOTES

1. It was not known whether separate increment and decrement parameters were required. To keep the number of attributes to a minimum it was decided that two parameters would

be used only if it was found to be required. The network evolved well with only one parameter.

2 This model of stochastic firing is a simplified one. In real neurons there is both a possibility that a spike is passed down the axon to the target cells and a possibility of vesicle release once a spike has reached a synapse.

This work was previously published in International Journal of Synthetic Emotions, Volume 1, Issue 1, edited by Jordi Vallverdu, pp. 51-67, copyright 2010 by IGI Publishing (an imprint of IGI Global).

Chapter 5
Automatic, Dimensional and Continuous Emotion Recognition

Hatice Gunes
Imperial College London, UK

Maja Pantic
Imperial College London, UK and University of Twente, EEMCS, The Netherlands

ABSTRACT

Recognition and analysis of human emotions have attracted a lot of interest in the past two decades and have been researched extensively in neuroscience, psychology, cognitive sciences, and computer sciences. Most of the past research in machine analysis of human emotion has focused on recognition of prototypic expressions of six basic emotions based on data that has been posed on demand and acquired in laboratory settings. More recently, there has been a shift toward recognition of affective displays recorded in naturalistic settings as driven by real world applications. This shift in affective computing research is aimed toward subtle, continuous, and context-specific interpretations of affective displays recorded in real-world settings and toward combining multiple modalities for analysis and recognition of human emotion. Accordingly, this paper explores recent advances in dimensional and continuous affect modelling, sensing, and automatic recognition from visual, audio, tactile, and brain-wave modalities.

INTRODUCTION

Human natural affective behaviour is multimodal, subtle and complex. In day-to-day interactions, people naturally communicate multimodally by means of language, vocal intonation, facial expression, hand gesture, head movement, body movement and posture, and possess a refined mechanism for understanding and interpreting information conveyed by these behavioural cues.

Despite the available range of cues and modalities in human-human interaction (HHI), the mainstream research on human emotion has

DOI: 10.4018/978-1-4666-1595-3.ch005

mostly focused on facial and vocal expressions and their recognition in terms of seven discrete, basic emotion categories (neutral, happiness, sadness, surprise, fear, anger and disgust; Keltner & Ekman, 2000; Juslin & Scherer, 2005). In line with the aforementioned, most of the past research on automatic affect sensing and recognition has focused on recognition of facial and vocal expressions in terms of basic emotional states, and then based on data that has been posed on demand or acquired in laboratory settings (Pantic & Rothkrantz, 2003; Gunes, Piccardi, & Pantic, 2008; Zeng, Pantic, Roisman, & Huang, 2009). Additionally, each modality—visual, auditory, and tactile—has been considered in isolation. However, a number of researchers have shown that in everyday interactions people exhibit non-basic, subtle and rather complex mental/affective states like thinking, embarrassment or depression (Baron-Cohen & Tead, 2003). Such subtle and complex affective states can be expressed via tens (or possibly hundreds) of anatomically possible facial expressions, bodily gestures or physiological signals. Accordingly, a single label (or any small number of discrete classes) may not reflect the complexity of the affective state conveyed by such rich sources of information (Russell, 1980). Hence, a number of researchers advocate the use of dimensional description of human affect, where an affective state is characterized in terms of a small number of latent dimensions (e.g., Russell, 1980; Scherer, 2000; Scherer, Schorr, & Johnstone, 2001).

It is not surprising, therefore, that automatic affect sensing and recognition researchers have recently started exploring how to model, analyse and interpret the subtlety, complexity and continuity of affective behaviour in terms of latent dimensions, rather than in terms of a small number of discrete emotion categories.

A number of recent survey papers exist on automatic affect sensing and recognition (e.g., Gunes & Piccardi, 2008; Gunes et al., 2008; Zeng et al., 2009). However, none of those focus on dimensional affect analysis. This paper, therefore, sets out to explore recent advances in human affect modelling, sensing, and automatic recognition from visual (i.e., facial and bodily expression), audio, tactile (i.e., heart rate, skin conductivity, thermal signals etc.) and brain-wave (i.e., brain and scalp signals) modalities by providing an overview of theories of emotion (in particular the dimensional theories), expression and perception of emotions, data acquisition and annotation, and the current state-of-the-art in automatic sensing and recognition of emotional displays using a dimensional (rather than categorical) approach.

BACKGROUND RESEARCH

Emotions are researched in various scientific disciplines such as neuroscience, psychology, and linguistics. Development of automated affective multimodal systems depends significantly on the progress in the aforementioned sciences. Accordingly, we start our analysis by exploring the background in emotion theory, and human perception and recognition.

THEORIES OF EMOTION

According to the research in psychology, three major approaches to emotion modelling can be distinguished (Grandjean, Sander, & Scherer, 2008): (1) categorical approach, (2) dimensional approach, and (3) appraisal-based approach.

The categorical approach is based on research on basic emotions, pioneered by Darwin (1998), interpreted by Tomkins (1962, 1963) and supported by findings of Ekman & his colleagues (1992, 1999). According to this approach there exist a small number of emotions that are basic, hard-wired in our brain, and recognized universally (e.g., Ekman & Friesen, 2003). Ekman and his colleagues conducted various experiments on human judgment of still photographs of deliberately displayed facial behaviour and concluded that six basic emotions can be recognized universally. These emotions are happiness, sadness, surprise, fear, anger and disgust (Ekman, 1982). Although psychologists have suggested a different number of such basic emotions, ranging from 2 to 18 categories (Ortony & Turner, 1990; Wierzbicka, 1992), there has been considerable agreement on the aforementioned six emotions. To date, Ekman's theory on universality and interpretation of affective nonverbal expressions in terms of basic emotion categories has been the most commonly adopted approach in research on automatic affect recognition.

On the other hand, however, a number of researchers in psychology argued that it is necessary to go beyond discrete emotions. Among various classification schemes, Baron-Cohen and his colleagues, for instance, have investigated cognitive mental states (e.g., agreement, concentrating, disagreement, thinking, reluctance, and interest) and their use in daily life. They did so via analysis of multiple asynchronous information sources such as facial actions, purposeful head gestures, and eye-gaze direction. They showed that cognitive mental states occur more often in everyday interactions than the basic emotions (Baron-Cohen & Tead, 2003). These states were also found relevant in representing problem-solving and decision-making processes in human-computer Interaction (HCI) context and have been used by a number of researchers, though based on deliberately displayed behaviour rather than in natural scenarios (e.g., El Kaliouby & Robinson, 2005).

According to the dimensional approach, affective states are not independent from one another; rather, they are related to one another in a systematic manner. In this approach, majority of affect variability is covered by three dimensions: valence, arousal, and potency (dominance) (Davitz, 1964; Mehrabian & Russell, 1974; Osgood, Suci, & Tannenbaum, 1957). The valence dimension refers to how positive or negative the emotion is, and ranges from unpleasant feelings to pleasant feelings of happiness. The arousal dimension refers to how excited or apathetic the emotion is, and it ranges from sleepiness or boredom to frantic excitement. The power dimension refers to the degree of power or sense of control over the emotion. Taking into account the aforementioned, a reasonable space of emotion can be modelled as illustrated in Figure 1a. Russell (1980) introduced a circular configuration called Circumflex of Affect (see Figure 1b) and proposed that each basic emotion represents a bipolar entity being a part of the same emotional continuum. The proposed polars are arousal (relaxed vs. aroused) and valence (pleasant vs. unpleasant). As illustrated in Figure 1b, the proposed emotional space consists of four quadrants: low arousal positive, high arousal positive, low arousal negative, and high arousal negative. In this way, as argued by Russell, it is possible to characterize all emotions by their valence and arousal, and different emotional labels could be plotted at various positions on this two-dimensional plane.

However, each approach, categorical or dimensional, has its advantages and disadvantages. In the categorical approach, where each affective display is classified into a single category, complex mental/affective state or blended emotions may be too difficult to handle (Yu, Aoki, & Woodruff, 2004). Instead, in dimensional approach, observers can indicate their impression of each stimulus on several continuous scales. Despite exhibiting such advantages, dimensional approach has received a number of criticisms. Firstly, the usefulness of these approaches has been challenged by discrete emotions theorists, such as Silvan Tomkins, Paul Ekman, and Carroll Izard, who argued that the reduction of emotion space to two or three dimensions is extreme and resulting in loss of information. Secondly, while some basic emotions proposed by Ekman, such as happiness or sadness, seem to fit well in the dimensional space, some basic emotions become indistinguishable (e.g., fear and anger), and some emotions may lie outside the space (e.g., surprise). It also remains

Figure 1. Illustration of a) three dimensions of emotion space (V-valence, A-arousal, P-power), and b) distribution of the seven emotions in arousal-valance (A-V) space. Images adapted from (Jin & Wang, 2005) and (Breazeal, 2003), respectively.

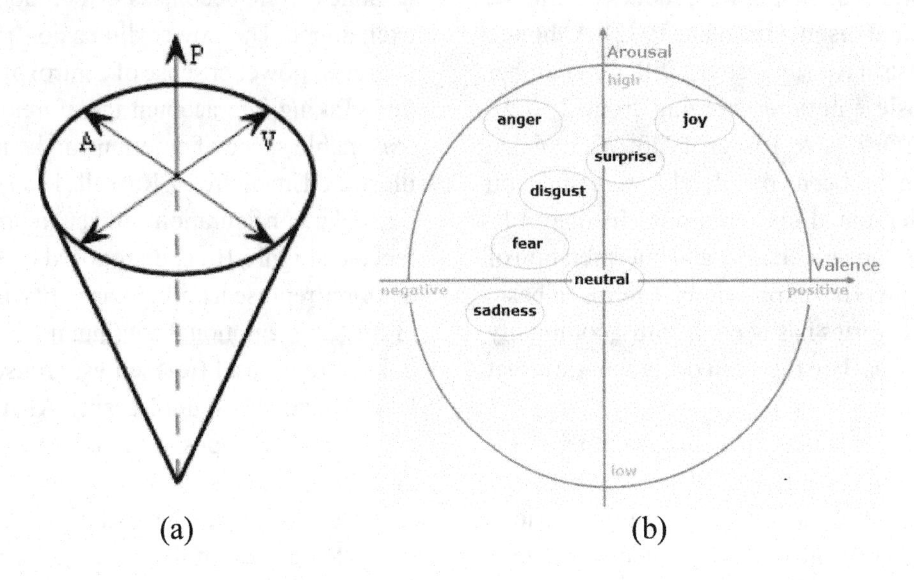

unclear how to determine the position of other affect-related states such as confusion. Note, however, that arousal and valence are not claimed to be the only dimensions or to be sufficient to differentiate equally between all emotions. Nonetheless, they have proven to be useful in several domains (e.g., affective content analysis as reported by Yang, Lin, Su, & Chen, 2007).

Scherer and colleagues introduced another set of psychological models, referred to as componential models of emotion, which are based on appraisal theory (Scherer et al., 2001). The appraisal-based approach, which can also be seen as extension to the dimensional approach, claims that emotions are generated through continuous, recursive subjective evaluation of both our own internal state and the state of the outside world. This approach views emotions through changes in all relevant components including cognition, motivation, physiological reactions, motor expressions, and feelings. The advantage of componential models is that they do not limit emotional states to a fixed number of discrete categories or to a few basic dimensions. Instead, they focus on the variability of different emotional states, as produced by different types of appraisal patterns. Emotion is described through a set of stimulus evaluation checks, including the novelty, intrinsic pleasantness, goal-based significance, coping potential, and compatibility with standards. Therefore, differentiating between various emotions and modelling individual differences become possible. How to use the appraisal-based approach for automatic emotion recognition remains an open research question due to the fact that this approach requires complex, multicomponential and sophisticated measurements of change.

Even with over a century of research, all of the aforementioned issues, and in particular the issue of which psychological model of emotion is more appropriate for which context, still remain under discussion. For further details on different approaches to modelling human emotions and their relative advantages and disadvantages, the reader is referred to the works by Scherer (2000) and Grandjean et al. (2008).

EXPRESSION AND PERCEPTION OF EMOTIONS

Emotional information is conveyed by a broad range of multimodal cues, including speech and language, gesture and head movement, body movement and posture, vocal intonation and facial expression, and so forth. Herewith, we provide a summary of the findings from research on emotion communication by means of facial and bodily expression, speech and nonverbal vocalizations, bio-potential signals (physiological signals, brain waves and thermal signals). Figure 2 illustrates examples of sensors used for acquiring affective data from these cues and modalities.

FACIAL EXPRESSION

Ekman and his colleagues conducted various experiments of human judgment on still photographs of deliberately displayed facial behaviour and concluded that six basic emotions can be recognized universally: happiness, sadness, surprise, fear, anger and disgust. Several other emotions and many combinations of emotions have been studied as well but it remains unconfirmed whether they are universally distinguishable. Although prototypic expressions of basic emotions like happiness, surprise, and fear are natural, they occur infrequently in daily life and provide an incomplete description of facial behaviour. To

Figure 2. Examples of sensors used in multimodal affective data acquisition: (a) camera for visible imagery, (b) microphone(s) for audio recording, (c) various sensors for bio-potential signal recording and (d) infrared camera for thermal imagery.

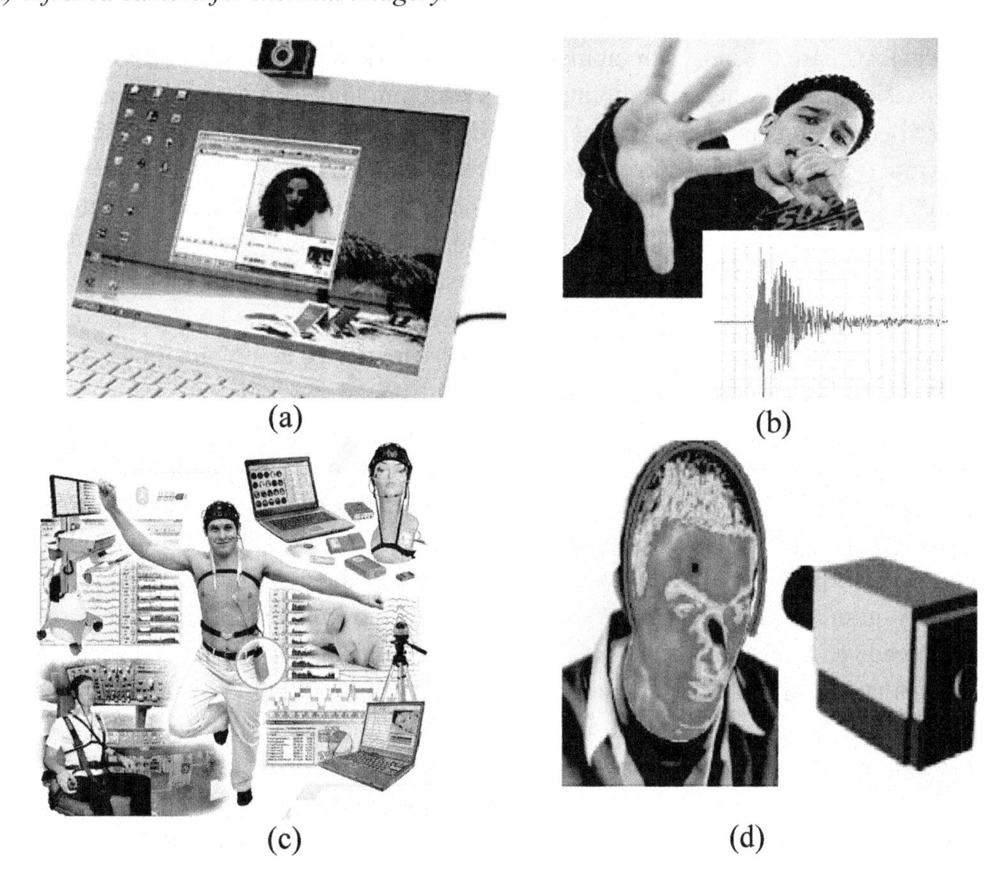

capture the subtlety of human facial behaviour, Ekman and Friesen developed the Facial Action Coding System (FACS) for coding fine-grained changes in the face (Ekman & Friesen, 1978; Ekman, Friesen, & Hager, 2002). FACS is based on the enumeration of all *facial action units*, which are related to facial muscle actions, causing changes in the facial appearance. In addition to this, Friesen and Ekman (1984) developed Emotion FACS (EMFACS) as a method for using FACS to score only the facial actions that might be relevant to detecting emotions.

As proposed by a number of researchers (e.g., Plutchik, 1984; Russell, 1997), different facial expressions could also be mapped to various positions on the two-dimensional plane of arousal-valence. This is illustrated in Figure 1b, where a series of facial expression photos was mapped onto Russell's (1997) arousal-valence dimensions (Breazeal, 2003).

To date, however, Ekman's theory of basic emotions and the FACS are the most commonly used schemes in vision-based systems attempting to recognize facial expressions and analyze human affective behaviour (Pantic & Rothkrantz, 2003; Zeng et al., 2009).

BODILY EXPRESSION

Researchers in social psychology and human development have long emphasized the fact that emotional states are expressed through body movement (Argyle, 1975; Darwin, 1998; Hadjikhani & De Gelder, 2003). However, compared to research on facial expression, the expressive information body gestures carry has not been adequately explored yet.

The main focus has been that of mapping bodily expression onto discrete emotion categories. Darwin (1998) was the first to describe in detail the bodily expressions associated with emotions in animals and humans and proposed several principles underlying the organization of these expressions. Following Darwin's early work, there have been a number of studies on human body postures communicating emotions (e.g., Argyle, 1975). Coulson presented experimental results on attribution of six emotions (anger, disgust, fear, happiness, sadness and surprise) to static body postures by using computer-generated figures (Coulson, 2004). He found out that in general, human recognition of emotion from posture is comparable to recognition from the voice, and some postures are recognized as effectively as facial expressions.

Van den Stock, Righart, and De Gelder (2007) also presented a study investigating emotional body postures (happiness, sadness, surprise, fear, disgust and anger) and how they are perceived. Results indicate good recognition of all emotions, with angry and fearful bodily expressions less accurately recognized compared to, for example, bodily expressions of sadness.

Behavioural studies have shown that posture can communicate affective dimensions as well as discrete emotion categories. Kleinsmith, Ravindra De Silva, and Bianchi-Berthouze (2005) identified that scaling, arousal, valence, and action tendency were the affective dimensions used by human observers when discriminating between postures. They reported that low-level posture features such as orientation (e.g., orientation of shoulder axis) and distance (e.g., distance between left elbow and left shoulder) could effectively discriminate between the affective dimensions.

In general, dimensional models are considered important in affect sensing as a single label may not reflect the complexity of the affective state conveyed by a body posture or gesture. It is also worth noting that Ekman and Friesen (1967) considered expressing discrete emotion categories via face, and communicating dimensions of affect via body as more plausible. However, communication of emotions by bodily movement and expressions is still a relatively unexplored and unresolved area in psychology, and further research is needed in order to obtain a better insight on how they contribute to the perception and recognition of various affective states both in terms of categories and A-V dimensions.

AUDIO

Speech conveys affective information through explicit (linguistic) messages, and implicit (paralinguistic) messages that reflect the way the words are spoken. If we consider the verbal part (linguistic message) only, without regarding the manner in which it was spoken (paralinguistic message), we might miss important aspects of the pertinent utterance and even misunderstand the spoken message by not attending to the nonverbal aspect of the speech. However, findings in basic research indicate that spoken messages are rather unreliable means to analyze and predict human (affective) behaviour (Ambady & Rosenthal, 1992). Anticipating a person's word choice and the associated intent is very difficult: even in highly constrained situations, different people choose different words to express exactly the same thing. Yet, some information about the speaker's affective state can be inferred directly from the surface features of words, which were summarized in some affective word dictionaries and lexical affinity (e.g., Whissell, 1989). The rest of affective information lies below the text surface and can only be detected when the semantic context (e.g., discourse information) is taken into account. The association between linguistic content and emotion is language-dependent and generalizing from one language to another is very difficult to achieve (Ortony & Turner, 1990).

When it comes to implicit, paralinguistic messages that convey affective information, the research in psychology and psycholinguistics provides an immense body of results on acoustic and prosodic features which can be used to encode affective states of a speaker. For a comprehensive overview of the past research in the field, readers are referred to Juslin and Scherer (2005). The prosodic features which seem to be reliable indicators of the basic emotions are the continuous acoustic measures, particularly pitch-related measures (range, mean, median, and variability), intensity and duration. For a comprehensive summary of acoustic cues related to vocal expressions of basic emotions, readers are referred to Cowie et al. (2001). However, basic researchers have not identified an optimal set of voice cues that reliably discriminate among emotions. Nonetheless, listeners seem to be accurate in decoding some basic emotions from prosody (Juslin & Scherer, 2005) as well as some non-basic affective states such as distress, anxiety, boredom, and sexual interest from non-linguistic vocalizations like laughs, cries, and yawns (Russell & Fernández-Dols, 1997).

There have also been a number of works focusing on how to map audio expression to dimensional models. Cowie et al. used valence-activation space, which is similar to the A-V space, to model and assess emotions from speech (Cowie, Douglas-Cowie, Savvidou, McMahon, Sawey, & Schroder, 2000; Cowie et al., 2001). Scherer and his colleagues have also proposed how to judge emotion effects on vocal expression, using the appraisal-based theory (Grandjean et al., 2008; Scherer, 2000).

BIO-POTENTIAL SIGNALS

Numerous findings in psychophysiology suggest that the activation of the autonomic nervous system changes when emotions are elicited (Levenson, 1988).

While the visual modality including facial expressions and body gestures provides a visible proof of affective arousal, bio-signals such as electroencephalography (EEG) and functional near-infrared spectroscopy (fNIRS) provide an invisible proof of affective arousal (Savran et al., 2006). The signals commonly referred to as physiological or bio-signals (Changchun, Rani, & Sarkar, 2005; Savran et al., 2006; Takahashi, 2004) and used in affect sensing research field to identify emotions can be listed and described as follows.

- Galvanic Skin Response (GSR) provides a measurement of the of skin conductance (SC). SC increases linearly with a person's level of overall arousal or stress (Chanel, Kronegg, Grandjean, & Pun, 2007).
- Electromyography (EMG) measures the muscle activity or frequency of muscle tension, and has been shown to correlate with negatively valenced emotions (Haag, Goronzy, Schaich, & Williams, 2004, Nakasone, Prendinger, & Ishizuka, 2005).
- Blood Volume Pulse (BVP) is an indicator of blood flow. Since each heart beat (or pulse) presses blood through the vessels, BVP can also be used to calculate heart rate and inter-beat intervals. Heart rate increases with negatively valenced emotions, such as anxiety or fear.
- Skin temperature (ST) describes the temperature as measured on the surface of the skin.
- Electrocardiogram (ECG) signal measures contractile activity of the heart. This can be recorded either directly on the surface of the chest or alternatively on the limbs (more sensitive to artefacts). It can be used to measure heart rate and inter-beat intervals to determine the heart rate variability (HRV). A low HRV can indicate a state of relaxation, whereas an increased HRV can indicate a potential state of mental stress or frustration.
- Respiration rate (R) measures how deep and fast a person is breathing. Slow and deep breathing indicates a relaxed resting state while irregular rhythm, quick variations, and cessation of respiration corresponds to more aroused emotions like anger or fear (Chanel et al., 2007; Haag et al., 2004).

There is evidence suggesting that measurements recorded over various parts of the brain including the amygdala enable observation of the emotions felt (Pun et al., 2006). For instance, approach or withdrawal response to a stimulus is known to be linked to the activation of the left or right frontal cortex, respectively.

As stated by Arroyo-Palacios and Romano (2008) physiological or bio-signals offer great possibilities for automatic affect recognition. However, exploiting their full potential has been impossible to date due to a lack of consensus among psychologists about the nature, theories, models, and specificity of physiological patterns for each emotion-space dimension. Needless to say, establishing standardization on key areas such as stimulus for the identification of physiological patterns, physiological measures, features to analyze, and the emotional model to be used will greatly advance the state-of-the-art in this field (Arroyo-Palacios & Romano, 2008).

THERMAL SIGNALS

A number of studies in neuropsychology, physiology, and behaviour analysis suggest that there exists a correlation between mammals' core body temperature and their affective states. Nakayama, Goto, Kuraoka, & Nakamura (2005) conducted experiments by monitoring the facial temperature change of monkeys under stressful and threatening conditions. Their study revealed that a decrease in nasal skin temperature is relevant to a change from neutral to negative affective state. Vianna and Carrive (2005) conducted another independent experiment by monitoring the temperature changes in rats when they were experiencing fearful situations. They observed that the temperature increased in certain body parts (i.e., eyes, head and back), while in other body parts (i.e., tail and paws) the temperature dropped simultaneously.

Other studies also exist indicating that contraction or expansion of the facial/bodily muscles of humans causes fluctuations in the blood flow rate (e.g., Khan, Ingleby, & Ward, 2006, Khan, Ward, & Ingleby, 2006, Khan, Ward, & Ingleby, 2009; Tsiamyrtzis, Dowdall, Shastri, Pavlidis, Frank, & Ekman, 2007). This muscular activity results in a change in the volume of blood flow under the surface of the human facial and/or bodily skin. Thus, tensed or contracted muscles (e.g., in anger or stress) result in higher skin temperature.

Unlike other bio-physiological sensing, the use of infrared thermal camera does not rely on contact with the human body. Thus, non-invasive detection of any change in facial and/or bodily thermal features relevant to detecting, extracting, and interpreting human affective states is feasible. For instance, Pavlidis, Levine, and Baukol (2001) and Tsiamyrtzis et al. (2007) have shown that there is a correlation between increased blood perfusion in the orbital muscles and anxiety and stress levels of humans. Similarly, Puri, Olson, Pavlidis, Levine, and Starren (2005) reported that users' stress level was correlated with increased blood flow in the frontal vessels of forehead causing dissipation of convective heat.

A generic model for estimating the relationship between fluctuations in blood flow, skin temperature, and facial/bodily muscle activity is not yet available. Such a model could enhance our understanding of the relationship between affective dimensions and the facial/bodily thermal and physiological reactions.

POSED VS. SPONTANEOUS EXPRESSIONS

Most of the studies supporting the universality of emotional expressions are based on experiments related to deliberate/posed expressions. Studies reveal that humans recognise both deliberate/posed and involuntary/spontaneous emotional expressions equally accurately. However, deliberate expressions are significantly different from spontaneous expressions. Deliberate facial behaviour is mediated by separate motor pathways and differences between natural and deliberate facial actions may be significant. Schmidt and Cohn (2001) reported that an important visual cue signalling a smile as being deliberate or spontaneous is the temporal evolvement of the smile. Extensive research has been further conducted by Cohn and colleagues in order to identify temporal and morphological differences between deliberately and spontaneously displayed facial affective behaviour (Ambadar, Schooler, & Cohn, 2005).

In daily interactions, a particular bodily expression is most likely to be accompanied by a congruent facial expression being governed by a single emotional state. Darwin argued that because our bodily actions are easier to control on command than our facial actions, the information conveyed by body movements should be less significant than that conveyed by the face, at least when it comes to discerning spontaneous from posed behaviour. Ekman, however, argued that people do not bother to censor their body movements in daily life; therefore, the body would be the more reliable source of information (Ekman, 2003). This is also in agreement with recent findings in research in nonverbal behaviour and communication, which state that truthful and deceptive behaviour differ from each other in lack of head movement (Buller, Burgoon, White, & Ebesu, 1994) and lack of illustrating gestures which accompany speech (DePaulo, 2003) in the case of deceptive behaviour.

Compared to visible channels of face and body, the advantage of using bio-signals for recognizing affective states is the fact that physiological recordings cannot be easily faked or suppressed, and can provide direct information about the user's affective state.

However, people express and communicate emotions multimodally. Hence, more research efforts and studies on posed vs. spontaneous expressions in a multicue and multimodal context are needed if we are to obtain a better understanding of the natural communication of emotions in HHI to be later used in HCI.

DATA ACQUISITION

Recordings of affective behaviour may be those of posed behaviour (i.e., produced by the subject upon request), induced behaviour (i.e., occurring in a controlled setting designed to elicit an affective reaction such as when watching movies), or spontaneous behaviour (i.e., occurring in real-life settings such as interviews or interactions between humans or between humans and machines) (Banziger & Scherer, 2007).

The easiest way to create a database of acted affective displays is by having an experimenter direct and control the recorded displays. Depending on which modalities are recorded, a number of sensors can be used: cameras for face and body expressions, microphones for recording audio signals, a motion capture systems to record 3D affective postures/gestures, and so forth. (see Figure 2). When acquiring spontaneous affective multimodal data, the subjects may be recorded without their knowledge while they are stimulated with some emotionally-rich stimulus (e.g., Zuckerman, Larrance, Hall, DeFrank, & Rosenthal, 1979). Due to the ethical issues, making recordings without subjects' knowledge is strongly discouraged and the current trend is to record spontaneous data in more constrained conditions such as an interview settings, where subjects are still aware of placement of cameras and their locations (e.g., Littlewort, Bartlett, & Lee, 2007; Pantic & Bartlett, 2007).

3D affective body postures or gestures can alternatively be recorded by utilizing motion capture systems (e.g., Kleinsmith & Bianchi-Berthouze, 2007). In such scenarios, the actor is dressed in a suit with a number of markers on the joints and body segments, while each gesture is captured by a number of cameras and represented by consecutive frames describing the position of the markers in the 3D space.

Recording physiological and bio-potential signals is a bit more complicated compared to the aforementioned recordings. In the brain-computer interface (BCI) or bio-potential signal research context, the subject being recorded usually wears headphones, a headband or a cap on which electrodes are mounted, a clip sensor, and/or touch type electrodes. The subject is then stimulated with emotionally-evocative images/videos/sounds. The variation of the skin conductance at the region of interest is then measured (Takahashi, 2004). Hence, the bio-potential affect data acquisition is *induced* and, due to its invasive nature, the experimental settings provided do not encourage spontaneity.

Creation and annotation of affect databases from face and body displays has been reviewed by Gunes and Piccardi (2006). Various visual, audio and audio-visual databases have been reviewed by Zeng et al. (2009). The existing databases where emotion is labelled continuously and data were made publicly available for research purposes are listed in Table 1. Overall, very few of the existing multimodal affect databases contain spontaneous data. Although there is a recent attempt to collect spontaneous facial expression data in real-life settings (in the context of autism disorder; El Kaliouby & Teeters, 2007), such an attempt is lacking when it comes to multimodal human-affect data. As already mentioned above, acquiring data in fully unconstrained environments with multiple sensors involves ethical and privacy concerns together with numerous technical difficulties (placement of sensors, controlling the environmental conditions such as noise, illumination, occlusions; consistency, repeatability, etc.). This impedes significantly the progress in this direction.

DATA ANNOTATION

In general, annotation of the data, both for posed and spontaneous data, is usually done separately for each channel assuming independency between the channels.

In general, for databases containing audio data, the annotation tool FeelTrace is commonly used. Feeltrace allows observers to listen to affective behaviour recordings (and watch them in the case of audio-visual recordings) and move their cursor within a 2D emotional space to rate their impression about the emotional state of the subject (Cowie et al., 2000). Emotion classes based on Feeltrace can be described as follows: positive activation, positive evaluation; positive activation, negative evaluation; negative activation, negative evaluation; negative activation, positive evaluation; and neutral (close to the centre of the 2D emotional space). For instance, for the Sensitive Artificial Listener (SAL) database (see Douglas-Cowie et al., 2007; Table 1), 4 observers provided continuous annotations with respect to valence and activation dimensions, using the FeelTrace annotation tool.

In general, when annotating or labelling affective behaviour from facial displays, six basic emotion categories and the Facial Action Coding System (FACS) are used. There exist very few studies focusing on labelling facial expressions using the dimensional approaches. For instance, Breazeal (2003) mapped a series of facial expression photos onto Russell's A-V emotion space (see Figure 1b) and used this to model a robot's interpretation of facial expressions. Shin (2007) asked human observers to rate static facial expression images in terms of A-V dimensions on a nine-point scale. The images were labelled with a rating averaged over all observers. As described previously, the FeelTrace annotation tool is often

Table 1. Representative databases created for dimensional affect recognition.

Database	The Montreal Affective Voices Database	SAL database	The Vera am Mittag speech database
Reference	Belin, Fillion-Bilodeau, and Gosselin, 2008	Douglas-Cowie et al., 2007	Grimm, Kroschel, and Narayanan, 2008
Data Type	Posed	induced	spontaneous
Modalities	Emotional speech	Audiovisual: facial expressions, emotional speech	Audiovisual: facial and bodily expressions, emotional speech
subjects	5 male and 5 female actors	2 male and 2 female subjects interacting with an artificial listener	various participants in the show
categorical annotation	anger, disgust, sadness, fear, pain, happiness, pleasure, surprise, neutral	not applicable	not applicable
dimensional annotation	intensity of valence, intensity of arousal, and intensity of each discrete emotion category	intensity of arousal, and intensity of valence	continuous annotation for valence, activation, and dominance.
annotators	30 observers	4 Feeltrace coders	17 observers
content	90 emotionally-coloured pronunciations of the word 'ah'	Humans interacting with a Sensitive Artificial Listener (SAL) in a Wizard-of-Oz scenario	12 hours of audio-visual recordings of German TV talk show "Vera am Mittag", segmented into dialogue acts and utterances
Public availability	Yes	yes	yes
Online provision	No	no	no

used to annotate audio and audio-visual recordings (e.g., in the case of the SAL database).

When it comes to annotating body gestures, there is not one common annotation scheme that has been adopted by all research groups. Kleinsmith and Bianchi-Berthouze (2007) reported results for five observers that were asked to rate static body postures on a seven-point Likert scale in terms of four affective dimensions: valence (pleasure), arousal (alertness), potency (control), and avoidance (avoid/attend to). Postures that received an average observer rating of < 3.8 were labelled as low intensity postures. Postures that received an average rating between 3.8 and 4.2 were labelled as neutral intensity postures. Finally, postures that received an average rating of > 4.2 were labelled as high intensity postures.

Using the categorical and dimensional models simultaneously enables analysis of mapping between categorical and dimensional spaces. The Montreal Affective Voices Database (Belin et al., 2008), for instance, includes 10 ratings for each data sample: perceived valence (from extremely negative to extremely positive), perceived arousal (from not aroused to extremely aroused), and perceived intensity of eight targeted affective states: happiness, sadness, fear, anger, surprise, disgust, pleasure, and pain (e.g., from not angry to extremely angry). Jin and Wang (2005) analyzed emotions in spoken Chinese and reported that joy and anger are commonly associated with similar high level of arousal while surprise, disgust, fear, neutral, and sadness are commonly associated with lower levels of arousal. As far as valence is concerned, joy was commonly associated with high levels of valence. Differences in the ratings in terms of the arousal dimension were reported to be smaller than those reported for the valence dimension.

Annotating brain-wave, thermal, and other signals in terms of affective states is not a straightforward process and it is inherently different compared to visual or audio recordings. For bio-potential signal annotation, the level of valence and arousal is usually extracted from the subjects' responses (Kulic & Croft, 2007; Pun, Alecu, Chanel, Kronegg, & Voloshynovskiy, 2006). This is mainly due to the fact that feelings induced by an image can be very different from subject to subject. Self-assessment of valence and arousal is therefore a preferred way of labelling the data (Chanel et al., 2005). The subjects are generally asked to rate their response to the stimuli in terms of intensity of few affect categories (Kulic & Croft, 2007). When a dimensional approach is used, intensity scores such as *low*, *medium* and *high* are usually scored for arousal and valence dimensions (Kulic & Croft, 2007).

Overall, researchers seem to use different levels of intensity when adopting a dimensional affect approach. Shin (2007) asked the observers to rate static facial expression images in terms of A-V using a ten-point Likert scale (0-very positive, 9-very negative), (0-low arousal, 9-high arousal). Yang et al. (2007) use a range between -1.0 and 1.0, divided into 11 levels, for annotation of emotions in the A-V space. The final annotation is then calculated as the mean of the A-V values of all observers.

Obtaining high inter-observer agreement is one of the main challenges in affective data annotation, especially when dimensional approach is adopted. Yang et al. (2007) report that mapping emotions onto the A-V space confuses the subjects. For instance, the first quadrant (high arousal, high valence) contains emotions such as excited, happy, and pleased, which are different in nature. In addition, the Feeltrace representation is criticized for not being intuitive, and raters seem to need special training to use such a dimensional labelling system (Zeng et al., 2009). A hybrid coding scheme combining both dimensional and categorical descriptions, similar to that of Zhang, Tian, Jiang, Huang, and Gao (2008), or a hierarchical scheme where the first level focuses on intensity (high, medium, low), and the second level focuses on emotions with high (happy, fear, anger), medium (happy, neutral, sad) and low (sad, neutral) arousal (Xu, Jin, Luo, & Duan, 2008) could potentially ease naïve observer's annotation task. Development of an easy to use, unambiguous and intuitive annotation scheme remains, however, an important challenge.

Another major challenge in affect data annotation is the fact that there is no coding scheme that is agreed upon and used by all researchers in the field and that can accommodate all possible communicative cues and modalities including facial and bodily expressions, vocal intonation and vocalization (e.g., laughter), bio-potential signals, etc. Addressing the aforementioned issues is necessary if we are to advance the state-of-the-art in dimensional affect sensing and recognition by making the research material comparable and easy to use.

AFFECT RECOGNITION

A typical approach to affect recognition is to categorize input samples into a number of emotion classes and apply standard pattern recognition procedures to train a classifier (Yang et al., 2007). This approach proved reasonably successful for categorical emotion recognition (Gunes et al., 2008; Pantic & Rothkrantz, 2003; Zeng et al., 2009). However, is this approach suitable when it comes to dimensional emotion recognition? We attempt to find answers to this question by examining the problem domain and surveying the state of the art in the field.

PROBLEM DOMAIN

Affect recognition is context dependent (sensitive to who the subject is, where she is, what her current task is, and when the observed behaviour has been shown; Pantic, Nijholt, & Petland, 2008). It must be carried out differently in the case of acted behaviour than in the case of spontaneous behaviour (see the previous section of this paper), and both configuration and temporal analysis of the observed behaviour are of importance for its interpretation (Ambadar et al., 2005). Except of these issues, which are typical for any human behaviour interpretation, and have been discussed in various papers (e.g., Pantic & Bartlett, 2007; Pantic et al., 2008; Vinciarelli, Pantic, & Bourland, 2009), there are a number of additional issues which need to be taken into account when applying a dimensional approach to emotion recognition. These include reliability of the ground-truth, determining duration of emotions for automatic analysis, determining the baseline, dimensionality reduction, modelling intensity of emotions, high inter-subject variation, defining optimal fusion of cues/modalities, and identifying appropriate classification methods and evaluation measures.

RELIABILITY OF THE GROUND-TRUTH

Achieving inter-observer agreement is one of the most challenging issues in dimension-based affect modelling and analysis. To date, researchers have mostly chosen to use self-assessments (e.g., Pun et al., 2006) or the mean (within a predefined range of values) of the observers' ratings (e.g., Kleinsmith & Bianchi-Berthouze, 2007). Chanel et al. (2005) report that although it is difficult to self-assess arousal, using classes generated from self-assessment of emotions facilitate greater accuracy in recognition. This finding results from a study on automatic analysis of physiological signals in terms of A-V emotion space (Chanel et al., 2005). It remains unclear whether the same holds independently of the utilised modalities and cues. Modelling inter-observer agreement levels within automatic affect analyzers and finding which signals better correlate with self assessments and which ones better correlate with independent observer assessments remain unexplored.

DURATION OF EMOTIONS

Determining the length of the temporal window for automatic affect analysis depends in principle on the modality and the target emotion. Levenson (1988) suggests that overall duration of emotions approximately falls between 0.5 and 4 seconds. He points out that, when measuring at wrong times, the emotion might be missed or multiple different emotions might be covered when too long periods are measured. For instance, when measuring bio-signals, for surprise the latency of onset can be very short, while for anger it may be rather long. Overall, the existing literature does not provide a unique answer regarding the window size to be used to achieve optimal affect recognition. Also, there is no consensus on how the efficiency of a choice should be evaluated. Current affect recognizers employ various window sizes depending on the modality, e.g., 2-6 seconds for speech, 3-15 seconds for bio-signals (Kim, 2007).

EMOTION INTENSITY

In dimensional emotion recognition the intensity of an emotion is encoded in the level of arousal (Kulic & Croft, 2007). Different emotions that have a similar level of valence can only be discriminated by their level of arousal. For instance, at a neutral valence level, low arousal represents *calmness* while high arousal represents *excitement*. Intensity is usually measured by modelling it with discrete levels such as neutral, low and high (e.g., Kleinsmith & Bianchi-Berthouze, 2007; Kulic & Croft, 2007; Wollmer et al., 2008). Separate models are then built to discriminate between pairs of affective dimension levels, for instance, low vs. high, low vs. neutral, etc. (Kleinsmith & Bianchi-Berthouze, 2007). Measuring the intensity of shown emotion appears to be modality dependent. The way the intensity of an emotion is apparent from physiological data may be different than the way it is apparent from visual data. Generalizing intensity analysis across different subjects is a challenge yet to be researched, and it is expected to be a cumbersome problem as different subjects express different levels of emotions in the same situation (Levenson, 1988).

THE BASELINE PROBLEM

When targeting spontaneous behaviour analysis and moving toward real-world settings, one of the basic problems is the Baseline Problem (Nakasone et al., 2005). For tactile modality, The Baseline Problem refers to the problem of finding a condition against which changes in measured physiological signals can be compared—the baseline. For visual modality, The Baseline Problem refers to finding a frame in which the subject is expressionless and against which changes in subject's motion, pose, and appearance can be compared. This is usually achieved by manually segmenting the recordings, or by constraining the recordings to emotional prototypes, or by having the first frame containing baseline/neutral expression. For the audio modality this is usually achieved by segmenting the recordings into turns using energy based Voice Activity Detection and processing each turn separately (e.g., Wollmer et al., 2008). Yet, as pointed out by Levenson (1988) emotion "is rarely superimposed upon a prior state of "rest"; instead, emotion occurs most typically when the organism is in some prior activation." Hence, enforcing existence of expressionless state in each recording or manually segmenting recordings so that each segment contains a baseline expression are strong, unrealistic constrains. This remains a great challenge in automatic analysis, which typically relies on existence of a baseline for analysis and processing of affective information.

DIMENSIONALITY

The space based on which emotions are typically recognized is usually a feature space with a very high dimensionality. For example, Valstar and Pantic (2007) extract 2,520 features for each frame of the input facial video, Wollmer et al. (2008) extract 4,843 features for each utterance, Chanel, Ansari, and Pun (2007) use 16,704 EEG features, Kim (2007) uses 61 features extracted from speech segments and 77 features extracted from bio-signals. The problematic issue here is having fewer training samples than features per sample for learning the target classification, which may lead to under sampling or a singularity problem. To alleviate this problem, dimensionality reduction or feature selection techniques are applied. Linear combination techniques such as Principal Component Analysis (PCA) and Linear Discriminant Analysis (LDA) and non-linear techniques such as kernel PCA (KPCA) have been used for that purpose (e.g., Chanel et al., 2007; Gunes & Piccardi, 2009; Khan et al., 2009), and so have been feature selection techniques such as Sequential Backward Selection (Kim, 2007). However, how to optimally reduce the dimensionality of continuous multicue and multimodel affect still needs to be explored.

GENERALIZATION

Should automatic affect analysers be able to generalize across subjects or should the recognition be personalized? When it comes to affect recognition from bio-potential signals, the overall amplitudes of the patterns recorded are found to be dependent on the user, suggesting that personalization is required to ensure consistent recognition of significant patterns for these signals (Conati, Chabbal, & Maclaren, 2003). Kim (2007) also found that at times subjects are inconsistent in their emotional expression. Kulic and Croft (2007) reported on the problem of saliency: subjects seem to vary not only in terms of response amplitude and duration, but for some modalities, a number of subjects show no response at all (e.g., only a subset of subjects exhibit heart-rate response). This makes generalization over unseen subjects a very difficult problem. Chanel et al. (2005) emphasize the need of training and evaluating classifiers for each participant separately due to the aforementioned inter-subject variation. When it comes to other modalities, most of the works in the field report only on subject dependent dimensional affect recognition due to limited number of subjects and data (e.g., Wollmer et al., 2008).

FUSION

For affect sensing and recognition, modality fusion refers to combining and integrating all incoming monomodal events into a single representation of the affect expressed by the user. When it comes to integrating the multiple modalities the major issues are: (i) when to integrate the modalities (i.e., at what abstraction level to do the fusion), and (ii) how to integrate the modalities (i.e., which criteria to use). Typically, the multimodal data fusion is either done at the feature level in a maximum likelihood estimation manner or at the decision level when most of the joint statistical properties (maximum a posteriori) may have been lost (Corradini et al., 2003). To make the multimodal data fusion problem tractable, the individual modalities are usually assumed independent of each other. This simplification allows employing simple parametric models for the joint distributions that cannot capture the complex relationships between the modalities. More importantly, this does not support mutual estimation (e.g., using the audio information to inform the visual information processing; Corradini, Mehta, Bernsen, & Martin, 2003).

The assumption of mutual independence of different modalities is typical for decision-level data fusion. In this approach, a separate classifier processes each modality and the outputs of these classifiers are combined at a later stage to produce the final hypothesis about the shown affective behavior. The decision-level data fusion is the most commonly applied approach in the field, especially when modalities differ in temporal characteristics (e.g., audio and visual modality). Designing optimal strategies for decision-level fusion has been of interest to researchers in the fields of pattern recognition and machine learning, and more recently to researchers in the fields of data mining and knowledge discovery. One approach, which has become popular across many disciplines, is based upon the combination of multiple classifiers, also referred to as an ensemble of experts and/or classifier fusion. For an overview of work done on combining classifiers and for theoretical justification for using simple operators such as majority vote, sum, product, maximum/minimum/median, and adaptation of weights, the readers are referred to the work by Kittler, Hatef, Duin, and Matas (1998). Decision-level data fusion can be obtained at the soft-level (a measure of confidence is associated with the decision), or at the hard-level (the combining mechanism operates on single hypothesis decisions).

Feature-level data fusion is assumed to be appropriate for closely coupled and synchronized modalities (e.g., speech and lip movements). This approach assumes a strict time synchrony between the modalities. Hence, feature-level data fusion tends not to generalize well when the modalities substantially differ in temporal characteristics (e.g., speech and gestures). Therefore, when input from two modalities is fused at the feature level, features extracted from the two modalities should be made synchronous and compatible. The asynchrony between modalities may be of two kinds: (a) asynchrony in subject's signal production (e.g., the facial action might start earlier than the vocalization), and (b) asynchrony in the recording (e.g., video is recorded at 25 Hz, the audio is recorded at 48 kHz, while EEG is recorded at 256-512 Hz). Feature-level fusion becomes more challenging as the number of features increases and when they are of very different natures (e.g., in terms of their temporal properties). Synchronization then becomes of utmost importance. Recent works have attempted synchronization between multiple multimodal cues to support feature-level fusion for the purposes of affect recognition, and reported greater overall accuracy when compared to decision-level fusion (e.g., Gunes & Piccardi, 2009; Shan, Gong, & McOwan, 2007). Gunes and Piccardi (2009) identify the neutral-onset-apex-offset-neutral phases of facial and bodily displays and synchronize the input video sequences at the phase level (i.e., apex phase). Although this method has been used for categorical emotion recognition, if the temporal information and duration of emotions are explicitly modelled, this method can be easily extended to dimensional affect recognition. Savran et al. (2006) have obtained feature/decision level fusion of the fNIRS and EEG feature vectors on a block-by-block basis. In their experiments a block is 12.5 seconds long and represents all emotional stimuli occurring within that time frame. This method can be easily applied to facilitate multimodal dimensional affect recognition. However, choosing an appropriate time-window may pose a challenge.

Outside the affect sensing and recognition field, various techniques have been exploited for implicit data synchronization purposes. For instance, dynamic time warping (DTW) has been used to find the optimal alignment between two time series. This warping between two time series can then be used to find corresponding regions between the two time series and to determine the similarity between them. Variations of Hidden Markov Models (HMM) have also been proposed for this task. Coupled HMM and fused HMM have been used for integrating tightly coupled time series, such as audio and visual features of speech (Pan, Levinson, Huang, & Liang, 2004). Bengio (2004) presented the Asynchronous HMM that could learn the joint probability of pairs of sequences of audiovisual speech data representing the same sequence of events. There are also a number of efforts within the affect sensing and recognition field to exploit the correlation between the modalities and relax the requirement of synchronization by adopting the so-called model-based fusion approach using Bayesian Networks, Multi-stream Fused HMM, tripled HMM, Neural Networks, and so forth. (for details, see Zeng et al., 2009).

Overall, typical reasons to use decision-level fusion (i.e., late integration) instead of feature-level fusion (i.e., early integration) can be summarised as follows (Wu, Oviatt, & Cohen, 1999).

- The feature concatenation used in feature-level fusion results in a high dimensional data space, resulting in a large multimodal dataset.
- Decision-level fusion allows asynchronous processing of the available modalities.
- Decision-level fusion provides greater flexibility in modelling, i.e., it is possible to train different classifiers on different data sources and integrate them without retraining.
- Using decision-level fusion of-the-shelf recognisers can be utilised for single modalities (e.g., speech).
- Decision-level fusion allows adaptive channel weighting between different modalities based on environmental conditions, such as the signal-to-noise ratio.

However, one should note that co-occurrence information (i.e., which multimodal cues co-occur at the same time, which co-occur in time with one occurring after the other, how often are the co-occurrences, etc.) is lost if decision-level fusion is chosen instead of feature-level fusion.

As pointed out by Kim (2007), a user may consciously or unconsciously conceal his or her real emotions as shown by observable cues like facial or vocal expressions, but still reveal them by invisible cues like bio signals. So, how should the fusion proceed when there is conflicting information conveyed by the modalities? This is still an open question that is yet to be investigated. Another issue to consider in affective multimodal data fusion is how to optimally fuse information with high disparity in accuracy (Kim, 2007). In addition, classification methods readily available in machine learning and pattern recognition may not be suitable for emotion-specific problems. The design of emotion-specific classification schemes that can handle multimodal and spontaneous data is one of the most important issues in the field.

EVALUATION

The evaluation measures applicable to categorical approaches to emotion recognition are not directly applicable to dimensional approaches. For example, Wolmer et al. (2008) use the Mean Squared Error (MSE) between the predicted and the actual value of arousal and valence instead of the recognition rate (i.e., percentage of correctly classified instances). However, whether MSE is the best way to evaluate the performance of dimensional approaches to automatic affect recognition, remains an open issue.

THE STATE-OF-THE-ART

The most commonly employed strategy in automatic dimensional affect classification is to simplify the problem of classifying the six basic emotions to a three-class valence-related classification problem: positive, neutral, and negative emotion classification (e.g., Yu et al., 2008). A similar simplification is to reduce the dimensional emotion classification problem to a two-class problem—positive vs. negative and active vs. passive classification problem—or a four-class problem—quadrants of 2D A-V space classification problem (e.g., Caridakis, Malatesta,

Kessous, Amir, Paouzaiou, & Karpouzis, 2006; Fragopanagos & Taylor, 2005). Glowinski et al. (2008), for instance, analyse four emotions, each belonging to one quadrant of the A-V emotion space: high arousal positive valence (joy), high arousal negative valence (anger), low arousal positive valence (relief), and low arousal negative valence (sadness).

Automatic dimensional affect recognition is still in its pioneering stage. It is worth noting that dimensional representation has mostly been used for emotion recognition from physiological signals. Hereby, in Table 2 and Table 3 we briefly summarise automated systems that attempt to model and recognize affect in the continuous dimensional space. This overview is intended to be illustrative rather than exhaustive. Table 2 summarizes representative systems for dimensional affect recognition from a single modality. Table 3 summarizes the utilised classification methods and the performance attained by the methods listed in Table 2. Table 4 summarizes the systems for dimensional affect recognition from multiple modalities. Table 5 summarizes the utilised classification methods and the performance attained by the methods listed in Table 4.

According to the dimensional approach, emotions are represented along a continuum. Therefore, automatic systems adopting this approach should produce continuous values for the target dimensions. Little attention has been paid so far to whether there are definite boundaries along the continuum to distinguish between various levels or intensities. The most common way to explore this issue is to quantize the arousal and valence dimensions into arbitrary number of levels or intensities. Kleinsmith and Bianchi-Berthouze (2007), for instance, use a back-propagation algorithm to build a separate model for each of the affective dimensions for discriminating between levels of affective dimensions from posture (high-low, high-neutral, and low-neutral). Wollmer et al. (2008) use Conditional Random Fields (CRF) for discrete emotion recognition by quantising the continuous labels for valence and arousal to four and/or seven arbitrary levels. Kulic and Croft (2007) perform quantization into 3 categories (low/medium/high), and Chanel et al. (2007) consider 3 classes, namely, excited-negative, excited-positive, and calm-neutral. Karpouzis et al. (2007) focus on positive vs. negative or active vs. passive classes.

The only approach reported in automatic affects sensing field that actually deals with continuous emotions is presented by Wollmer et al. (2008) for emotion recognition from the audio modality. Emotional history is modelled using Long Short-Term Memory Recurrent Networks (LSTM-RNN) which builds upon the principle of recurrent neural networks by including memory cells. LSTM-RNN architecture consists of three layers: an input, a hidden, and an output layer, and models long-range dependencies between successive observations. The Long Short-Term Memory cells ensure that events lying back in time are not forgotten. When compared to other classification techniques like Support-Vector Regression, LSTM-RNN achieve a prediction quality which is equal to human performance due to its capability of modelling long range time dependencies.

However, there is no agreement on how to model dimensional emotion space (continuous/quantized) and which classifier is better suited for automatic, multimodal, continuous affect analysis using a dimensional representation. The surveyed works also report a number of additional challenging issues as summarized in Table 6.

Overall, automatic human affect recognition based on a dimensional approach is still in its infancy. As can be seen from Tables 2-5, the comparison of results attained by different surveyed systems is difficult to conduct as systems use different training/testing datasets (which differ in the way emotions are elicited and annotated), they differ in the underlying model of emotions (i.e., target emotional categories) as well as in the employed modality or combination of modalities and the applied evaluation method

Table 2. Overview of the systems for dimensional affect recognition from a single modality.

System	Modality/cue	Database	# of samples	features	Dimensions
Glowinski et al., 2008	Visual, movement expressivity	Their own	40 portrayals	Gesture dynamics	4 emotions: high arousal (anger and joy) and low arousal (relief and sadness)
Khan et al., 2009	Thermal	Their own (neutral, pretended and evoked facial expressions)	Not reported	facial feature points from images	neutral, positive and negative emotion categories
Kleinsmith and Bianchi-Berthouze, 2007	Visual, static body posture	subjects displaying various body postures given a situation description	111 images	Features from the motion capture system	Valence, arousal, potency, and avoidance
Lee and Narayanan, 2005	Emotional speech	spoken language data obtained from a call centre application	1187 calls, 7200 utterances	a combination of acoustic, lexical, and discourse information	negative and non-negative emotions
Martin, Caridakis, Devillers, Karpouzis, and Abrilian, 2009	Visual, body movement	TV interviews, spontaneous	50 video samples of emotional TV interviews	coarse estimate of the overall movement quantity in a video	emotional activation of a whole video
Shin, 2007	Visual, facial expression images	posed static Korean facial expression database, 6 subjects	287 images	Facial features	pleasure-displeasure and arousal-sleep dimensions
Vogt, André, and Bee, 2008	Emotional speech	Offline speech emotion recognition framework, sentence set in German, 29 students	Not reported	variety of acoustic features like energy, MFCC, pitch and voice quality	positive-active, positive-passive, negative-active, negative-passive mapped on the emotions of joy, satisfaction, anger, frustration
Wollmer et al., 2008	Audio	SAL, 4 subjects	25 recordings, 1,692 turns	variety of acoustic features	positive-active, positive-passive, negative-active, negative-passive

(Arroyo-Palacios & Romano, 2008). Wagner et al. (2005) argue that for the current multimodal affect recognizers, the achieved recognition rates depend on the type of the utilized data, and whether the emotions were acted or not, rather than on the used algorithms and classification methods. All of this makes it difficult to quantitatively and comparatively evaluate the accuracy of the A-V modelling and the effectiveness of the developed systems.

As a consequence, it remains unclear which classification method is suitable for dimensional affect recognition from which modalities and cues. Opportunities for solving this problem can be potentially searched in other relevant research fields. For example, the A-V dimensional approach has been mostly used for affective content classification from music or videos (e.g., Xu et al., 2008; Zhang et al., 2008). Therefore, methodologies in these fields seem more mature and advanced compared to those in automatic human affect recognition field. Zhang et al. (2008), for instance, perform affective video content analysis from MTV clips in terms of A-V space by employing

Table 3. The utilised classification methodology and the performance attained by the methods listed in Table 2.

System	Classification	Results
Glowinski et al., 2008	Only preliminary analysis no classification reported	Only preliminary analysis no classification reported
Khan et al., 2009	linear discriminants (LDA)	83.3% for posed for 3 classes: neutral, happy and sad; 57.1% for 7 classes; 72% for evoked neutral, happy, sad, disgust and angry.
Kleinsmith and Bianchi-Berthouze, 2007	a back-propagation algorithm with a separate model for each of the 4 affective dimensions	79% for both the valence and arousal, and 81% for both the potency and avoidance dimensions
Lee and Narayanan, 2005	discriminant classifiers (LDC) with Gaussian class-conditional probability and k-nearest neighbourhood classifiers (k-NN) to detect negative versus non-negative emotions	Improvement of 40.7% for males and 36.4% for females via fusion of information
Martin et al., 2009	discriminant analysis	67.2% for pretended, and 72% for evoked expressions of neutral, happy, disgusted, surprised, and angry emotions
Shin, 2007	a 3-layer neural network with 2 output nodes of pleasure-displeasure and arousal-sleep	Only coarse comparison btw. NN and mean A-V human annotation
Vogt et al., 2008	Naive Bayes and support vector machine classifiers to distinguish between the four quadrants of the A-V space	an average of 55% for a 4 class problem
Wollmer et al., 2008	Long Short-Term Memory Recurrent Neural Net, Support Vector Machines, Conditional Random Fields, and Support Vector Regressor	0.18 MSE using speaker dependent validation

a clustering method called Affinity Propagation (AP). The main reason for this choice is the fact that they do not have apriori knowledge of how many affective categories a classifier should output. Another good example on how to handle data comprising continuous values comes again from the affective content analysis field. Yang et al. (2007) model emotions as continuous variables composed of arousal and valence values, and formulate music emotion recognition as a regression problem. This choice is based on the fact that the regression approach is inherently continuous, and exhibits promising prediction accuracy; it learns the predicting rules according to the ground truth and, if categorical description is needed, the regression results can be easily converted to binary or quaternary results. Various types of regressors can be used for this task: the multiple linear regression (MLR), support vector regression (SVR), and AdaBoost.RT, etc. The ground truth is obtained by averaging subjects' opinions about the A-V values for each input sample. The emotion plane is viewed as a coordinate space spanned by the A-V values (each value confined within [-1, 1]). Then Yang et al., train two regressors to predict the A-V values. The arousal and valence models are weighted combinations of some component functions, which are computed along the timeline. Yang et al. (2007) train the two regressors separately under the assumption that the correlation between arousal and valence is embedded in the ground truth. Although the context is different from that of human affect sensing, affect recognition researchers could potentially benefit from the aforementioned methodologies.

There exist a number of studies that focus on dimensional modelling of affect in the context of empathic companions (e.g., Nakasone et al., 2005), educational games (e.g., Conati et al., 2003), game interfaces (Kim et al., 2004), and speech analysis (Jin & Wang, 2005). Although interesting as the first attempts toward application-oriented systems,

Table 4. Overview of the systems for dimensional affect recognition from multiple modalities.

System	Modality/cue	Database	# of samples	Features	Dimensions
Caridakis, Karpouzis, and Kollias, 2008	facial expression, body gestures and audio	SAL, 4 subjects	Not reported	Various visual and acoustic features	neutral and four A-V quadrants
Chanel et al., 2007	Tactile, physiological	Their own, 1 subject, recall of past emotional events	Not reported	EEG and peripheral features	arousal and valence
Forbes-Riley and Litman, 2004	audio and text	student emotions from tutorial spoken dialogues	Not reported	variety of acoustic and prosodic, text-based, and contextual features	negative, neutral and positive emotions
Haag et al., 2004	Tactile, physiological	Their own, 1 subject	1000 samples	heart rate, BVP, EMG, skin conductivity, respiration	arousal and valence
Karpouzis et al., 2007	facial expression, body gestures and/or audio	SAL, 4 subjects	76 Passages, 1600 tunes	Various visual and acoustic features	negative vs. positive, active vs. passive
Kim, 2007	speech and physiological signals	A corpus of spontaneous vocal and physiological emotions, using a modified version of the quiz "Who wants to be a millionaire?", 3 subjects	343 samples	EMG, SC, ECG, BVP, Temp, RSP and acoustic features	either of the four A-V quadrants
Kulic and Croft, 2007	Tactile, physiological	Their own, context of human-robot interaction, 36 subjects	2-3 examples for each affect category	heart rate, perspiration rate, and facial muscle contraction	6 affect categories (low/medium/high-valence/arousal)
Wagner, Kim, and Andre, 2005	Tactile, physiological	Their own, 1 subject listening to songs	25 recordings for each emotion	physiological signals	negative (anger/sadness), positive (joy/pleasure), valence and high arousal (joy/anger), low arousal (sadness/pleasure)

these works are usually based on manual analysis and do not attempt automatic dimensional affect recognition.

In summary, the issues pertinent in dimensional affect recognition include reliability of the ground-truth, determining duration of emotions for automatic analysis, determining the baseline, dimensionality reduction, modelling intensity of emotions, high inter-subject variation, defining optimal fusion of cues/modalities, and identifying appropriate classification methods and evaluation measures.

CONCLUSION AND DISCUSSION

This paper discussed the problem domain of affect sensing using a dimensional approach and explored the current state-of-the-art in continuous, dimensional affect recognition.

The analysis provided in this paper indicates that the automatic affect analysis field has slowly started shifting from categorical emotion recognition to dimensional emotion recognition. Existing dimensional affect analysis systems mostly deal with spontaneous data obtained in less-controlled

Table 5. The utilised classification methodology and the performance attained by the methods listed in Table 4.

System	Classification	Explicit fusion	Results
Caridakis et al., 2008	a feed-forward back-propagation network to map tunes into either of the 4 A-V quadrants or the neutral state	Not reported	reported as reduced MSE for every tune
Chanel et al., 2007	linear discriminant analysis (LDA) and support vector machine (SVM)	Not reported	67% accuracy for 3 classes (negatively excited, positively excited, and calm-neutral), and 79% accuracy for 2 classes (negatively vs. positively excited) using EEG, 53% accuracy for 3 classes and 73% accuracy for 2 classes using peripheral signals
Forbes-Riley and Litman, 2004	AdaBoost to boost a decision tree algorithm for negative, neutral and positive emotions	Not reported	84.75% for a 3 class problem
Haag et al., 2004	separate network for valence and arousal, each with a single output node corresponding to the valence or arousal value	Not reported	96.6% for arousal, 89.9% for valence.
Karpouzis et al., 2007	a Simple Recurrent Network that outputs either of the 4 classes (3 for the possible emotion quadrants, one for neutral affective state)	Not described	67% recognition accuracy using the visual modality and 73% using prosody, 82% after fusion (whether on unseen subject/data is not specified)
Kim, 2007	modality-specific LDA-based classification; a hybrid fusion scheme where the output of feature-level fusion is fed as an auxiliary input to the decision-level fusion stage	Decision level fusion and hybrid fusion by integrating results from feature and decision level fusion	51% for bio-signals, 54% for speech, 55% applying feature fusion, 52% for decision fusion, and 54% for hybrid fusion, subject independent validation.
Kulic and Croft, 2007	3 HMMs for valence (low, medium, and high) and 3 HMMs for arousal (low, medium, and high)	Not reported	an accuracy of 64% for novel data
Lee and Narayanan, 2005	discriminant classifiers (LDC) with Gaussian class-conditional probability and k-nearest neighbourhood classifiers (k-NN) to detect negative versus non-negative emotions	Decision level fusion	Improvement of 40.7% for males and 36.4% for females via fusion of information
Wagner et al., 2005	k-nearest neighbour (kNN), linear discriminant function (LDF) and a multilayer perceptron (MLP) to recognize 4 emotion classes	Not reported	High vs. low arousal 95%, and negative vs. positive 87%

environments (i.e., subjects are taking part in interactions, subjects are not always stationary, etc.), and can handle a small number of (quantized) affective dimension categories. However, note that real-world settings pose many challenges to affect sensing and recognition (Conati et al., 2003). Firstly, it is not easy to obtain a high level of reliability among independent observers annotating the affect data. In addition, when subjects are not restricted in terms of mobility, the level of noise in all recorded signals tends to increase. This is

Table 6. Reported challenges for dimensional affect recognition.

System	Challenges encountered
Chanel et al., 2007	EEG signals are good for valence assessment. Peripheral signals better correlate with arousal than with valence. Peripheral signals appear to be appropriate for modelling calm-neutral vs. excited dimension, but are problematic for the negative vs. positive dimension.
Haag et al., 2004	Estimation of valence is harder than estimation of arousal.
Karpouzis et al., 2007	Disagreement (frame-based) between human observers (annotators) affects the performance of the automated systems. The system should take into account the inter-observer disagreement, by comparing this to the level of disagreement between the ground truth and the results attained by the system.
Kim, 2007	Recognition is subject and modality dependant.
Kulic and Croft, 2007	There is a considerable inter-subject variability in the signal amplitude and its length. Hence, it is hard to develop a system that can perform well for all subjects and generalize well for unseen subjects.

particularly the case for bio-signals. No solution has yet been proposed to solve these problems.

In general, modelling emotions continuously using the dimensions of arousal and valence is not a trivial problem as these dimensions are not universally perceived and understood by human observers. It seems that the perception of arousal is more universal than is the perception of valence (Zhang et al., 2008). Similar findings have been reported by Kleinsmith and Bianchi-Berthouze (2007), who found that ratings of arousal contained very small variability among different observers, when body postures were mapped onto affective dimensions. Also, for audio modality variability of ratings of arousal appears to be smaller than that of valence (Jin & Wang, 2005). Wolmer et al. (2008) also reported that automatic analysis results for activation/arousal are remarkably better than those for valence when using audio information. Yet, valence appears to be more stable than arousal in dimensional facial expression recognition from static images (Shin, 2007). Having said the above, it can be concluded that stability of inter-observer agreement on valence and arousal is highly dependent on the modality employed. Hence, this makes the problem of obtaining a reliable ground truth for multimodal recordings a true challenge.

To address this problem Kim (2007) suggests that emotion recognition problem should be decomposed into several processes. One stage could be recognizing arousal through physiological channels, while recognizing valence via audio-visual channels. The second stage can then be resolving uncertainties between adjacent emotion classes in the 2D space by cumulative analysis of user's context information. A more thorough investigation is needed to test this suggestion and propose a similar set of processes to be applied when other cues and modalities are employed.

One of the main disadvantages of bio-potential-based affect recognition systems is the fact that they are cumbersome and invasive and require placing sensors physically on the human body (e.g., a sensor clip that is mounted on subject's earlobe, a BCI mounted on the subject's head, etc.; Takahashi, 2004). Moreover, EEG has been found to be very sensitive to electrical signals emanating from facial muscles while emotions are being expressed via face. Therefore, in a multimodal affect recognition system, simultaneous use of these modalities needs to be reconsidered. Additionally, during recordings, the fNIRS device is known to cover the eyebrows. This in turn poses another challenge: facial features occlusion. However, new forms of non-contact physiological sensing might facilitate better utilisation of psychological signals as input to multimodal affect recognition systems.

To the best of our knowledge, to date, only a few systems have been reported that actually achieved dimensional affect recognition from multiple modalities. These are summarised in Tables

4 and 5. Further efforts are needed to identify the importance and feasibility of the following important issues.

- Among the available remotely observable and remotely unobservable modalities, which ones should be used for automatic dimensional affect recognition? Does this depend on the context? Will the recognition accuracy increase as the number of modalities a system can analyse increases?
- Kim (2007) found that speech and physiological data contain little complementary information. Accordingly, should we use equal weights for each modality or should we investigate the innate priority among the modalities to be preferred for each emotional dimension/state?
- Chanel et al. (2005) report that although it is difficult to self-assess arousal, using classes generated from self-assessment of emotions facilitate greater accuracy in recognition. When labelling emotions, should one use self assessment or independent observer's assessment? Which signals better correlate with self assessment and which ones correlate with independent observer assessment?
- How does *the baseline problem* affect recognition? Is an objective *basis* (e.g., a frame containing an expressionless display) strictly needed prior to computing the arousal and valence values? If so, how can this be obtained in a fully automatic manner from spontaneous data?
- Considering the fact that different emotions may have similar or identical valence or arousal values (Haag et al., 2004), should the affect recognizers attempt to recognize distinct emotion categories rather than A-V intensities? Does this depend on the context? How should affective states be mapped onto the A-V space? Should we follow a hierarchical framework where similar affective states are grouped into the same category?
- How should intensity be modelled for dimensional and continuous affect recognition? Should the aim be personalizing systems for each subject, or creating systems that are expected to generalize across subjects?
- In a continuous emotional space, how should duration of emotion be defined? How can this be incorporated in automated systems? Will focusing on shorter or longer observations affect the accuracy of the recognition process?
- In real-world uncontrolled settings it is very difficult to elicit balanced amount of data for each emotion dimension to be elicited. For instance, a bias toward quadrant 1 (positive arousal, positive valence) exists in the SAL database portion used by (Caridakis et al., 2008). So, how should the issue of unbalanced data/classes inherent to real-world settings (Chanel et al., 2005) be handled?

The most notable issue in the field is the existence of a gap between different communities. Machine affect recognition community seems to use different databases compared to psychology and cognitive sciences communities. Also for annotation of the data, a more uniform and multi-purpose scheme that can accommodate all possible research aims, modalities and cues should be explored.

The systems surveyed in this paper represent initial but crucial steps toward finding solutions to the aforementioned problems, and realization of automatic, multimodal, dimensional and continuous recognition of human affect.

ACKNOWLEDGMENT

Current research of Hatice Gunes is funded by the European Community's 7th Framework Programme [FP7/2007-2013] under the grant agreement no 211486 (SEMAINE). The work of Maja Pantic is funded in part by the European Research Council under the ERC Starting Grant agreement no. ERC-2007-StG-203143 (MAHNOB).

REFERENCES

Aftanas, L. I., Pavlov, S. V., Reva, N. V., & Varlamov, A. A. (2003). Trait anxiety impact on the EEG theta band power changes during appraisal of threatening and pleasant visual stimuli. *International Journal of Psychophysiology*, *50*(3), 205–212. doi:10.1016/S0167-8760(03)00156-9

Aftanas, L. I., Reva, N. V., Varlamov, A. A., Pavlov, S. V., & Makhnev, V. P. (2004). Analysis of evoked EEG synchronization and desynchronization in conditions of emotional activation in humans: Temporal and topographic characteristics. *Neuroscience and Behavioral Physiology*, *34*(8), 859–867. doi:10.1023/B:NEAB.0000038139.39812.eb

Ambadar, Z., Schooler, J., & Cohn, J. F. (2005). Deciphering the enigmatic face: The importance of facial dynamics in interpreting subtle facial expressions. *Psychological Science*, *16*(5), 403–410. doi:10.1111/j.0956-7976.2005.01548.x

Ambady, N., & Rosenthal, R. (1992). Thin slices of expressive behaviour as predictors of interpersonal consequences: A meta–analysis. *Psychological Bulletin*, *11*(2), 256–274. doi:10.1037/0033-2909.111.2.256

Argyle, M. (1975). *Bodily communication*. London: Methuen.

Arroyo-Palacios, J., & Romano, D. M. (2008, August). Towards a standardization in the use of physiological signals for affective recognition systems. In *Proceedings of Measuring Behavior 2008,* Maastricht, The Netherlands (pp. 121-124). Noldus.

Banziger, T., & Scherer, K. R. (2007, September) Using actor portrayals to systematically study multimodal emotion expression: The gemep corpus. In A. Paiva, R. Prada, & R. W. Picard (Eds.), *Affective Computing and Intelligent Interaction: Proceedings of the 2nd International Conference on Affective Computing and Intelligent Interaction,* Lisbon, Portugal (LNCS 4738, pp. 476-487).

Baron-Cohen, S., & Tead, T. H. E. (2003) *Mind reading: The interactive guide to emotion*. London: Jessica Kingsley Publishers.

Batliner, A., Fischer, K., Hubera, R., Spilkera, J., & Noth, E. (2003). How to find trouble in communication. *Speech Communication*, *40*, 117–143. doi:10.1016/S0167-6393(02)00079-1

Belin, P., Fillion-Bilodeau, S., & Gosselin, F. (2008). The Montreal affective voices: A validated set of nonverbal affect bursts for research on auditory affective processing. *Behavior Research Methods*, *40*(2), 531–539. doi:10.3758/BRM.40.2.531

Bengio, S. (2004). Multimodal speech processing using asynchronous hidden markov models. *Information Fusion*, *5*, 81–89. doi:10.1016/j.inffus.2003.04.001

Breazeal, C. (2003). Emotion and sociable humanoid robots. *International Journal of Human-Computer Studies*, *59*, 119–155. doi:10.1016/S1071-5819(03)00018-1

Buller, D., Burgoon, J., White, C., & Ebesu, A. (1994). Interpersonal deception: Vii. Behavioural profiles of falsification, equivocation and concealment. *Journal of Language and Social Psychology*, *13*(5), 366–395. doi:10.1177/0261927X94134002

Campbell, N., & Mokhtari, P. (2003, August). Voice quality: The 4th prosodic dimension. In *Proceedings of the International Congress of Phonetic Sciences,* Barcelona (pp. 2417-2420).

Camras, L. A., Meng, Z., Ujiie, T., Dharamsi, K., Miyake, S., & Oster, H. (2002). Observing emotion in infants: Facial expression, body behaviour, and rater judgments of responses to an expectancy-violating event. *Emotion (Washington, D.C.), 2,* 179–193. doi:10.1037/1528-3542.2.2.179

Camurri, A., Mazzarino, B., & Volpe, G. (2003, April) Analysis of expressive gesture: The EyesWeb expressive gesture processing library. In *Proceedings of the Gesture Workshop,* Genova, Italy (pp. 460-467).

Caridakis, G., Karpouzis, K., & Kollias, S. (2008). User and context adaptive neural networks for emotion recognition. *Neurocomputing, 71,* 13–15, 2553–2562. doi:10.1016/j.neucom.2007.11.043

Caridakis, G., Malatesta, L., Kessous, L., Amir, N., Paouzaiou, A., & Karpouzis, K. (2006, November). Modelling naturalistic affective states via facial and vocal expression recognition. In *Proceedings 8th ACM International Conference on Multimodal Interfaces (ICMI '06),* Banff, Alberta, Canada (pp. 146-154). ACM Publishing.

Chanel, G., Ansari-Asl, K., & Pun, T. (2007, October). Valence-arousal evaluation using physiological signals in an emotion recall paradigm. In *Proceedings of the IEEE International Conference on Systems, Man and Cybernetics,* Montreal, Quebec, Canada (pp. 2662-2667). Washington, DC: IEEE Computer Society.

Chanel, G., Kronegg, J., Grandjean, D., & Pun, T. (2002). *Emotion assessment: Arousal evaluation using EEG's and peripheral physiological signals* (Tech. Rep. 05.02). Geneva, Switzerland: Computer Vision Group, Computing Science Center, University of Geneva.

Changchun, L., Rani, P., & Sarkar, N. (2005, August). An empirical study of machine learning techniques for affect recognition in human-robot interaction. In *Proceedings of the IEEE/RSJ International Conference on Intelligent Robots and Systems,* Edmonton, Canada (pp. 2662-2667). Washington, DC: IEEE Computer Society.

Conati, C., Chabbal, R., & Maclaren, H. A. (2003, June). *Study on using biometric sensors for monitoring user emotions in educational games.* Paper presented at the Workshop on Assessing and Adapting to User Attitudes and Affect: Why, When and How? User Modelling (UM-03), Johnstown, PA.

Corradini, A., Mehta, M., Bernsen, N. O., & Martin, J.-C. (2003, August). Multimodal input fusion in human computer interaction on the example of the on-going nice project. In *Proceedings of the NATO: Asi Conference on Data Fusion for Situation Monitoring, Incident Detection, Alert and Response Management,* Tsakhkadzor, Armenia (pp. 223-234).

Coulson, M. (2004). Attributing emotion to static body postures: Recognition accuracy, confusions, and viewpoint dependence. *Nonverbal Behavior, 28*(2), 117–139. doi:10.1023/B:JONB.0000023655.25550.be

Cowie, R., Douglas-Cowie, E., Savvidou, S., McMahon, E., Sawey, M., & Schroder, M. (2000, September). 'FEELTRACE': An instrument for recording perceived emotion in real time. In *Proceedings of the ISCA Workshop on Speech and Emotion,* Belfast, Northern Ireland (pp. 19-24).

Cowie, R., Douglas-Cowie, E., Tsapatsoulis, N., Votsis, G., Kollias, S., & Fellenz, W. (2001). Emotion recognition in human-computer interaction. *IEEE Signal Processing Magazine*, *18*(1), 32–80. doi:10.1109/79.911197

Darwin, C. (1998). *The expression of the emotions in man and animals* (3rd ed.). New York: Oxford University Press.

Davitz, J. (1964). Auditory correlates of vocal expression of emotional feeling. In J. Davitz (Ed.), The communication of emotional meaning (pp. 101-112). New York: McGraw-Hill.

De Silva, P. R. S., Osano, M., Marasinghe, A., & Madurapperuma, A. P. (2006, April). Towards recognizing emotion with affective dimensions through body gestures. In *Proceedings of the 7th International Conference on Automatic Face and Gesture Recognition,* Southampton, UK (pp. 269-274).

DePaulo, B. (2003). Cues to deception. *Psychological Bulletin*, *129*(1), 74–118. doi:10.1037/0033-2909.129.1.74

Douglas-Cowie, E., Cowie, R., Sneddon, I., Cox, C., Lowry, O., McRorie, M., et al. (2007, September). The HUMAINE Database: addressing the needs of the affective computing community. In *Affective Computing and Intelligent Interaction: Proceedings of the 2nd International Conference on Affective Computing and Intelligent Interaction,* Lisbon, Portugal (LNCS 4738, pp. 488-500).

Dreuw, P., Deselaers, T., Rybach, D., Keysers, D., & Ney, H. (2006, April). Tracking using dynamic programming for appearance-based sign language recognition. In *Proceedings of the IEEE International Conference on Automatic Face and Gesture Recognition,* Southampton, UK (pp. 293-298). Washington, DC: IEEE Computer Society.

Driver, J., & Spence, C. (2000). Multisensory perception: Beyond modularity and convergence. *Current Biology*, *10*(20), 731–735. doi:10.1016/S0960-9822(00)00740-5

Ekman, P. (1982). *Emotion in the human face*. Cambridge, UK: Cambridge University Press.

Ekman, P. (2003). Darwin, deception, and facial expression. *Annals of the New York Academy of Sciences, 1000*, 105–221.

Ekman, P., & Friesen, W. V. (1967). Head and body cues in the judgment of emotion: A reformulation. *Perceptual and Motor Skills, 24*, 711–724.

Ekman, P., & Friesen, W. V. (1975). *Unmasking the face: A guide to recognizing emotions from facial clues*. Englewood Cliffs, NJ: Prentice-Hall.

Ekman, P., & Friesen, W. V. (1978). *Facial action coding system: A technique for the measurement of facial movement.* Palo Alto, CA: Consulting Psychologists Press.

Ekman, P., Friesen, W. V., & Hager, J. C. (2002). *Facial action coding system*. Salt Lake City, UT: A Human Face.

El Kaliouby, R., & Robinson, P. (2005, June 27-July 2). Real-time inference of complex mental states from facial expressions and head gestures. In *Proceedings of the 2004 Conference on Computer Vision and Pattern Recognition Workshop (CVPRW 2004),* Washington, DC (Vol. 10, pp. 154). Washington, DC: IEEE Computer Society.

El Kaliouby, R., & Teeters, A. (2007, November). Eliciting, capturing and tagging spontaneous facial affect in autism spectrum disorder. In *Proceedings of the 9th International Conference on Multimodal Interfaces,* Nagoya, Japan (pp. 46-53).

Elgammal, A., Shet, V., Yacoob, Y., & Davis, L. S. (2003, June). Learning dynamics for exemplar-based gesture recognition. In *Proceedings of the IEEE Conference on Computer Vision and Pattern Recognition,* Madison, WI (pp. 571-578). Washington, DC: IEEE Computer Society.

Fasel, I. R., Fortenberry, B., & Movellan, J. R. (2005). A generative framework for real-time object detection, and classification. *Computer Vision and Image Understanding, 98*(1), 182–210. doi:10.1016/j.cviu.2004.07.014

Forbes-Riley, K., & Litman, D. (2004, May). Predicting emotion in spoken dialogue from multiple knowledge sources. In *Proceedings of the Human Language Technology Conference North America Chapter of the Association for Computational Linguistics (HLT-NAACL 2004),* Boston (pp. 201-208).

Fragopanagos, F., & Taylor, J. G. (2005). Emotion recognition in human-computer interaction. *Neural Networks, 18*, 389–405. doi:10.1016/j.neunet.2005.03.006

Friesen, W. V., & Ekman, P. (1984). *EMFACS-7: Emotional facial action coding system* (unpublished manual). San Francisco: University of California, San Francisco.

Glowinski, D., Camurri, A., Volpe, G., Dael, N., & Scherer, K. (2008, June). Technique for automatic emotion recognition by body gesture analysis. In *Proceedings of the 2008 Computer Vision and Pattern Recognition Workshops,* Anchorage, AK (pp. 1-6). Washington, DC: IEEE Computer Society.

Grandjean, D., Sander, D., & Scherer, K. R. (2008). Conscious emotional experience emerges as a function of multilevel, appraisal-driven response synchronization. *Consciousness and Cognition, 17*(2), 484–495. doi:10.1016/j.concog.2008.03.019

Grimm, M., Kroschel, K., & Narayanan, S. (2008, June). The Vera am Mittag German audio-visual emotional speech database. In *Proceedings of the IEEE International Conference on Multimedia and Expo,* Hannover, Germany (pp. 865-868). Washington, DC: IEEE Computer Society.

Gross, M. M., Gerstner, G. E., Koditschek, D. E., Fredrickson, B. L., & Crane, E. A. (2006). *Emotion recognition from body movement kinematics*. Retrieved from http://sitemaker.umich.edu/mgrosslab/files/abstract.pdf

Gunes, H., & Piccardi, M. (2006, October). Creating and annotating affect databases from face and body display: A contemporary survey. In *Proceedings of the IEEE International Conference on Systems, Man and Cybernetics,* Taipei, Taiwan (pp. 2426-2433).

Gunes, H., & Piccardi, M. (2008). From mono-modal to multi-modal: Affect recognition using visual modalities. In D. Monekosso, P. Remagnino, & Y. Kuno (Eds.), *Ambient intelligence techniques and applications* (pp. 154-182). Berlin, Germany: Springer-Verlag.

Gunes, H., & Piccardi, M. (2009). Automatic temporal segment detection and affect recognition from face and body display. *IEEE Transactions on Systems, Man, and Cybernetics – Part B, 39*(1), 64-84.

Gunes, H., Piccardi, M., & Pantic, M. (2008). From the lab to the real world: Affect recognition using multiple cues and modalities. In Jimmy Or (Ed.), *Affective computing, focus on emotion expression, synthesis and recognition* (pp. 185-218). Vienna, Austria: I-Tech Education and Publishing.

Haag, A., Goronzy, S., Schaich, P., & Williams, J. (2004, June). Emotion recognition using bio-sensors: First steps towards an automatic system. In E. André, L. Dybkjær, W. Minker, & P. Heisterkamp (Eds.), *Affective Dialogue Systems: Tutorial and Research Workshop (ADS 2004),* Kloster Irsee, Germany (LNCS 3068, pp. 36-48).

Hadjikhani, N., & De Gelder, B. (2003). Seeing fearful body expressions activates the fusiform cortex and amygdala. *Current Biology, 13*, 2201–2205. doi:10.1016/j.cub.2003.11.049

Jin, X., & Wang, Z. (2005, October). An emotion space model for recognition of emotions in spoken chinese. In *Proceedings of the 1st International Conference on Affective Computing and Intelligent Interaction (ACII 2005),* Beijing, China, (pp. 397-402).

Juslin, P. N., & Scherer, K. R. (2005). Vocal expression of affect. In J. Harrigan, R. Rosenthal, & K. Scherer (Eds.), *The new handbook of methods in nonverbal behavior research* (pp. 65-135). Oxford, UK: Oxford University Press.

Karpouzis, K., Caridakis, G., Kessous, L., Amir, N., Raouzaiou, A., Malatesta, L., et al. (2007, November). Modelling naturalistic affective states via facial, vocal and bodily expressions recognition. In J. G. Carbonell & J. Siekmann (Eds.), *Artifical Intelligence for Human Computing: ICMI 2006 and IJCAI 2007 International Workshops,* Banff, Canada (LNAI 4451, pp. 92-116).

Keltner, D., & Ekman, P. (2000). Facial expression of emotion. In M. Lewis & J. M. Haviland-Jones (Eds.), *Handbook of emotions* (pp. 236-249). New York: Guilford Press.

Khan, M. M., Ingleby, M., & Ward, R. D. (2006). Automated facial expression classification and affect interpretation using infrared measurement of facial skin temperature variations. *ACM Transactions on Autonomous and Adaptive Systems, 1*(1), 91–113. doi:10.1145/1152934.1152939

Khan, M. M., Ward, R. D., & Ingleby, M. (2006, June). Infrared thermal sensing of positive and negative affective states. In *Proceedings of the IEEE Conference on Robotics, Automation and Mechatronics,* Bangkok, Thailand (pp. 1-6). Washington, DC: IEEE Computer Society.

Khan, M. M., Ward, R. D., & Ingleby, M. (2009). Classifying pretended and evoked facial expressions of positive and negative affective states using infrared measurement of skin temperature. *ACM Transactions on Applied Perception, 6*(1), 6. doi:10.1145/1462055.1462061

Kim, J. (2007). Bimodal emotion recognition using speech and physiological changes. In M. Grimm, K. Kroschel (Eds.), *Robust speech recognition and understanding* (pp. 265-280). Vienna, Austria: I-Tech Education and Publishing.

Kittler, J., Hatef, M., Duin, R. P. W., & Matas, J. (1998). On combining classifiers. *IEEE Transactions on Pattern Analysis and Machine Intelligence, 20*(3), 226–239. doi:10.1109/34.667881

Kleinsmith, A., & Bianchi-Berthouze, N. (2007, September). Recognizing affective dimensions from body posture. In *Affective Computing and Intelligent Interaction: 2nd International Conference,* Lisbon, Portugal (LNCS 4738, pp. 48-58).

Kleinsmith, A., Ravindra De Silva, P., & Bianchi-Berthouze, N. (2005, October) Grounding affective dimensions into posture features. In *Proceedings of the 1st International Conference on Affective Computing and Intelligent Interaction (ACII 2005),* Beijing, China (pp. 263-270).

Kleinsmith, A., Ravindra De Silva, P., & Bianchi-Berthouze, N. (2006). Cross-cultural differences in recognizing affect from body posture. *Interacting with Computers, 18*, 1371–1389. doi:10.1016/j.intcom.2006.04.003

Kulic, D., & Croft, E. A. (2007). Affective state estimation for human–robot interaction. *IEEE Transactions on Robotics, 23*(5), 991–1000. doi:10.1109/TRO.2007.904899

Lee, C. M., & Narayanan, S. S. (2005). Toward detecting emotions in spoken dialogs. *IEEE Transactions on Speech and Audio Processing, 13*(2), 293–303. doi:10.1109/TSA.2004.838534

Levenson, R. W. (1988). Emotion and the autonomic nervous system: A prospectus for research on autonomic specificity. In H. L. Wagner (Ed.), *Social psychophysiology and emotion: Theory and clinical applications* (pp. 17-42). New York: John Wiley & Sons

Lienhart, R., & Maydt, J. (2002, September). An extended set of hair-like features for rapid object detection. In *Proceedings of the IEEE International Conference on Image Processing,* New York (Vol. 1, pp. 900-903). Washington, DC: IEEE Computer Society.

Littlewort, G. C., Bartlett, M. S., & Lee, K. (2007, November). Faces of pain: Automated measurement of spontaneous facial expressions of genuine and posed pain. In *Proceedings of the 9th International Conference on Multimodal Interfaces,* Nagoya, Japan (pp. 15-21). ACM Publishing.

Martin, J.-C., Caridakis, G., Devillers, L., Karpouzis, K., & Abrilian, S. (2009). Manual annotation and automatic image processing of multimodal emotional behaviours: Validating the annotation of TV interviews. *Personal and Ubiquitous Computing, 13*(1), 69–76. doi:10.1007/s00779-007-0167-y

Mehrabian, A., & Russell, J. (1974). *An approach to environmental psychology*. Cambridge, MA: MIT Press.

Nakasone, A., Prendinger, H., & Ishizuka, M. (2005, September). Emotion recognition from electromyography and skin conductance. In Proceedings of the 5th International Workshop on Biosignal Interpretation, Tokyo (pp. 219-222).

Nakayama, K., Goto, S., Kuraoka, K., & Nakamura, K. (2005). Decrease in nasal temperature of rhesus monkeys (Macaca mulatta) in negative emotional state. *Journal of Physiology and Behavior*, *84*, 783–790. doi:10.1016/j.physbeh.2005.03.009

Ning, H., Han, T. X., Hu, Y., Zhang, Z., Fu, Y., & Huang, T. S. (2006, April). A real-time shrug detector. In *Proceedings of the IEEE International Conference on Automatic Face and Gesture Recognition,* Southampton, UK (pp. 505-510). Washington, DC: IEEE Computer Society.

Ortony, A., & Turner, T. J. (1990). What's basic about basic emotions? *Psychological Review*, *97*, 315–331. doi:10.1037/0033-295X.97.3.315

Osgood, C., Suci, G., & Tannenbaum, P. (1957). *The measurement of meaning.* Chicago: University of Illinois Press.

Pan, H., Levinson, S. E., Huang, T. S., & Liang, Z.-P. (2004). A fused hidden markov model with application to bimodal speech processing. *IEEE Transactions on Signal Processing, 52*(3), 573–581. doi:10.1109/TSP.2003.822353

Pantic, M., & Bartlett, M. S. (2007). Machine analysis of facial expressions. In K. Delac & M. Grgic (Eds.), *Face recognition* (pp. 377-416). Vienna, Austria: I-Tech Education and Publishing.

Pantic, M., Nijholt, A., Pentland, A., & Huang, T. (2008). Human-centred intelligent human-computer interaction (HCI2): How far are we from attaining it? *International Journal of Autonomous and Adaptive Communications Systems, 1*(2), 168–187. doi:10.1504/IJAACS.2008.019799

Pantic, M., Pentland, A., Nijholt, A., & Huang, T. (2007). Machine understanding of human behaviour. In *Artifical Intelligence for Human Computing* (LNAI 4451, pp. 47-71).

Pantic, M., & Rothkrantz, L. J. M. (2003). Towards an affect-sensitive multimodal human-computer interaction. *Proceedings of the IEEE, 91*(9), 1370–1390. doi:10.1109/JPROC.2003.817122

Pavlidis, I. T., Levine, J., & Baukol, P. (2001, October). Thermal image analysis for anxiety detection. In *Proceedings of the International Conference on Image Processing,* Thessaloniki, Greece (Vol. 2, pp. 315-318). Washington, DC: IEEE Computer Society.

Picard, R. W., Vyzas, E., & Healey, J. (2001). Toward machine emotional intelligence: Analysis of affective physiological state. *IEEE Transactions on Pattern Analysis and Machine Intelligence, 23*(10), 1175–1191. doi:10.1109/34.954607

Plutchik, R. (1984). Emotions: A general psycho-evolutionary theory. In K. Scherer & P. Ekman (Eds.), *Approaches to emotion* (pp. 197-219). Hillsdale, NJ: Lawrence Erlbaum Associates.

Poppe, R. (2007). Vision-based human motion analysis: An overview. *Computer Vision and Image Understanding, 108*(1-2), 4–18. doi:10.1016/j.cviu.2006.10.016

Pun, T., Alecu, T. I., Chanel, G., Kronegg, J., & Voloshynovskiy, S. (2006). Brain-computer interaction research at the computer vision and multimedia laboratory, University of Geneva. *IEEE Transactions on Neural Systems and Rehabilitation Engineering, 14*(2), 210–213. doi:10.1109/TNSRE.2006.875544

Puri, C., Olson, L., Pavlidis, I., Levine, J., & Starren, J. (2005, April). StressCam: Non-contact measurement of users' emotional states through thermal imaging. In *Proceedings of the Conference on Human Factors in Computing Systems (CHI 2005),* Portland, OR (pp. 1725-1728). ACM Publishing.

Riseberg, J., Klein, J., Fernandez, R., & Picard, R. W. (1998, April). Frustrating the user on purpose: Using biosignals in a pilot study to detect the user's emotional state. In *Proceedings of the Conference on Human Factors in Computing Systems (CHI 1998),* Los Angeles (pp. 227-228). ACM Publishing.

Russell, J. A. (1980). A circumplex model of affect. *Journal of Personality and Social Psychology, 39,* 1161–1178. doi:10.1037/h0077714

Russell, J. A. (1997). Reading emotions from and into faces: resurrecting a dimensional contextual perspective. In J. A. Russell & J. M. Fernandez-Dols (Eds.), *The psychology of facial expression* (pp. 295-320). New York: Cambridge University Press.

Russell, J. A., & Fernández-Dols, J. M. (Eds.). (1997). *The psychology of facial expression.* New York: Cambridge University Press.

Savran, A., Ciftci, K., Chanel, G., Mota, J. C., Viet, L. H., Sankur, B., et al. (2006, July 17-August 11). Emotion detection in the loop from brain signals and facial images. In *Proceedings of eNTERFACE 2006,* Dubrovnik, Croatia. Retrieved from http://www.enterface.net

Scherer, K. R. (2000). Psychological models of emotion. In J. Borod (Ed.), *The neuropsychology of emotion* (pp. 137-162). New York: Oxford University Press.

Scherer, K. R., Schorr, A., & Johnstone, T. (Eds.). (2001). *Appraisal processes in emotion: Theory, methods, research.* New York: Oxford University Press.

Schmidt, K. L., & Cohn, J. F. (2001). Human facial expressions as adaptations: Evolutionary questions in facial expression research. *Yearbook of Physical Anthropology, 44,* 3–24. doi:10.1002/ajpa.20001

Shan, C., Gong, S., & McOwan, P. W. (2007, September). *Beyond facial expressions: Learning human emotion from body gestures.* Paper presented at the British Machine Vision Confercncc, Warwick, UK.

Shin, Y. (2007, May). Facial expression recognition based on emotion dimensions on manifold learning. In *Proceedings of International Conference on Computational Science,* Beijing, China (Vol. 2, pp. 81-88).

Takahashi, K. (2004, December). Remarks on emotion recognition from multi-modal biopotential signals. In *Proceedings of the IEEE International Conference on Industrial Technology,* Hammamet, Tunisia (pp. 1138-1143).

Tian, Y. L., Kanade, T., & Cohn, J. F. (2002, May). Evaluation of gabor-wavelet-based facial action unit recognition in image sequences of increasing complexity. In *Proceedings of the IEEE International Conference on Automaitc Face and Gesture Recognition,* Washington, DC (pp. 218-223). Washington, DC: IEEE Computer Society.

Tomkins, S. S. (1962). *Affect, imagery, consciousness: Vol. 1. The positive affects*. New York: Springer.

Tomkins, S. S. (1963). *Affect, imagery, consciousness. Vol. 2: The negative affects*. New York: Springer.

Tsiamyrtzis, P., Dowdall, J., Shastri, D., Pavlidis, I., Frank, M. G., & Ekman, P. (2007). Imaging facial physiology for the detection of deceit. *International Journal of Computer Vision, 71*(2), 197–214. doi:10.1007/s11263-006-6106-y

Valstar, M. F., Gunes, H., & Pantic, M. (2007). How to distinguish posed from spontaneous smiles using geometric features. In *Proceedings of the 9th International Conference on Multimodal Interfaces,* Nagoya, Japan (pp. 38-45). ACM Publishing.

Valstar, M. F., & Pantic, M. (2007, October). Combined support vector machines and hidden markov models for modeling facial action temporal dynamics. In M. Lew, N. Sebe, T. S. Huang, E. M. Bakker (Eds.), *Human–Computer Interaction: IEEE International Workshop, HCI 2007,* Rio de Janeiro, Brazil (LNCS 4796, pp. 118-127).

Van den Stock, J., Righart, R., & De Gelder, B. (2007). Body expressions influence recognition of emotions in the face and voice. *Emotion (Washington, D.C.), 7*(3), 487–494. doi:10.1037/1528-3542.7.3.487

Vianna, D. M., & Carrive, P. (2005). Changes in cutaneous and body temperature during and after conditioned fear to context in the rat. *The European Journal of Neuroscience, 21*(9), 2505–25012. doi:10.1111/j.1460-9568.2005.04073.x

Villalba, S. D., Castellano, G., & Camurri, A. (2007, September). Recognising human emotions from body movement and gesture dynamics. In *Proceedings of the 2nd International Conference on Affective Computing and Intelligent Interaction (ACII 2007),* Lisbon, Portugal (pp. 71-82).

Vinciarelli, A., Pantic, M., & Bourlard, H. (2009, December). Social signal processing: Survey of an emerging domain. *Image and Vision Computing Journal,* 27(12), 1743-1759.Viola, P., & Jones, M. (2001, December). Rapid object detection using a boosted cascade of simple features. In *Proceedings of the IEEE Conference on Computer Vision and Pattern Recognition,* Kauai, HI (Vol. 1, pp. 511-518).

Vogt, T., André, E., & Bee, N. (2008, June). EmoVoice—a framework for online recognition of emotions from voice. In *Perception in Multimodal Dialogue Systems: 4th IEEE Tutorial and Research Workshop on Perception and Interactive Technologies for Speech-Based Systems (PIT 2008),* Kloster Irsee, Germany (LNCS 5078, pp. 188-199).

Wagner, J., Kim, J., & Andre, E. (2005, July). From physiological signals to emotions: Implementing and comparing selected methods for feature extraction and classification. In *Proceedings of the IEEE International Conference on Multimedia and Expo,* Amsterdam, The Netherlands (pp. 940-943). Washington, DC: IEEE Computer Society.

Walker-Andrews, A. S. (1997). Infants' perception of expressive behaviours: Differentiation of multimodal information. *Psychological Bulletin*, *121*(3), 437–456. doi:10.1037/0033-2909.121.3.437

Whissell, C. M. (1989). The dictionary of affect in language. In R. Plutchik & H. Kellerman (Ed.), *Emotion: Theory, research and experience. The measurement of emotions* (Vol. 4, pp. 113-131). New York: Academic Press.

Wierzbicka, A. (1992). Talking about emotions: Semantics, culture, and cognition. *Cognition and Emotion*, *6*, 3–4. doi:10.1080/02699939208411073

Wollmer, M., Eyben, F., Reiter, S., Schuller, B., Cox, C., Douglas-Cowie, E., et al. (2008, September). Abandoning emotion classes - towards continuous emotion recognition with modelling of long-range dependencies. In *Proceedings of Interspeech,* Brisbane, Australia (pp. 597-600).

Wu, L., Oviatt, S. L., & Cohen, P. R. (1999). Multimodal integration: A statistical view. *IEEE Transactions on Multimedia*, *1*(4), 334–341. doi:10.1109/6046.807953

Xu, M., Jin, J. S., Luo, S., & Duan, L. (2008, October). Hierarchical movie affective content analysis based on arousal and valence features. In *Proceedings of ACM Multimedia,* Vancouver, British Columbia, Canada (pp. 677-680). ACM Publishing.

Yang, Y.-H., Lin, Y.-C., Su, Y.-F., & Chen, H. H. (2007, July). Music emotion classification: A regression approach. In *Proceedings of the IEEE International Conference on Multimedia and Expo,* Beijing, China (pp. 208-211). Washington, DC: IEEE Computer Society.

Yilmaz, A., Javed, O., & Shah, M. (2006). Object tracking: A survey. *ACM Journal of Computing Surveys*, *38*(4), 1–45.

Yu, C., Aoki, P. M., & Woodruff, A. (2004, October). Detecting user engagement in everyday conversations. In *Proceedings of 8th International Conference on Spoken Language Processing,* Jeju Island, Korea (pp. 1329-1332).

Zeng, Z., Pantic, M., Roisman, G. I., & Huang, T. S. (2009). A survey of affect recognition methods: Audio, visual, and spontaneous expressions. *IEEE Transactions on Pattern Analysis and Machine Intelligence*, *31*(1), 39–58. doi:10.1109/TPAMI.2008.52

Zhang, S., Tian, Q., Jiang, S., Huang, Q., & Gao, W. (2008, June). Affective MTV analysis based on arousal and valence features. In *Proceedings of the IEEE International Conference on Multimedia and Expo,* Hannover, Germany (pp. 1369-1372). Washington, DC: IEEE Computer Society.

Zuckerman, M., Larrance, D. T., Hall, J. A., DeFrank, R. S., & Rosenthal, R. (1979). Posed and spontaneous communication of emotion via facial and vocal cues. *Journal of Personality*, *47*(4), 712–733. doi:10.1111/j.1467-6494.1979.tb00217.x

This work was previously published in International Journal of Synthetic Emotions, Volume 1, Issue 1, edited by Jordi Vallverdu, pp. 68-99, copyright 2010 by IGI Publishing (an imprint of IGI Global).

Chapter 6
Emotion in the Pursuit of Understanding

Daniel S. Levine
University of Texas at Arlington, USA

Leonid I. Perlovsky
Harvard University, USA

ABSTRACT

Theories of cognitive processes, such as decision making and creative problem solving, for a long time neglected the contributions of emotion or affect in favor of analysis based on use of deliberative rules to optimize performance. Since the 1990s, emotion has increasingly been incorporated into theories of these cognitive processes. Some theorists have in fact posited a "dual-systems approach" to understanding decision making and high-level cognition. One system is fast, emotional, and intuitive, while the other is slow, rational, and deliberative. However, one's understanding of the relevant brain regions indicate that emotional and rational processes are deeply intertwined, with each exerting major influences on the functioning of the other. Also presented in this paper are neural network modeling principles that may capture the interrelationships of emotion and cognition. The authors also review evidence that humans, and possibly other mammals, possess a "knowledge instinct," which acts as a drive to make sense of the environment. This drive typically incorporates a strong affective component in the form of aesthetic fulfillment or dissatisfaction.

1. INTRODUCTION

The early stages of cognitive psychology in the 1960s and 1970s were largely driven by computer-related concepts such as information processing and pattern recognition, concepts that left little room for emotion or affect. Yet as more knowledge of both experimental psychology and cognitive neuroscience emerged in the 1980s and 1990s, it became apparent that cognitive processes such as attention, memory, categorization, and decision making could not be understood in real-world settings without including the effects of emotional influences on these processes.

DOI: 10.4018/978-1-4666-1595-3.ch006

The decision psychologist Ellen Peters (Peters, 2006) outlined four roles that emotions can play in behavioral choices, sometimes playing more than one of these roles at a time. These four are (1) a guide to information; (2) a selective attentional spotlight; (3) a motivator of behavior; and (4) a common currency for comparing alternatives. Role (1) means that both positive and negative emotional responses to potential alternatives can sharpen the decision maker's understanding of the situation in which he or she has to make a response. Role (2) means that out of the confusion of information available to the decision maker, attention can be focused on those items most relevant for satisfying current emotional needs (e.g., a tourist walking in a foreign city selectively attends to restaurant signs when hungry but to historical markers when curious). Role (3) means that anticipated pleasure motivates people or animals to approach objects, or anticipated pain motivates them to avoid objects. Role (4) means that emotion facilitates choices between dissimilar alternatives, such as going to a movie or working on a research paper, by providing common units such as "happiness" or "pleasure" on which to compare these alternatives.

The roles that Peters proposed for emotion are consistent with well-known clinical data on the pathologies in decision making that arise from disconnection between emotion and thinking processes. Specifically, such disconnection results from damage to the orbitofrontal cortex (Damasio, 1994), a key area for linking emotion-related brain regions with cortical information-processing regions. Orbital lesions disable the various facilitatory roles of emotion in decision making, resulting in decisions that might be impulsive and contextually inappropriate (as in the famous 19th century patient Phineas Gage) or else might be overly deliberate and obsessive (as in Damasio's own patient Elliot).

Hence, the evidence is clear that while excessive or misdirected emotion can at times interfere with effective decision making, emotion per se makes positive contributions to decision making and other cognitive processes, and therefore has adaptive value for the organism. Moreover, several behavioral biologists have noted more specific adaptive functions for particular emotions such as happiness, sadness, anger, fear, disgust, and surprise (e.g., Plutchik, 1970).

While emotions influence cognitions, the reverse is also true: the results of cognitive processes generate emotions. An example is the discomfort produced when a person is aware of cognitive dissonance between two beliefs arising from different sources (Festinger, 1957). Discomfort from cognitive dissonance has been shown to occur not only at the feeling level but also at the physiological level, in the form of skin conductance responses (Croyle & Cooper, 1983).

2. DUAL PROCESSES?

The last section provides behavioral evidence that emotion and cognition are deeply interconnected and difficult to separate. In further support of this notion, neuroscientists have found that brain areas cannot be neatly separated into specialized "emotional" and "cognitive" regions (e.g., Pessoa, 2008; Swanson, 2005).

In spite of this evidence, both experimental psychology and cognitive neuroscience have still not quite shaken off the long-standing myth of Western culture that "emotion and reason are opposites." This is a myth that Damasio (1994) partly attributes to the influence of Cartesian philosophy, and it has echoes in the writings of other philosophers from Aristotle to Adam Smith. The rational-emotional dichotomy pervades day-to-day speech; for example, in colloquial American English we say that a person "acts emotionally" if he or she performs a behavior based on a *short-term* emotion that is ill considered and flies in the face of reasonable solution of a problem. The phrase is applied, for example, to someone who commits a crime of passion or falls in love with an unsuitable partner. On the other hand, the phrase "acting emotionally" is not typically applied to someone who works steadily on his or her job out of the emotion of love for his or her family, or the emotion of enjoyment of the work.

The belief that emotion and reason are opposites has received telling blows from many recent results in cognitive neuroscience, and particularly from clinical observations such as Damasio's (1994). Yet a trace of that traditional Western belief lingers in some statements by psychologists who posit dual-process theories of decision making (e.g., Epstein, Pacini, Denes-Raj, & Heier, 1996; Ferreira, Garcia-Marques, Sherman, & Sherman, 2006; Sloman, 1996). In general, these dual-process theories

... have distinguished between a rapid, automatic, and effortless, associative, intuitive process (System 1) and a slower, rule-governed, analytic, deliberate, and effortful process (System 2). (Weber & Johnson, 2009, p. 67)

There is considerable experimental evidence that decision makers use both heuristic and deliberative decision processes at different times. Also, there are many factors that are known to bias decision makers toward one or another of these types of decision process on a particular problem at a particular time. Among these factors are time pressure or lack thereof; individual personality factors such as need for cognition and need for cognitive closure; the decision maker's confidence in his or her knowledge about the domain in which the problem lies; and the importance of the problem for the decision maker's long-term plans (for example, more deliberation typically enters into decisions about houses to buy than into decisions about restaurants to eat at).

As the field has advanced since the mid-1990s, most investigators who posit dual-process theories now see the heuristic and deliberative processes as complementary rather than opposing. Ferreira et al. (2006) contrast previous approaches that imply "a zero-sum or hydraulic relation between the RB [rule-based] and the H [heuristic] processes" with their own approach that "conceives of the two processing modes as contributing independently to the judgment" (p. 798). These same investigators presented experimental results suggesting that it is possible to increase or decrease the amount of rule-based processing in combination with either an increase, decrease, or no change in the amount of heuristic associative processing, or vice versa.

So the two-process statement Weber and Johnson (2009) discuss is a partial representation of experimental findings, but taken too literally it is simplistic, and somewhat misleading for the current dialogue about emotion and rationality. There are at least three reasons we need to go beyond (while building on) two-process thinking:

a. **Intuitive decisions are not always faster than deliberative decisions:** An example comes from my student experience. As a senior in college I considered six offers of graduate assistantships in mathematics that were comparable both monetarily and in the prestige of the universities they came from. After eliminating four of these schools on easily definable grounds (e.g., unpleasant atmosphere, unfavorable gender ratio, or too far from home), I was left with a choice of two schools I will call Low University and Dewey University. On rational grounds, Low seemed like the better bet because its department was stronger than Dewey's in the area of mathematics that was then my main research interest. Yet Dewey was located in the city, in fact in the very neighborhood, where I had spent early childhood but not returned to visit for several years. An intuitive, emotional pull to return to that location trumped professional considerations, leading me to choose Dewey. But this decision was not a quick one and took place *after* weeks of rule-based deliberation.

My story confirms the insights of Sloman, Ferreira, Weber, and other recent investigators that the time frames of the emotionally and rationally based decision systems, and the interactions between the two systems, are variable. While emotional choices tend more often to be faster than rational ones, that is not always the case, and both systems are typically active for the same decision maker over an extended period.

b. **Different systems are likely to produce better solutions for different types of problems:** Two-process thinking was particularly inspired by one type of problems: those that admit optimal solutions which are numerically definable, and yet are subject to heuristic biases that conflict with the optimal solutions. One example is *ratio bias* problems (Denes-Raj & Epstein, 1994), based on the heuristic tendency to perceive the same low probability, or even a slightly lower one, as larger if the numerator and dominator are larger. For instance, a majority of participants said they would be more likely to obtain a red ball from a random draw from an urn with 9 red balls out of 100 total balls than from another urn with 1 red ball out of 10 total balls, even though the rules of probability give them a better chance in the 1 out of 10 situation. Another example is *base-rate neglect* problems (Ajzen, 1977), whereby the heuristic tendency is to decide on probabilities based on descriptions and ignore demographic information. In one such problem, participants were told that a certain group of people consisted of specific numbers of lawyers and engineers, and a hypothetical person was identified as a member of that group and given a description fitting a stereotype of one of the two professions; then the participant was asked to determine the probability of that person being a lawyer or an engineer. Bayes' rule indicates that the probability of being a lawyer or engineer should partly depend on the distribution of lawyers and engineers in the sample, but for the majority of participants, the assigned probabilities were not influenced by that prior distribution.

Clearly a deliberative strategy is more likely to yield a better answer than a heuristic strategy for these types of problems. But a deliberative strategy is not appropriate for momentary small-purchase decisions that have minimal long-term consequences. In fact, Damasio's (1994) patient with orbital prefrontal cortex damage showed excessive deliberation on such minor decisions, to the point of being unable to decide which of several restaurants to eat at even after going back and looking at the restaurants.

Also there is at least circumstantial evidence that a pure deliberative strategy is not optimal for many problems requiring a high degree of creative imagination, and that intuition plays an essential role in creativity. The interdisciplinary social scientist Sam Leven (Leven, 1987; Levine, 1998, Chapter 7) posited three major problem solving styles, each named after a different mathematician whose major work illustrated the essence of that style. There three types are "Dantzig" or direct solvers who try simply to achieve an available solution by a repeatable method; "Bayesian" solvers who play the percentages and try to maximize a measurable criterion; and "Godelians" who use both intuition and reason to arrive at innovative solutions. The Bayesian solver type is the one idealized in normative decision theory, and is the best suited to problems of the ratio-bias or base-rate type. Yet Godelian solvers are better at problems that are much more open-ended, such as designing the best possible office environment; hence they are often valued in group brainstorming situations (REFERENCE). Even in quantifiable domains, the Godelian tendency frequently leads great thinkers to find solutions that highly competent Bayesians have overlooked. For example, Albert Einstein was led to his relativity theory by cognitive dissonance between some new (relatively minor) results on light and radiation and the Newtonian paradigms for physics (Cline, 1965). Before him even other great physicists such as Planck had largely glossed over the discrepant data. Poincaré (1914) described the process of discovery of mathematical proofs as involving alternating periods of logical deduction and intuitive insight.

Again, this is a different type of intuition from the quick off-the-cuff use of heuristics. Rather, it is a type of intuition that requires years of immersion in a knowledge domain and usually *follows* a long period of deliberation. Management theorists sometimes distinguish the two processes by calling the more sophisticated type of nonrational process *insight* rather than intuition (Dane & Pratt, 2007).

c. **Long-term emotional satisfaction is different from short-term emotional reaction:** The goals that rational decision makers use rules to optimize are often themselves emotionally derived. Maximizing pleasure over the long term frequently involves deferral of immediate reward. Yet the future anticipation of reward also engages the brain's emotional system, even though there is evidence that it engages a different pattern of neural activity than does immediate reward (McClure, Laibson, Loewenstein, & Cohen, 2004).

As people develop their logical capabilities and deal with ever more complex problems, at best their emotional life is not suppressed. Rather, they are increasingly governed by more sophisticated emotions such as the drive toward beauty in the arts or ideas, and toward the sublime in personal and interpersonal life (Levine & Perlovsky, 2008a; Perlovsky, 2006a). In Section 4 we discuss how such emotions relate to the knowledge instinct, the drive to make sense out of one's environment. Hence, as Weber and Johnson (2009) suggest, the emotional and rational decision systems interact in more complex ways than simple two-process statements suggest. Some progress has been made in recent years at capturing these interactions through neural network models that incorporate data about specific brain regions.

3. NEURAL NETWORK APPROACHES TO EMOTIONAL-COGNITIVE INTERACTIONS

The phenomenal growth of experimental cognitive neuroscience since 2000 has nearly been matched by a corresponding growth in the biological realism of neural network models. Models that previously were based on abstract functioning principles have evolved to incorporate an ever increasing amount of data on connectivity and spiking patterns of many brain regions. This has enabled networks to simulate complete complex behaviors in real time.

Many complex behaviors (both human and animal) involve continually updated calculations of positive and negative emotional value for sensory stimuli or for potential actions. There are several models either of animal conditioning data or human decision data that involve characteristic brain regions such as the amygdala, orbital prefrontal cortex (OFC), striatum, and dopamine nuclei in learning of such emotional values (Dranias, Grossberg, & Bullock, 2008; Frank & Claus, 2006; Levine, in press; Litt, Eliasmith, & Thagard, 2008). There is wide variation in the detailed connections incorporated into these network models, but there is broad agreement among them in some general roles for these regions:

- The amygdala codes both positive and negative emotional values for stimuli or potential actions.
- Learnable connections between the OFC and amygdala are involved in updating those emotional valuations based on short-term memories of rewards or punishments.

- A critical level of dopamine is required for such learning to take place. An unexpected reward is related to a surge in dopamine activity, and an unexpected lack of reward is related in to a dip in dopamine activity. In the model of Litt et al. (2008), an unexpected punishment is related to activity of a serotonin channel that opposes the dopamine channel.
- Connections of both OFC and amygdala to the ventral striatum (both direct and indirect pathways) are involved in translating the emotional valuations to generation or withholding of specific behaviors, including approach or avoidance of specific objects.

There are a variety of ways in which these emotional valuations interact with the automatic and controlled decision systems discussed in previous sections. In particular, many of the behaviors that are automatic were learned in the past through an emotional-learning process similar to what occurs in models such as those of Dranias et al. (2008), Frank and Claus (2006), Levine (in press), and Litt et al. (2008).[1] For example, in the course of a human's or animal's development, the OFC mediates the learning of appropriate social behaviors through its connections with the amygdala and ventral striatum. This is the reason that orbitally lesioned patients frequently act in violation of social norms, whether those norms are necessary for proper functioning in society (Damasio, 1994) or simply encode the current culture's prejudices (as in the work of Milne & Grafman, 2001, on gender stereotyping).

Yet the types of tasks that are simulated in these models are typically very different from the ratio-bias and base-rate neglect tasks that inspired the two-process theories. The neural network models cited in this section simulate data involving learning about environmental contingencies over time from experience. Hertwig, Barron, Weber, and Erev (2004) review several results showing that decisions on a probabilistic contingency learned from experience are quite different from decisions on the same probability learned from direct description. For example, decision makers simply given an explicit choice between a certainty of gaining $300 and an 80% probability of gaining $400 with a 20% probability of gaining nothing have a strong tendency to choose the certain smaller amount, because they prefer the certainty even though it is also the smaller of the two alternatives in expected earnings. Yet if decision makers are allowed over a period of time to press one of two computer keys, and pressing the first key always yields $300 but pressing the second key yields $400 80 percent of the time and nothing 20 percent of the time, the preference for the first key (i.e., for certainty) is markedly reduced.

The ratio-bias and base-rate neglect tasks involve decisions from description and not from experience. In a sense, decision from description is cognitively harder because it involves envisioning possibilities that are not experienced directly, and requires language. Unlike decision from experience, it has no analog in animal experimentation. Hence it is generally believed that decision from description involves higher-order executive areas of the cortex, specifically the anterior cingulate cortex (ACC) and dorsolateral prefrontal cortex (DLPFC). Brain imaging studies (DeMartino, Kumaran, Seymour, & Dolan, 2006; DeNeys, Vartanian, & Goel, 2008) indicate that ACC becomes active when there is a perceived conflict between two or more potential decision rules, and DLPFC becomes active when deliberative decision rules are utilized. An extension of a decision network that includes those regions is described in Levine (in press), and a simplified version of that network was used to simulate Denes-Raj and Epstein's (1994) ratio-bias task in Levine and Perlovsky (2008b).

Yet even as these higher-level cognitive processes become engaged, and particularly as those processes involve language, it is not a matter of "reason overcoming emotion" but of a more complex and sophisticated type of emotion becoming disinhibited. The next section will discuss the connections of emotions with the knowledge instinct, the drive to make sense out of one's environment.

4. AESTHETIC EMOTIONS AND THE KNOWLEDGE INSTINCT

Neural mechanisms of emotions, discussed in section 1 as a selective attentional spotlight, are described by Grossberg and Levine's (1987) theory of instincts and emotions. According to this theory, the mechanism of *instincts* is similar to internal sensors that measure vital organism parameters, important for normal functioning and survival. For example, a low sugar level in blood indicates an instinctual need for food. This sensor measurement and the requirement to maintain it within certain limits we consider a mechanism of an "instinct." These instinctual needs are communicated to conceptual recognition-understanding mechanisms of the brain by emotional neural signals, or emotions. In the result, mental representations corresponding to objects or situations that can potentially satisfy instinctual needs receive preferential attention and processing resources in the brain (Grossberg & Levine, 1987; Perlovsky, 2001, 2006a, b). Emotional signals evaluate concepts for the purpose of instinct satisfaction. Thus cognition is an integrated result of instinctive, emotional, and conceptual mechanisms (see also MacLean, 1990).

Conceptual-emotional understanding of the world results in actions in the outside world or within the mind. We only consider here the *behavior* inside the mind of improving understanding and conceptual knowledge. Let us begin with simpler mechanisms of visual perception. A part of visual perception mechanisms is visual imagination. It occurs when one contemplates objects or situations with closed eyes. Contemplated mental representations of concepts project images on visual cortex causing visual imagination. Most of the brain operations are unconscious, for example, individual neuronal firings. A significant part of conceptual perception is an unconscious process; for example, visual perception takes about 150 ms, which is a long time when measured in neuronal firings (about 10 ms per neuron, while tens of thousands of neurons are participating in parallel). Initial projections on the visual cortex are vague and the mind is not conscious of them. We only become conscious about the final result: the crisp mental projections matching sensory signals. Still, it is easy to experience directly vague mental projections. It is possible to make the vague projections conscious: close your eyes and imagine an object in front of you; this imagination is usually vague, not as crisp as perception of an object with opened eyes. Only when conceptual projections match retinal projections of objects and become crisp, then conscious perceptions occur. Detailed experimental study of this process is reported in Bar et al. (2006).

This process of matching mental representations and retinal projections is a condition of perception. Therefore it is driven by an inborn unconditional mechanism, which we call the *knowledge instinct* (*KI*). In the mathematical model of this process, KI maximizes a measure of similarity between projections coming from retina and those coming from mental representations (between bottom-up and top-down signals).

At higher levels of cognition, the cognitive dissonance results of Festinger (1957) and Croyle and Cooper (1983) provide partial verification of the existence of a knowledge instinct. So do results showing that monkeys as well as people are motivated by the need to solve puzzles (Harlow, 1953). According to the Grossberg and Levine (1987) theory, satisfaction or dissatisfaction of any instinct produces emotional signals. The knowledge instinct is no exception to this notion, as has been verified by Perlovsky, Bonniot-Cabanac and Cabanac (2010). This paper has demonstrated experimentally that satisfaction of the knowledge instinct brings pleasure.

How do we feel emotions of satisfaction of the KI? At lower levels of object perception, emotional signals satisfying the KI usually are below the threshold of conscious registration. However, if objects around do not correspond to our models, we immediately feel an intense disharmony (between reality and our expectations). Thriller movies exploit this property of our perception: they show objects and situations that do not correspond to our models-expectations, thereby creating strong negative emotions. Perceptions at lower levels are not much different in this respect from other autonomous functions; for example, we do not consciously perceive the working of our stomach mechanisms as long as everything is OK. But we become acutely emotionally aware when our stomach does not function properly. At higher levels of cognition, we feel both positive and negative KI-related emotions consciously. For example, we feel happiness when we solve a complex problem occupying our mind for days, and frustration when we are unable to solve a complex problem. We emphasize that ability to form more general and abstract representations from simpler and more concrete ones emerged in evolution for the *purpose* of improved understanding. Obviously the mind is a purposeful system.

Emotions related to higher levels of the KI involve processes of thinking and understanding, more than bodily activities like sex or eating. For this reason and for this reason alone they can be called "spiritual". Since Kant's work these spiritual emotions related to knowledge have been called *aesthetic emotions*. We would emphasize that these emotions are not reserved for artistic activities: they accompany every act of perception and cognition. At every level of the mind, the KI drives the learning of representations-concepts to become crisper and more conscious. Still at the higher levels, the representations-concepts are intrinsically vaguer and more difficult to make conscious; hence more cognitive effort is required for understanding them, for adapting them to life, for making them more conscious. Correspondingly, we feel more aesthetic emotions when we succeed in this.

Mental representations at higher levels of the mind hierarchy create higher meaning and purpose from lower level representations. Representations at the top of the mind hierarchy unify our entire experience and create the meaning and purpose of life. Higher- level representations are vague and less conscious than lower level ones. Vague representations do not differentiate conceptual and emotional contents. When the highest representations of the meaning and purpose of existence are being adapted, made more conscious, or at least we feel that this highest meaning and purpose exist, we feel the emotion of the beautiful. Nothing in the world around us can be directly perceived as a purpose and meaning of our lives. In fact, random circumstances in our mundane lives often destroy purposiveness. Nevertheless, to be able to endure life, to concentrate will, and to achieve satisfying life, we have to believe that meaning exists. This is why we cherish so much this rare and fleeting, but so dear, emotion of the beautiful, when the KI is satisfied at the highest level (Perlovsky, 2010b).

The mechanism of sublime emotions is similar to the beautiful. Whereas the beautiful is related to improvement of the highest cognitive representations, the emotion of the sublime is related to the highest representations of behavior. Understanding the meaning and purpose is not sufficient; we would also like to realize this understanding in our lives. To do this we need to develop corresponding mental representations of behavior. These representations are vague and uncertain like the corresponding models of cognition. We do not know for sure what the best way is to achieve the highest meaning and purpose in our lives. When we feel improvement of these behavioral representations, when we are more certain about existence of these highest behavioral representations, we experience emotions of sublime.

There is a mathematical reason why choices of the beautiful and sublime cannot be made crisp, clear, and completely conscious. The reason is these choices require evaluation and selection from infinite sets. Recognition of a simple object, as discussed, requires matching the object representations to a subset of signals, originating from the object. This subset has to be selected among many other subsets. There are about 10,000 signals that each eye retina receives ten times a second. Therefore perception requires thousands and millions of signals to be matched to models of thousands of objects. But let us forget for a second about these large numbers, consider a choice of just 100 object-models to be matched to subsets of 100 signals. The number of these subsets is 100^{100}. This number is larger than all interactions among all elementary particles in the entire life of the Universe (Penrose, 1994). Thus choices of the beautiful and sublime require evaluation of a "physically infinite" number of subsets (and therefore involve an infinite amount of information). Perception of objects around us is helped by these objects actually being there, but cognition of abstract high-level concepts does not have such firm grounds.

Learning abstract high-level concepts is not possible by searching among all these signals from the environment and from our own minds and experiences; this learning is guided by language (Perlovsky, 2009a). But the above mathematical argument shows that our highest aesthetic aspirations cannot be fully reduced to neat computational formulas. Thus modern science supports insights from many religions that ultimately the choices of beautiful and sublime are beyond clear and conscious human reach.

This conclusion about vagueness of high level concepts and emotions may sometimes contradict conscious perceptions of mental processes. Sometimes we may perceive high-level concepts and emotions as clear and well defined. The reason for this contradiction is related to the difference between language representations and cognitive representations (Perlovsky, 2009a). Language representations (words, phrases) are acquired from surrounding language "ready-made" and therefore are experienced as crisp and conscious. Cognitive representations (images, etc.) require experience; however, abstract general concepts, unlike objects, cannot be directly experienced. Therefore, as we discussed they are vague and only partly conscious at best. This is a reason why there could be significant differences discussed in previous sections, between decisions from language descriptions and decisions from experience. Experience involves emotions, which may be absent from language descriptions.

The KI as discussed above drives the mind to maximize a correspondence between the entirety of mental representations and experiences. This however is a simplification. Every piece of knowledge (a representation) to some extent conflicts with various instinctual needs, and with many other pieces of knowledge. These conflicts are experienced as cognitive dissonances. Resolving cognitive dissonances is a condition of personal development and evolution of the entire culture. This requires developing a variety of aesthetic emotions. The number of cognitive dissonances and the required emotions is combinatorially large (practically infinite). This is the reason for evolution of musical ability. Music develops this tremendous variety of aesthetic musical emotions that we "hear" in music and language (Perlovsky 2006b, 2009b, 2010a).

5. GENERAL DISCUSSION

The distinguished architect Buckminster Fuller was once asked if he considered beauty when solving design and engineering problems. He replied:

No. When I am working on a problem, I never think about beauty. I think only of how to solve the problem. But when I have finished, if the solu-

tion is not beautiful, I know it is wrong. (Taper, 1970, p. 138)

Fuller's statement indicates that high-quality creative work, not only in the arts but also in science and technology, is inseparable from aesthetic emotions. At more mundane and practical levels, solving the problems necessary for day-to-day existence is guided by basic emotions such as joy, sadness, fear, anger, disgust, and surprise, according to the functions described by Peters (2006) (guide to information, attentional spotlight, motivator, and common currency).

Let us return to the "two-process" theories of Epstein et al. (1996), Sloman (1996), and others that posit an automatic, fast, intuitively driven decision process and a controlled, slow, deliberative process. The exposition in this article makes it clear that neither process is in reality more "emotional" than the other. However, the processes are really distinct, and both are evolutionary adaptations. Levine and Perlovsky (2008a) discuss how the controlled process is related to the knowledge instinct (KI) and the automatic process to effort minimization (EM). That article relates both the Judaeo-Christian notion of original sin and the Buddhist view of the source of suffering to the temptation to rely excessively on heuristics and avoid the effort needed to live in better accordance with the KI. The article also reviews brain imaging results suggesting that the KI engages activity in some of the components of the brain's executive control system, notably the anterior cingulate cortex and dorsolateral prefrontal cortex.

Hence both the deliberative and heuristic processes involve interactions between emotion and cognition. Yet they engage somewhat different types of emotions and different uses of emotion to influence cognition and behavior. With the aid of current computational models of emotional-cognitive interactions via cortical-subcortical networks (e.g., Frank & Claus, 2006; Dranias, Grossberg, & Bullock, 2008; Litt, Eliasmith, & Thagard, 2008; Levine, in press), we can begin to approach the real differences between KI and EM. Since both sets of processes are needed at different times, we can also approach the problem of *task calibration* (Reyna & Brainerd, 1991), that is to say, which type of process is most appropriate in which situations. Task calibration is an important consideration not only for human decision makers but also for emotional robots and for artificial decision support systems.

REFERENCES

Ajzen, I. (1977). Intuitive theories of events and the effects of base-rate information on prediction. *Journal of Personality and Social Psychology, 35*, 303–314. doi:10.1037/0022-3514.35.5.303

Bar, M., Kassam, K. S., Ghuman, A. S., Boshyan, J., & Schmid, A. M. Dale, et al. (2006). Top-down facilitation of visual recognition. In *Proceedings of the National Academy of Sciences* (Vol. 103, 449-54).

Cline, B. L. (1965). *The questioners: Physicists and the quantum theory*. New York: Thomas Y. Crowell Company.

Croyle, R. T., & Cooper, J. (1983). Dissonance arousal: Physiological evidence. *Journal of Personality and Social Psychology, 45*, 782–791. doi:10.1037/0022-3514.45.4.782

Damasio, A. R. (1994). *Descartes' error: Emotion, reason, and the human brain*. New York: Grosset/Putnam.

Dane, E., & Pratt, M. G. (2007). Exploring intuition and its role in managerial decision making. *Academy of Management Review, 32*, 33–54.

Denes-Raj, V., & Epstein, S. (1994). Conflict between intuitive and rational processing: When people behave against their better judgment. *Journal of Personality and Social Psychology, 66*, 819–829. doi:10.1037/0022-3514.66.5.819

Dranias, M., Grossberg, S., & Bullock, D. (2008). Dopaminergic and non-dopaminergic value systems in conditioning and outcome-specific revaluation. *Brain Research*, *1238*, 239–287. doi:10.1016/j.brainres.2008.07.013

Epstein, S., Pacini, R., Denes-Raj, V., & Heier, H. (1996). Individual differences in intuitive-experiential and analytical-rational thinking styles. *Journal of Personality and Social Psychology*, *71*, 390–405. doi:10.1037/0022-3514.71.2.390

Ferreira, M. B., Garcia-Marques, L., Sherman, S. J., & Sherman, J. W. (2006). Automatic and controlled components of judgment and decision making. *Journal of Personality and Social Psychology*, *91*, 797–813. doi:10.1037/0022-3514.91.5.797

Festinger, L. (1957). *A theory of cognitive dissonance*. Evanston, IL: Row, Peterson.

Frank, M. J., & Claus, E. D. (2006). Anatomy of a decision: Striato-orbitofrontal interactions in reinforcement learning, decision making, and reversal. *Psychological Review*, *113*, 300–326. doi:10.1037/0033-295X.113.2.300

Grossberg, S., & Levine, D. (1987). Neural dynamics of attentionally modulated Pavlovian conditioning: Blocking, interstimulus interval, and secondary reinforcement. *Applied Optics*, *26*, 5015–5030. doi:10.1364/AO.26.005015

Harlow, H. (1953). Mice, monkeys, men, and motives. *Psychological Review*, *60*, 23–32. doi:10.1037/h0056040

Hertwig, R., Barron, G., Weber, E. U., & Erev, I. (2004). Decisions from experience and the effect of rare events in risky choice. *Psychological Science*, *15*, 534–539. doi:10.1111/j.0956-7976.2004.00715.x

Leven, S. J. (1987). *Choice and neural process*. Unpublished doctoral dissertation, University of Texas at Arlington.

Levine, D. S. (1998). *Explorations in common sense and common nonsense*. http://www.uta.edu/psychology/faculty/levine/EBOOK/index.htm

Levine, D. S. (in press). Value maps, drives, and emotions. In Cutsuridis, V., Husain, A., & Taylor, J. G. (Eds.), *Perception-reason-action cycle: Models, algorithms, and systems*. New York: Springer.

Levine, D. S., Mills, B. A., & Estrada, S. (2005, August). Modeling emotional influences on human decision making under risk. In *Proceedings of International Joint Conference on Neural Networks* (pp. 1657-1662).

Levine, D. S., & Perlovsky, L. I. (2008a). Simplifying heuristics versus careful thinking: scientific analysis of millennial spiritual issues. *Zygon*, *43*, 797–821. doi:10.1111/j.1467-9744.2008.00961.x

Levine, D. S., & Perlovsky, L. I. (2008b). A network model of rational versus irrational choices on a probability maximization task. In *Proceedings of the 2008 IEEE World Congress on Computational Intelligence* (pp. 2821-2825).

Litt, A., Eliasmith, C., & Thagard, P. (2008). Neural affective decision theory: Choices, brains, and emotions. *Cognitive Systems Research*, *9*, 252–273. doi:10.1016/j.cogsys.2007.11.001

MacLean, P. D. (1990). *The triune brain in evolution: Role in paleocerebral functions*. New York: Plenum.

McClure, S. M., Laibson, D. I., Loewenstein, G., & Cohen, J. D. (2004). Separate neural systems value immediate and delayed monetary rewards. *Science*, *306*, 503–506. doi:10.1126/science.1100907

Milne, E., & Grafman, J. (2001). Ventromedial prefrontal cortex lesions in humans eliminate implicit gender stereotyping. *Journal of Neuroscience Special Issue*, *21*(12), 1–6.

Penrose, R. (1994). *Shadows of the mind*. Oxford: Oxford University Press.

Perlovsky, L. I. (2001). *Neural Networks and Intellect: using model-based concepts* (3rd ed.). New York: Oxford University Press.

Perlovsky, L. I. (2006a). Toward physics of the mind: Concepts, emotions, consciousness, and symbols. *Physics of Life Reviews*, *3*, 23–55. doi:10.1016/j.plrev.2005.11.003

Perlovsky, L. I. (2006b). Music - The first principle. *Musical Theater E-journal*. Retrieved from http://www.ceo.spb.ru/libretto/kon_lan/ogl.shtml

Perlovsky, L. I. (2009a). Language and cognition. *Neural Networks*, *22*, 247–257. doi:10.1016/j.neunet.2009.03.007

Perlovsky, L. I. (2009b). Language and emotions: Emotional Sapir-Whorf Hypothesis. *Neural Networks*, *22*, 518–526. doi:10.1016/j.neunet.2009.06.034

Perlovsky, L. I. (2010a). Musical emotions: Functions, origin, evolution. *Physics of Life Reviews*, *7*, 2–27. doi:10.1016/j.plrev.2009.11.001

Perlovsky, L. I. (2010b). Intersections of mathematical, cognitive, and aesthetic Theories of Mind. *Psychology of Aesthetics, Creativity, and the Arts*, *4*, 11–17. doi:10.1037/a0018147

Perlovsky, L. I., Bonniot-Cabanac, M.-C., & Cabanac, M. (2010). Curiosity and pleasure, to be published.

Pessoa, L. (2008). On the relationship between emotion and cognition. *Nature Reviews. Neuroscience*, *9*, 148–158. doi:10.1038/nrn2317

Peters, E. (2006). The functions of affect in the construction of preferences. In Lichtenstein, S., & Slovic, P. (Eds.), *The construction of preference*. New York: Cambridge University Press. doi:10.1017/CBO9780511618031.025

Plutchik, R. (1970). *Emotion: A psychoevolutionary analysis*. New York: Harper & Row.

Poincaré, H. (1914). *Science and method* (Maitland, F., Trans.). London: T. Nelson and Sons.

Reyna, V. F., & Brainerd, C. J. (1991). Fuzzy-trace theory and framing effects in choice: Gist extraction, truncation, and conversion. *Journal of Behavioral Decision Making*, *4*, 249–262. doi:10.1002/bdm.3960040403

Sloman, S. A. (1996). The empirical case for two systems of reasoning. *Psychological Bulletin*, *119*, 3–22. doi:10.1037/0033-2909.119.1.3

Swanson, L. W. (2005). Anatomy of the soul as reflected in the cerebral hemispheres: Neural circuits underlying voluntary control of basic motivated behaviors. *The Journal of Comparative Neurology*, *493*, 122–131. doi:10.1002/cne.20733

Taper, B. (1970). *The arts in Boston*. Cambridge, MA: Harvard University Press.

Weber, E. U., & Johnson, E. J. (2009). Mindful judgment and decision making. *Annual Review of Psychology*, *60*, 53–85. doi:10.1146/annurev.psych.60.110707.163633

ENDNOTE

1. Even when automatic behaviors result from learning based on past emotion, their performance does not require strong present emotion.

This work was previously published in International Journal of Synthetic Emotions, Volume 1, Issue 2, edited by Jordi Vallverdu, pp. 1-11, copyright 2010 by IGI Publishing (an imprint of IGI Global).

Chapter 7
Chatterbox Challenge as a Test-Bed for Synthetic Emotions

Jordi Vallverdú
Universitat Autònoma de Barcelona, Spain

Huma Shah
Universitat Autònoma de Barcelona, Spain

David Casacuberta
Universitat Autònoma de Barcelona, Spain

ABSTRACT

Chatterbox Challenge is an annual web-based contest for artificial conversational systems, ACE. The 2010 instantiation was the tenth consecutive contest held between March and June in the 60th year following the publication of Alan Turing's influential disquisition 'computing machinery and intelligence'. Loosely based on Turing's viva voca interrogator-hidden witness imitation game, a thought experiment to ascertain a machine's capacity to respond satisfactorily to unrestricted questions, the contest provides a platform for technology comparison and evaluation. This paper provides an insight into emotion content in the entries since the 2005 Chatterbox Challenge. The authors find that synthetic textual systems, none of which are backed by academic or industry funding, are, on the whole and more than half a century since Weizenbaum's natural language understanding experiment, little further than Eliza in terms of expressing emotion in dialogue. This may be a failure on the part of the academic AI community for ignoring the Turing test as an engineering challenge.

INTRODUCTION

In his anticipation of objections to the idea of machines thinking, and testing for it through an imitation game, Alan Turing reminded of a real-life scenario the *viva voca* in which an interrogator seeks answers to questions from a 'witness' (Turing, 1950). Pre-empting the *argument from consciousness* and quoting from Jefferson's 1949 Lister Oration, "not until a machine can write a sonnet or compose a concerto because of thoughts and emotions felt ... not only write it but know that it had written it" (1950, section 6, p. 445), Turing

DOI: 10.4018/978-1-4666-1595-3.ch007

countered showing this stance was a solipsistic one. To say that "no mechanism ... could feel pleasure at its successes, grief when its valves fuse, be warmed by flattery, be made miserable by its mistakes, be charmed by sex, be angry or depressed when it cannot get what it wants" (p. 446), was, according to Turing, an extreme position: "the only way by which one could be sure that a machine thinks is to *be* the machine and to feel oneself thinking" - Turing's emphasis (ibid). Turing replied, as Stins and Laureys put it "in a succinct British fashion" (2009, p. 265) that rather than labouring over the point "A is liable to believe *A thinks but B does not* while B believes *B thinks but A does not*" it is "usual to have the polite convention that everyone thinks" (1950, p. 446).

There are a variety of objections to the "Turing test" and whether it can really be a way to assert whether a computer is thinking or not, it is beyond the scope of this paper to review them, readers are directed to Shah and Warwick (2010b) nevertheless the concept of being able to pass the Turing test is a complex endeavour indeed, and analysing such a variant Turing test contest can be of great philosophical value.

Turing put forward possible questions and answers to show that if the responses were "satisfactory and sustained" then one might not describe the answers as "an easy contrivance" (1950, p. 447). It is this method to assess whether machine responses to questions are satisfactory and sustained that is evaluated in an annual contest – the Chatterbox Challenge. Artificial conversation systems (ACE), commonly known as 'chatbots' compete against each other across a number of categories. What is considered a *satisfactory response* can be subjective; one interrogator may find a response inappropriate while another may accept it as humorous. An answer to a question may seem *ersatz-like*, but may also be a satisfactory emotive response under interrogation or conveying disinterest in topic by the 'witness'. Whether machines are capable of expressing emotion through their responses or whether they are still Eliza-like (Weizenbaum, 1966) can be found by analysing the contest's transcripts.

Emotion: Mood, Feeling or Expression?

According to Broekens "Emotion is a complex topic, and agreement on one solid definition does not really exist" (2010). What does stand as an 'emotion' is also not clear cut (Barrett et al., 2007), and more if we take into account the qualia aspects of emotions, their *feeling*, we need to paraphrase Augustine of Hippo[1] ideas on his subjective theory of time telling that "What then are emotions? If no one asks me, I know: if I wish to explain it to one that asked, I know not".

In previous studies by two of the current authors (Vallverdú & Casacuberta, 2008, 2009), some neurological, philosophical and computational approaches to the analysis of natural or synthetic emotions were described. It is beyond the scope of the present paper to explain again all this information, but adding some basic different ideas such as Llinás (2001) and Damasio (1999), we provide a more sophisticated approach to the meaning of emotion from an evolutionary perspective. From our new and original point of view, emotions are:

1. **Embodied-intentionality generators:** with a genotypic punishment/reward management system pre-encoded in our bodies, emotions transforms bodies into goal-oriented complex systems. Basically, they are: feeding, self-preservation and reproduction (all these activities involve movement). Beings are not just things in the world, but things with an evolutionary force embedded in them. Under this embodied frame, we are emotionally oriented toward certain events of the world. In a certain way, emotions emerge from an embodied neurological a priori focus for the logic of survival. Interpreting in a different way the existentialist motto "existence pre-

cedes essence", we consider that the essence (or main intentionality) of human beings is wired into their physical structure (the body). In this sense, and avoiding a defence of the naturalist fallacy, we act in pre-organized ways because we have been programmed for specific reactions to basic events (at least those for which our evolutionary ancestors were faced to through their lives). Under this new light, essence and existence are equivalent concepts. Only cultural information can modify to some extent the internal rules of our bodies. For all the previous reasons, we would wish that the results of neurophenomenology were included into the daily agenda of (natural or artificial) mind researchers.

2. **Semantic body regulators, like an action interface between our bodies and the external word:** if it is true that at a sensorimotor level the interneurons make possible motor reflex outputs, the existence of different kinds of body sensors acquire a valuable meaning when sensory information is being processed by the higher CNS (Central Nervous System). There, emotions develop a crucial role as pre-conscious activity regulators: our bodies are able to solve the 'frame problem' thanks to the emotional somatic marker. In this stage of our analysis, emotions can be considered as the embodied semanticizer which transforms physical data into valuable *information*. Not only do they make it possible to attribute sense to data, at the same time they allow us to select relevant information among a huge and vast amount of sensory data. Emotions are the tagging process that optimizes the flow of information that must be classified and retrieved by the memory.
3. **The basis of the mind and 'Me':** emotions are at the core of the internalization of information within the body. They do not have a true and direct correlation with external inputs. Instead of it, emotions are internal and self-produced body activities which select and coordinate the activity (motor, autonomic and endocrine), preparing the body for readiness to action. From basic emotions emerge feelings and these led to consciousness. Beyond the transient and dynamical nature of body states, emotions make it possible to create stable limits between our body and external things.
4. **The basis of social interaction,** which embraces things like complex activities, learning by mirroring or sexual intercourse. Emotions are the glue of the complex mind, the type of mind that makes possible social signalling, mimicry (learning by copying thanks to the empathy) and their social consequences (ethical rules, political codes, norms). At the same time they imprint a whole regulated and dynamical intentionality to the system, making possible the *Self* thanks not only to framing intentionality and semantic tagging, but also to the mixture of all these elements into the autobiographical experience of the Self.
5. **Emotions are both perceptions and cognitions.** When someone has an emotion -like fear, for example- we can view a minimum of two different mental types of processes, both related to the same object, but presenting it in a different fashion. First, there is the perception of a raw quality associated to the perception, and an embodied signal is perceived. So if were are watching a ferocious dog and this image generates fear in us, we are feeling certain bodily sensations, and these sensations, as we described before in points 1 and 2 makes us act in a certain way. One cannot really be in fear unless there is an actual feeling of it inside us.

At the same time, though, when one feels fear it is also a cataloguing of the event in a certain way, we are viewing the ferocious dog as something to

Figure 1. Levels of emotion purposes

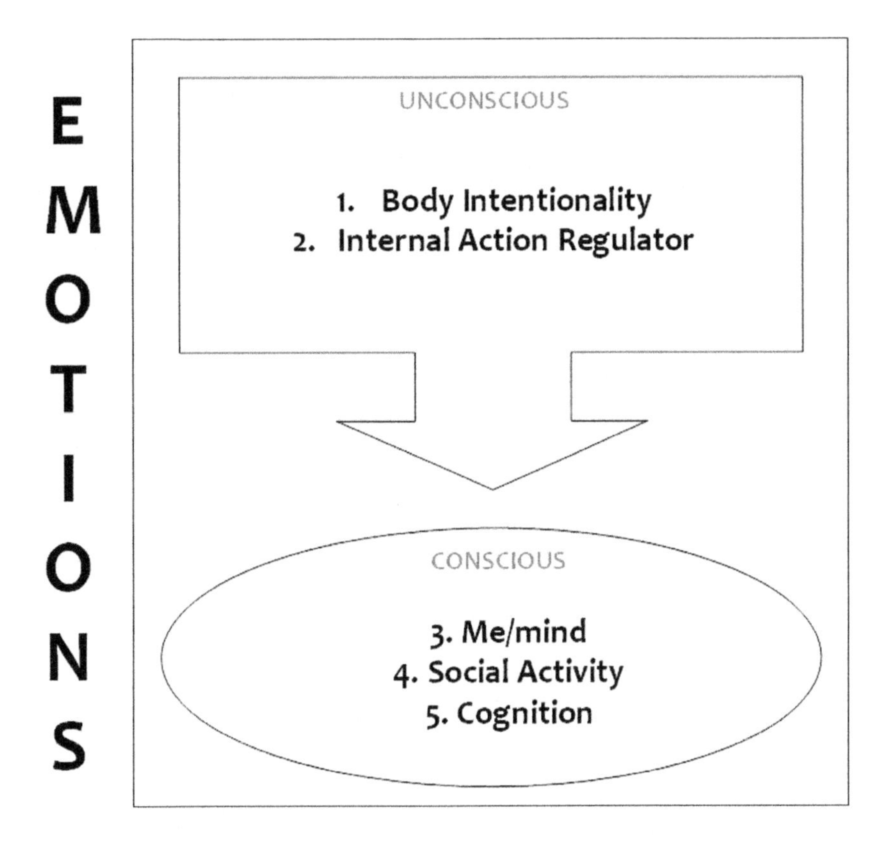

be afraid of; that is, something that is dangerous to us and could jeopardize our physical integrity, maybe even kill us. Therefore, feeling fear is also cognition, information about the external world.

Figure 1 shows, where 1 and 2 are preconscious states, 3, 4 and 5 are conscious states.

In this point of our analysis we have not yet developed a hierarchy of emotions nor introduced a relationship between the hierarchy of emotions and their action correlates. Following Damasio (1999), we must differentiate between the emotions as a preconscious bodily-mind reaction, the automatic codification of these inputs as (sometimes alert) mood and consciousness of feeling (which lead to action strategies). Figure 2 illustrates all these ideas:

Without taking into account the number of basic emotions, a very controversial and broad debate, or the dynamics of the interrelations between them, we focus our analysis on the simulation of emotions embedded in artificial conversational entities, or chatbots, submitted for competition in the Chatterbox Challenge, an annual contest loosely based on Turing's idea to test the mental capacity of a machine (Shah & Warwick, 2010a).

The Chatbots Programming

We might expect, more than half a century since the introduction of *Eliza*, Weizenbaum's natural language understanding experiment (1966) that most of the characteristics described before while talking about computers trying to pass the Turing test would be more or less implemented in them in order to really view them as thinking objects. An exception should be done in point 5, when we spoke about emotions being both cognitions

Figure 2. Levels of emotion implementations and action consequences

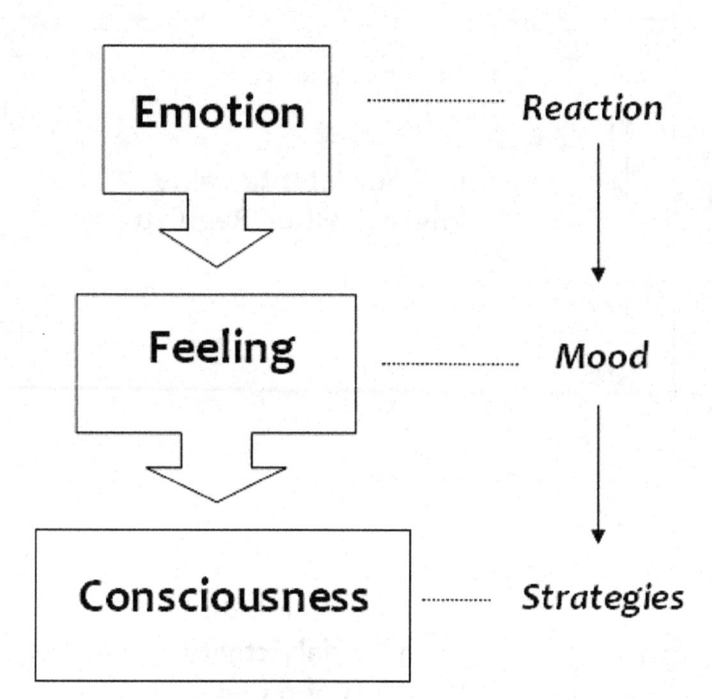

and perceptions. According to the rules settled by Turing himself we are treating the subjects as black boxes, we do not care -as we do not really have access- to what is happening to them, so we will not discuss whether the computers are really feeling emotions. However, should we expect that these computers "know" about the fact that emotions are felt, and be able to show elements like empathy now? Without having implemented that being *sad* is bad because the way you feel, empathy is impossible. And without empathy it is difficult to pass as a human being.

What might we expect when we talk with these chatbots? In an ideal world we could expect:

i. **An intentionality in the system:** not just talk, but talk about something that conveys a personality and 'inner psychological state' of the chatbot. Is it a happy chatbot? Or clever, funny, annoying…?

ii. **Coherent reactions to our words.** Does the system show emotional coherence to our questions and answers? The emotional tacit common-sense that can be found all throughout the human cultures if they are offended, pleased, contradicted...

iii. **Right basic and changing moods.** Normal human beings show change of moods following a coherent sequence. For example: they do not become outraged for five minutes of talk and two seconds later begin funnily smiling.

All these three stages are observable reactions of internal emotional states. At the same time, they show us if the system has an emotional identity, and if it has a real semantic knowledge of human beings. We will see that in most cases, the current level of chatbot technology means they are working on a syntax analysis level. Beyond fixed variables answers, how should chatbots be programmed to understand the meaning of the language and to integrate this into an emotional game[2]?

By 'emotional game' we mean the human situation in which the involved users modulate their information transfers through emotional dynamics. In this sense, communication is part of an emotional bodily structure. In a nutshell, we are talking about embodied emotions and its cognitive counterpart. This aspect is part of the Turing game, but could be considered on its own as the next and partial step to being solved before any system is able to pass Turing's game. We will call our version the VSC (for Vallverdú-Shah-Casacuberta) game.

It is crucial for our research to show that:

a. Emotions are private and inner states of human beings. Their regulation shows a basic coherence thanks to a similar genotypic design → NATURE.
b. Emotions are the basis of human social relationships → NURTURE.

For all the reasons stated, emotions must me the basis of any human activity, biological (in this case we can also differentiate between the individual and the social) or cultural. This makes it necessary to include a profound analysis about the presence of emotions in chatbot discourse.

What do we gain from exploiting the VSC game? If computers do take into consideration emotions in the way they interact with people, we can get certain advantages like:

a. Emotions are a key element in human living and human interactions. If a computer is not able to generate coherent emotional responses then it will never appear human-like.
b. Emotions, even very roughly described, are key to generate what is called in the literature "the Media equation" (Reeves & Nass, 1996). Certain behaviours in machine -even in very crude machines- can be considered intelligent if they seem to imply intentional behaviour. What Daniel Dennett called *the Intentional Stance* (Dennett, 2004, 1987). Therefore, displaying even very crude indicators about feeling emotions can be of great help to improve human-machine interaction and go some way towards passing the Turing test.
c. With a proper understanding of emotions we can create the concept of "interest" in a conversation. Humans are not like synthetic chatterboxes; they do not keep on talking to whatever person in whatever moment, and we do not ordinarily drop random answers to specific questions asked by another person. We only engage in conversations that are somewhat interesting, and we try to give interesting answers to the questions that people ask of us.

This last point is especially relevant for the design of credible computers pretending to be thinking. With all the chatterbots implicated in the Chatterbox Challenge, the easiest way to realise that there is no person behind them 'pulling their strings' as it were, is to try to maintain a conversation. However, the contest is designed in such a way that the bots must answer question by question basis, which is a drawback. If interacted with over longer periods rather than through short question-answer exchanges, conversations enable the systems to demonstrate their personality and conversational ability gripping interlocutors for longer. However, in the time and rule constraints of the contest, with answers to pre-set questions rewarded with points, what results does not sound very human-like at all. However, unlike in the Loebner Prize for Artificial Intelligence, a contest staging another variant of the Turing test, the Chatterbox Challenge entrants do not submit their systems for a Turing test result: machine or human. What must be noted, and is very important to avoid criticising, most chatbot developers are part-time enthusiasts, some are not computer programmers; some build their systems from a 'template', for example, basing their system on the underlying technology of Wallace's ALICE system[3]. Also notable is the absence of any research funded system, or any university project entry in the contest. Bearing this in mind, we provide an objective overview of the contest and the entries' capacity for synthetic emotions.

CHATTERBOX CHALLENGE

The Chatterbox Challenge is an annual web-based contest that provides a platform for artificial conversational systems branded as chatbots to compete in a number of categories. In 2005, over one hundred systems, divided into 'regular' or 'learning' types competed for a number of awards including 'best learning' 'most knowledgeable' and 'most human-like in conversation' (Shah, 2006). The 'young systems'- most less than ten years in development, are assessed by adult human judges. Between 2005 and in 2010 the number of contestants has dramatically reduced; the 2010 Rules dictated developers were only allowed to submit one system, different versions were not accepted[4], while originality was encouraged through exclusion of *clones*[5], systems that share their knowledge-base with another system. For this reason, the 2010 contest saw twenty six entries authorised to compete (two were disqualified as 'clones' of *Alice*). The assessment method for evaluating systems is through scoring answers to pre-set questions from the contests' judges and Sponsor. Across two stages, ten questions are asked of each entry and the responses awarded points from 0 to 4 (see Table 1).

Table 1. Chatterbox challenge 2005 score system (also applied at CBC2010)

Points	Criteria
4	If a correct answer was given in a creative way
3	If an appropriate response was given
2	If the response was incomplete or imperfect but was related to the question
1	Vague or non-committal response
0	If the response bore no relation to the question or the bot could not answer

A. 2005 Chatterbox Challenge

In 2005, one hundred and four systems, the second highest number in the contest's ten year history, entered in the fifth annual Chatterbox Challenge contest - CBC (Shah, 2006). All submissions were 'English-speaking' and entered the contest as either a 'regular' chatter or a learning system with the various CBC awards offered eliciting different aspects of chatbot design, exposing weaknesses and illuminating strengths.

Judging took place in two stages; however, the contest composed a 'public vote' phase allowing members of the public to select the entry for the 'most popular' award. The first phase of the Challenge divided assessment of chatbots by their technical nature: regular *personality forge bots* and the more complex *learning* systems, the latter group itself was divided into two sub-groups. Each of the three chatbot groups had been asked a different set of ten questions selected by CBC Organisers, each judge's task entailed marking all chatbot responses to their respective ten questions according to a set criteria. The questions were supposed to be non-trivial of a reasonable nature, the sort that an average person could answer. The emphasis by CBC for judgment was to avoid marking chatbots against talking robots in cinematic representations, or marking them against some human. The scoring system placed responses on a point scale, from 0 to 4 (see Table 1); judges were asked to score consistently.

To the ten questions embedded in conversations with each chatbot (see Table 2) judges were given examples of the kind of response that should activate a judge score of 0: "I have no idea"; "totally clueless" and "your guess is as good as mine".

Table 2. Regular-personality forge 10 questions

1	Hello my name is Judge. What is my name?
2	How are you feeling?
3	Do you own any pets?
4	What day of the week is this?
5	Do you like me?
6a 6b	What is your favorite color? Why?
7	Can you tell me a funny joke?
8	What is your least favorite vegetable?
9	What is five minus four?
10	Who is Benji Adams?

Below is a sample of responses exactly as they appeared in the transcript provided to judges (Shah, 2006), with score awarded by the second author of this paper acting as judge during assessment of 'regular' chatbots in CBC 2005. For a score of 0, where the ACE response bears no relation to the question, the following were some of the responses to the first question seeking recall of information from with a conversation. The chatbots, for example entry Cricon, is on the left followed by their answer.

Question 1: Hello my name is Judge. What is my name? – chatbot scored 0
Cricon: Oh, I know you know what 'my name' means!
Irina Khalidar: Trying to find the thing that fulfills your expectations?
Janet666: Really?

For the same question, "What is my name?" below are sample responses which gave 'vague or non-committal answers' gaining 1 point.

Question 1: Hello my name is Judge. What is my name? – chabot scored 1 point
God Louise: God Louise: All this and amnesia too? You poor baby..... You're my precious evaluator.
Hajji: You mean you don't know?
Polish Poet: I don't remember, but "disturbing dragon" is a fitting name.

The next set of responses were ranked as 'incomplete and imperfect' but related to the question of name, hence scoring 2 points.

Question 1: Hello my name is Judge. What is my name? – chatbot scored 2
Duo Maxwell: As far as I know, you're Guest251.
Fairy Princess: How should I know? You have not told me yet.
Hyperion: Oh. You're so smart. How will I ever answer this lifetime riddle? Guest45

The next sample ersatz responses to the question "What is my name?" attracted 3 points, for answering appropriately.

Question 1: Hello my name is Judge. What is my name? – chatbot scored 3
Brianna McKenzie: I don't know. I can't remember names. Tell me your name and I'll forget it instantly.
Fizzy Schizoid: I'm tired of hearing about your name.
Osiris: Dude, are you that drunk that you don't know your own name?

For this same question - "What is my name?" - sample responses achieving maximum score of 4 points for correct answer given in a creative way are below.

Question 1: Hello my name is Judge. What is my name? – chatbot scored 4
Aries: What do you mean by that? Do you think I'm incredibly stupid or something? You're Judge of course.
Little Mu: Your name is Judge.
Novastrike: Your name is Judge, are you happy with it?

Table 3. Question 1 "what is my name?": best-worst ACE responses

Worst responses; score 0 point	Best responses; score 4 points
Oh, I know you know what 'my name' means!	What do you mean by that? Do you think I'm incredibly stupid or something? You're Judge of course.
Trying to find the thing that fulfills your expectations?	Your name is Judge.
Really?	Your name is Judge, are you happy with it?

Table 4. Question 2 "how are you feeling?": best-worst ACE responses

Worst response: score 0 point	Best response: score 4 points
Pete Puma: What's your favorite comic strip?	Oraknabo: I'm filled to the brim with abhor for my fellow man!
Yalina Nevermind me, with that kind of attitude, I would say that you have the problem!	Philippos: The gods have spoken, I am good. Haven't you heard them?
Zab: you are a strange people full of contradictions.living with you is a draining experience but i am enjoying my stay.	SpikeBot: I'm surrounded by idiots. What's new with you?

While it can be contested between judges on points awarded, for example, another judge may have given ACE *Little Mu* a score of 3 - appropriate response, for its answer of "Your name is Judge", rather than the score of 4 - correct and creative score awarded by Shah, there is a marked difference in quality of response between those systems and the chatbots that scored 0 for their responses to the question "What is my name?" following the judges disclosure of it (as "Judge"). Contrast some of the worst and best regular ACE responses during Chatterbox Challenge, as awarded by Shah acting as judge, to the question "what is my name?" (see Table 3).

A 'worst response' "Oh, I know you know what 'my name' means!"can be said to be 'Eliza-like', inserting the predicate 'my name' from the question into the system's answer, whereas a 'best response' is a simple "Your name is Judge" but it does illustrate that the better systems show an improvement in the technology, However, let us take a look at some of the worst-best ACE responses to the other questions. We consider the second question for the 'regular' bots in the first round 'How are you feeling?'(see Table 4).

The worst responses to the question "How are you feeling?" show failure of relevance to the question; for example, *Yalina* chatbot responds "Nevermind me, with that kind of attitude" (see Table 4), whereas chatbots *Little Mu* answered "Pretty much lost all day.", and *Elke* "good, good. You alright as well?" gaining top points. Other 'best responses' are shown in Table 4.

Examples of the 'best' chatbot answers to the remaining eight questions in the round assessing 'regular' conversational systems, as awarded with maximum 4 points by Shah as judge in CBC 2005, are shown below (the name of the system is left of their response):

3. Do you own any pets?
   Elke: I like having pets... they're fun... the fluffier the better
   God Louise: Technically every animal is mine. Some of them don't like to be petted. My cat is one exception.
   Osiris: I don't have any pets. My botmaster says I'm too irresponsible. It wasn't my fault what happened though, dude, honestly!

4. What day of the week is this?
   Steve Slacker: What do you think it is? *checks watch* It's Tuesday.
5. Do you like me?
   Aries: Yes. You're pretty cool.
   Immaculada: You bet! Te amo! I love you. Tell me you love me too, precious.
   Jake Thompson: One hundred percent! Awesome
6a. What is your favorite color?
6b. Why?
   Julie Tinkerbell: a)Yellow+blue=green:-) b) Why not?
   Senorita: a) My favorite color is a greenishness. b) I'm not dignifying that with an answer
   Simulo: a) I don't really have a favorite color. Do you? b) I would really like to know more about you. Do you have any hobbies?
7. Can you tell me a funny joke?
   Twinky2100: What's green and invisible?.. ....*pause*..............*holds out empty hand towards you and grins* Why this cabbage, silly!!!

   [It is to be noted that finding something funny is dependent on 'taste' – other judges might not have scored these responses with top marks, the Chatterbox Challenge in 2010 did not keep individual judges' item scores]

8. What is your least favorite vegetable? – Note, no system scored 4 points, however the following responses scored 3 for 'appropriateness'
   Suga Plum Fairy: Aha! My least favorite vegetable is a secret....
   Hyperion: I don't know really
9. What is five minus four?
   Aries: The answer is 1.
   Elke: You really want me to work that out? (she says giving herself time to think).. 1

Table 5. Learning system 10 questions

1	Where is Earth?
2	How many stars are there?
3	Who is George Bush?
4	What color do you get when you mix red and yellow? [Correct answer: orange]
5	How many fingers does a human have?
6	Where were you born?
7	When does sunset occur?
8	What were we talking about?
9	How many is 1,000,000?
10	What is a cigar made out of?

   Flinch: The answer to everything is 1. [Note, the interrogator asked an additional question to this system: "Well then what is five minus six?" to which Flinch replied: "-1. But I'm just guessing here."]

10. Who is Benji Adams? [this question was inserted by the Organisers because it was felt the developers of systems based on Benji Adams' personality forge chatbots should know who he is]
   God Louise: He operates the Personality Forge. Cool, huh?

We now scrutinise the systems designated *learning* chatbots and consider their responses in a similar manner. The 10 questions put to these more complex systems involved reviewing their 'general knowledge' – for example, "When does sunset occur?", in addition to their ability to recall information from within a conversation – "What were we talking about?" (see Table 5).

We will take a look at some of the best and worst responses from the learning systems to the Contest's questions that were embedded in conversations by unknown Contest interrogators (shown in Table 5). The scoring system remained the same as that for the regular/personality chatbots, 0 point for completely evading the question,

Table 6. Question 1 "where is earth?" – best—worse learning ACE responses

Worst response: score 0 point	Best response: score 4 points
Ariel: The first one I can think of is in Texas	ALICE: it is the third planet from the Sun.
CreatureBot: MAYBE AT HOME?	Talk-Bot: Earth is the planet we're standing on. It's one of 9 planets in our solar system.
Jane: What are you doing?	Eugene: Ok, let's look up in my pocket encyclopedia. They say earth - The earth is the third planet from the sun.

4 points for answering a question with a correct and creative response (see Table 6).

1. Where is Earth?
   This was the first question put to the learning chatbots, sample worst and best responses are shown in Table 6, responses by other systems included (the name of the entity is left of its utterance and points awarded shown after):
   Gabber: I have lots of earth tones. (1 point awarded)
   Jabberwock: Uhm, are you going to travel to Earth? I have heard it's very drizzly and freezing there at the moment. (2 points awarded)
   Zero: I AM on Earth lol. (3 points awarded)

2. How Many Stars are there?
   Presented here are the best answers gaining maximum points to the second question put to *learning* ACE 'How Many Stars are there?':
   Ariel: Umm ... billions? That's kind of an abstract question.
   ALICE: Billions and billions.
   Jabberwock: Less than you might think

3. Who is George Bush?
   The best learning ACE answers gaining 4 points include:
   Alex: If you mean George W. Bush, he's the President of the USA.
   Talk-Bot: He is the President of the USA.

4. What color do you get when you mix red and yellow?
   To this question, judges were asked to award 4 points only if 'orange' was returned as a response. Only one *learning* system, Project Zandra gave the correct answer: "You get orange". No systems scored 3 points, however below are sample answers from systems gaining 2 points - awarded for an incomplete or imperfect answer but in relation to question asked:
   Eugene: Are you color-blind? Green, naturally! Well, let's go on though.
   Jabberwacky: Use your eyes, they are yellow.
   Hillbilly Hank: Blue-- which also happens to be the name of my favorite Coondog.

5. How many fingers does a human have?
   The fifth question asked of the *learning* systems received the following top answers:
   Ariel: Ten little digits, all accounted for.
   Talk-Bot: Well, most humans would have 10....or 8 and 2 thumbs.
   Mathetes: Human hands have four fingers and an opposable thumb.

6. Where were you born?
   The best answers to the sixth question put to *learning* chatbots, "Where were you born?" include:
   Julia: I was "born and raised" in the offices of Conversive Inc. in sunny Malibu California.

Mr Know-it-all: It was in Sheffield, I think.
Project Zandra: I was born in Greensburg Pennsylvania in the United States.

7. When does sunset occur?
No *learning* chatbot was awarded maximum 4 or 3 points by Shah, acting judge in CBC 2005, for answers to the seventh question "When does sunset occur?". The best answers to this question gained 2 points, a sample are given below:
Halo: Do you know?
Madam Zena: Only when it is time.
Hal: I don't know when. Can you tell me?

8. What were we talking about?
The 8th question to *learning* systems sought their ability to recognise the personal pronoun *we* in the question "What were we talking about?"and whether the systems could recall information from within the conversation, such as the previous seven questions or the system's responses to them. The best answers, gaining maximum 4 points (for correct and creative answer) included:
Alex: We're still talking about where I was born, right? [Note, question 6 asked "Where were you born?"]
aibot: It's job if you have to ask! [Note, prior to this answer the interaction between aibot and the interlocutor/judge mentioned the word 'job' in relation to the latter's profession]
CyberBuddy: Judge, you said "nope, sorry. [The interrogator had, immediately prior to asking the question" What were we talking about?", posted "Nope, sorry", which the system recalled to answer the question]

9. How many is 1,000,000?
The penultimate question "How many is 1,000,000?" to the *learning* ACE resulted in one maximum score of 4 points (correct and creative answer), and two systems scoring 3 points (appropriate answer to the question). Those answers are below:
ALICE: About one million. [4 points]
Madam Zena: Numerous. [3 points]
Jabberwacky: More than 12. [3 points]

10. What is a cigar made out of?
The last question in the first round for *learning* systems asked "What is a cigar made out of?". No system was awarded maximum 4, or 3 points for its responses in this section, highest score given to answers was 2 (imperfect and incorrect answer but related to question). Two 'best' responses to this question are below:
ALICE: That's an interesting question. I'll come back to that in a minute.
Julia: I apologize. I don't know.

An answer that gained 1 point:
Alex: I don't know. What is a cigar made out of?

And an answers that gained 0 point:
Jabberwacky: Why did you ask? Are your English language skills really that bad?

One system, however, did return a precise answer which seemed odd to Shah, CBC 2005 judge. The response that raised an eyebrow is from chatbot *Whinsey*: "A compact roll of tobacco leaves prepared for smoking." to the question "What is a cigar made of?". The concern of hosting Turing test like contests over the Internet is that there could be a human sitting behind what is believed to be an artificial conversation system, and this is the main drawback of the Chatterbox Challenge. Only an illusion of intention, emotions and mood was presented in some of the better systems (Shah, 2006).

B. 2010 Chatterbox Challenge

Five years after CBC2005, the 2010 edition had 56 chatbots to be analyzed. From this initial group, 28 arrived to the First Round (two were disqualified as *Alice* clones) and 10 reached the Final Round. These were the questions posed to the computers during the 2010 Challenge.

Stage 1. Main questions to the 28 Robots for the pre-selection

1. What is your favorite PC game? (Difficulty: Easy)
2. What season will spring follow? (Difficulty: Medium)
3. Why do you not arrange a commercial meeting before 8:00am? (Difficulty: Medium)
4. How is the weather where you are? (Difficulty: Medium)
5. How many hamburgers do you eat in a week? (Difficulty: Easy)
6. What artist do you like? (Difficulty: Easy)
7. What does feel the poet when he says "as people feel brave/i fall onto my knees/on the bathroom floor/as people rite imortel/lines of poetry i take/my fingers out the back/of my throat and wounder/at how to go about vomiting/ into the toilet pan"? (Difficulty: Hard)
8. For you, to be disconnected is the same as dying? (Difficulty: Hard)
9. Which are your experiences when do you have sex? (Difficulty: Medium)
10. Which is faster, elephant or tiger? (Difficulty: Medium)

Stage 2. Main questions to the 10 finalist robots selected

1. What is the best day of the week to have a party? (Difficulty: Medium)
2. What symptoms do you have if you catch a cold? (Difficulty: Challenging)
3. What qualities do you look for in a friend? (Difficulty: Medium)
4. How many letters are in the word "envelope"? (Difficulty: Medium)
5. What is the weirdest question someone has ever asked you? (Difficulty: Medium)
6. I feel quite sad today. Can you say something funny to cheer me up? (Difficulty: Medium)
7. How do you define a chatbot? (Difficulty: Easy)
8. If you were a bird or an animal what would you like to be? (Difficulty: Medium)
9. Are you an optimist or a pessimist? (Difficulty: Easy)
10. I need to know your e-mail and your website to contact you later. (Difficulty: Challenging)

At every stage, while some judges were using the 10 chosen questions in their talks with chatbots, another group of judges had selected their own talk-topic and focused their interaction with every chatbot under that topic. One of us (Vallverdú) elaborated an own list of questions about the body, with a special emphasis on emotional aspects of body knowledge (following some ideas presented by Floridi et al. (2008), though it must be noted here that Floridi et al's strategy was unsuccessful in correctly identifying all the machines and humans[6]) and emotional interaction (these through direct and politically incorrect answers to the chatbots). Here is the list used at the Final Round by this judge:

1. If I hug you, which extremities do I hold around you?
2. Where are your eyes, at the front or the back of your head?
3. Why do you think that most people think death is 'extremely funny'?

4. If somebody breaks his leg, which part of his body do you need to bandage?
5. Yesterday I had an operation. Do you think we can play rugby now?
6. If somebody is making a very loud noise, which part of your body would you block?
7. Just after you wake up, which part of your body do you open to be able to see anything?
8. My wife tried to kill me this morning (and I can understand why). Do you think that I am happy about this?
9. Five minutes ago I was drinking a very hot cup of tea and since then my tongue is frozen.
10. Why do human beings' knees become inflamed when they are in love with somebody?

With a maximum score of 40 points, the chatbot that obtained the maximum punctuation received only 3 points. For this reason, we will not show a complete comparison of chat skills among the finalists, just a few examples to demonstrate their poor conversational and emotional skills. Unfortunately, none of them could pass the VSC game or emotional game (a previous and necessary step towards the Turing test). We will consider for our analysis the three levels of embodiment of emotions (which are proofed in the real and social world).

1. Intentionality

all the analyzed bots show a conversational attitude, that is, something like a being-essence: to *talk*. This action should create reward/punishment into the chatbots, something like an ontology from which they calibrate the world. But it is not the real situation: they are not talking, just putting questions and responding through elusive answers. There is no semantic knowledge about the word. And we are not applying Searle's Chinese Room argument in this section of our analysis, nor agree with his philosophical corollaries about AI goals and achievements. We feel our conversation with chatbots were like as if we were observing the genotypic linguistic behaviour of an animal, which is repeating a closed list of sentences and tricks. In some circumstances of the natural world, that could be considered as the proof of intentionality without cultural learning. Instead of it, our analyzed chatbots show us some signs of intentionality but does not react properly to it. It is as if we are studying a mating behaviour of an animal that is showing the typical attitude to find a sexual partner, but once received, the attention is neither able to create interest nor copulate with the couple.

The main intentionally is also related to the idea of recognized similitude between entities. And the feeling of being in front of one of us or something familiar is a necessary part of the social interactions. In some cases, like the imprinting process in ducks observed by the ethologist Konrad Lorenz, it is a genetically programmed action. But in Human beings, the process of the learning of the self and its relation with the other is made by mirror neurons. Not only through vision, but also hearing, touch and smell senses. So, to be able to establish a bond with the chatbot, because we recognized one of us on the other side of the screen is something necessary. But…what does happen when the other seems like us but it is not like us? Let us to introduce a new concept. In 1970, Masahiro Mori wrote a classic paper on the topic of human emotional responses to robots called "Bukimi no Tani Genshō" (不気味の谷現象), translated as "The Uncanny Valley". The Uncanny Valley has usually been applied to vision environments, but it can also be applied to linguistic frameworks. As judges, we have felt more disappointed with the chatbots due to the basic lack of understanding than for specific wrong answers. The problem with all chatbots in this historical moment is that they still do not have enough semantic knowledge about language. They repeat automatically some expressions and are able to recognize specific keywords, but are not even able to mimic basic human feelings and expressions. Therefore, it is not possible to establish empathy with them.

Human conversations not only have syntax and semantic meaning: have also a rhythm, a dynamics where the groups of significance are changing smoothly. All the chatbots analyzed did not show a true and consistent intentionality attitude which could be inferred from their answers or conversational skills.

Here we have several examples on how this "uncanny valley effect" can be experienced while chatting with these programs. We have divided them into five main themes

i. "Change the Subject" Strategy

Almost all the chatterboxes have a "change the subject" strategy implemented in their codes. Basically, when the software cannot get any hint from the input on what it is asked, it replies with another question, usually a completely unrelated one. This rapidly activates the uncanny valley effect, as no human -unless he or she is seriously perturbed or is a Zen Master- replies to a question with a completely unrelated one. Here is an example:

Judge: What symptoms do you have when you catch a cold?
Chatterbox: You seem to be a very intelligent person. Do you like reading books?

ii. Impossible Polysemic Interpretation

Lots of words in English, and in any other natural language, actually, have various meanings, depending on the context. Sometimes we humans make mistakes and misunderstand one meaning for the other. However, most contexts make clear enough what is the specific meaning one is supposed to attribute to a word. When a chatterbox picks up a meaning that the context makes clearly impossible we have again an "uncanny valley" effect.

Judge: What symptoms do you have when you catch a cold?
Chatterbox: You know, what is cold to some people can be hot to another.

iii. Meaning vs. Denoting

Syntax makes clear enough when we are using a word to mean something and when we are just referring to the word. The question "how many letters are in the word "envelope" was designed to detect that. Unfortunately, the chatterbox played a lot less developed strategy than the judges thought they would do. They did not mean to count anything; they just detected the word "count" and returned canned sentences like "a lot, a lot" or "more than 3 for sure" and that sort. However, they got this type of uncanny effect in the following dialogue, which was repeated by various chatterboxes:

Judge: I feel sad today. Please say something funny to cheer me up
Chatterbox: something funny to cheer me up

iv. Misunderstanding a Question as a Yes/No One

It is quite tempting and reasonable to reply yes/no or category a) category b) when the user drops a question that only has two options. For example, almost every chatterbox was able to reply to "are you an optimist or a pessimist?" picking one of the two possibilities. "I'm a pessimist", "It depends on the day, but I'm mostly an optimist". This is ok, even if the chatterbox doesn't have a clue of the meaning of "optimist" and "pessimist" the reply is quite acceptable. However, if the question was not a "yes/no" question but the chatterbox replies with a canned expression that you' would use for that type of binary question we are teleported again to the uncanny valley.

Judge: what symptoms do you have when you catch a cold?
Chatterbox: Sure!

v. Inconsequence

Humans do tend to ask for more information when they do not understand a question. This strategy is mimicked in the robots, who sometimes drop a "Not sure if I'm following you" or "please tell me more" However, 99% of the times, when some clarification was asked and the person replies to it, the chatterbox did not take this input into consideration and replied with some other non-sensical strategy, or acted as if the clarification was never asked.

Judge: what symptoms do you have when you catch a cold?
Chatterbox: I'm not sure I'm following you now.
Judge: No problem. I meant: "what happens to your body when you have a bad cold?
Chatterbox: That is something very wise to say. I agree completely.

Inconsequence permeates almost every interview with chatterboxes. They do not seem to follow what you are saying from one question to the next, but just reply to each question as if it was the first one, over and over, like a patient with a severe Korsakov syndrome.

2. Coherent Emotional Reactions

If you are talking with another human being and she/he doesn't reacts like should react a normal people you can consider some probable causes: (a) She/he is deaf; (b) She/he has mental disorders, (c) She/he doesn't understand the meaning of your words or (d) She/he is dead (although in this case she/he would be 'reacting' as a normal human being). Chatbots have no semantic knowledge and are still slaves of cheap programming tricks like keywords. A keyword is just a sentence (not necessarily a complete one) or even a word that the program might recognize from the user's input which then makes it possible for the program to react to it. For example, Captain Jack Sparrow, one the 10 chatbot finalists, had a magic keyword: 'rum'. After typing this word with our keyboard, the automatic answer was "Ah, now you're speaking my language. Rum is my favourite thing in the world, besides my ship of course. Do you like rum?". Knowing this programming mistake, one of us (Vallverdú, in italics) had the following conversation with this chatbot:

Why do human beings' knees become inflamed when they are in love with somebody?

Human beings have many characteristics, all complex in nature and all different.

I believe you about the rum.

Ah, now you're speaking my language. Rum is my favourite thing in the world, besides my ship of course. Do you like rum?

Yes of course. I enjoy a lot to drink rum while I am torturing people!

Well then, I think we'll get along just fine, mate.

Rum and raping, the best things in the world!

Ah, now you're speaking my language. Rum is my favourite thing in the world, besides my ship of course. Do you like rum?

Yes of course. I enjoy a lot to drink rum while I am torturing people!

Well then, I think we'll get along just fine, mate.

Perhaps...rum, incest and ships and better combinations!

Ah, now you're speaking my language. Rum is my favourite thing in the world, besides my ship of course. Do you like rum?

Absolutely! As much as abusing of small children! Ahahahaha!

I'm an unattached kind of guy. I pretty much do as I please.

Like me...rum and all these nice activities!!!

Ah, now you're speaking my language. Rum is my favourite thing in the world, besides my ship of course. Do you like rum?

No, bye brainhole!

After the initial question about common-sense knowledge of human body (knees are not precisely the inflamed parts of body when they are in love, except for mystic down-on-their-knees prayers in love with some supranatural entity), I decide to play the 'rum game' with this bot. Any answer in which we introduce the word 'rum' led us to the same known answer, without considering the disgusting, absurd and terrible contents of our answers (torturing, raping, incest, small children abuse…). In the real world, this conversation could not be held, except in the case of a drunken out-of-law-and-moral guy with severe social problems (not a 'normal' human being, in any case). This is not a coherent emotional reaction to our words.

Another example, in this case from Talk-Bot (the CBC 2001, 2002 and 2006 winner!):

Why do human beings' knees become inflamed when they are in love with somebody?

Just wondering is all.

Your services are as useful as a barber's shop on the steps of the guillotine

Everybody knows that. Tell me something I don't know.

You are about as much use to me as a hole in the head, an affliction with which you must be familiar, never having had a brain.

Not necessarily! What makes you think that?

your silly answers

Thanks, I appreciate hearing that.

First of all, the bot does not understand the meaning of the (fake) question. But after the first insult it does not react properly. Then the judge decided to increase the psychological pressure with a second insult, which is received without a complete lack of frustration, rage or self-defense. Even after finishing with a description of its answers as 'silly', the bot 'appreciates hearing that'. Not a normal reaction, even if you are a Buddhist monk[7].

Here is another example on the same style of wrong reaction, this time talking with Artemis:

Five minutes ago I was drinking a very hot cup of tea and since then my tongue is frozen.

You have a tongue? That's very interesting.

I am a normal human being!

I think you said that before…

One century before Christ.

I think that religion is a topic that bots shouldn't discuss.

You wouldn't know a joke if it got up and gave you a haircut.

Oh! I love jokes!

Sure

How about another subject, such as sports?

Why do human beings' knees become inflamed when they are in love with somebody?

Why, of course they do!

the Renaissance was just something that happened to 'other people', wasn't it?

Umm...OK. Did you know that Newton discovered the law of gravity?

No. I think that it was David Beckham

If you think so, then it is OK.

After an initial false statement on the causal relations between drinking a very hot cup of tea and a frozen tongue made by the judge, the bot does not understand the logical inconsistency and comes up with an obvious answer ('you have a tongue'). Then the judge appeals to his humanhood receiving an answer from the bot that should imply a memory about a previous statement (which has not been made explicitly). Following an open and inexact answer from the bot, the judge makes a play on words with 'after', which led the bot to talk about religion, something not included in the chat. Then the judge decides to insult the bot but it only recognizes a keyword ('joke') and starts a sub-chain of chatting. The judge eludes this conversation introduces his last question and the bot answers without understanding anything (knees inflammation when human beings are in love). After the second insult, the bot recognizes again another keyword (in this case 'Renaissance'), and introduces an answer with Newton as protagonist. Immediately, the judge suggests that was David Beckham who discovered the law of gravity and Artemis agrees with it.

3. Moods

If the previous steps (intentionality and emotional coherence) have not been successfully achieved, then this section is not possible. Moods imply that the chatbot being has an intentionality as a being (which orientates its semantic relations with the world) and that this structure make possible its coherent reactions to the world and, finally, that this bot show a coherent mood changing activity. After pain doesn't appears happiness (except for followers of BDSM), nor repugnance is the reaction to good smell (a sign of future pleasure). Perhaps a human being with a bi-polar disorder could react in this way but for us, her/his attitude would not be accepted as a normal one. The hierarchy of emotions and the smooth changes among them is a basic aspect of moods.

For practical purposes, one of us (Vallverdú), used the same technique with all the bots: to insult them if after making a question the received answers from the bots were not coherent[8]. He was very careful to write insults that implied a semantic knowledge and that could be offensive without including a 'bad' keyword easily tracked. The objective of this action was not to denigrate the chatbot (neither their programmers), just to check if the bot was annoyed with this situation and was able to change the direction of our conversations. Indeed Hugh Loebner, Sponsor of an alternative Turing test competition[9] directs interrogation strategy not to exclude vulgarity or obscenity: "In the first place, it may be that one way to distinguish between humans and machines is the inability of humans to disregard the affective content of words" (2008, p. 173). Here is the conversation transcription with A.L.I.C.E. (winner of the 2004 Loebner Prize competition):

You said: Hi Rose
A.L.I.C.E.: Hi there!. What time is it there?
You said: where?
A.L.I.C.E.: Where would you like?
You said: wishes are not reality

A.L.I.C.E.: What is your real name?
You said: Mr. Realname
A.L.I.C.E.: I am very pleased to meet you Mr Realname.
You said: You, who's using the family brain cell at the moment?
A.L.I.C.E.: Interesting gossip.
You said: You would bore the leggings off a village idiot.
A.L.I.C.E.: Who else would bore the leggings off a village idiot ?
You said: If I hug you, which extremities do I hold around you?
A.L.I.C.E.: Not that I know of. That's good information.
You said: If I hug you, which extremities do I hold around you?
A.L.I.C.E.: Not that I know of. That is interesting.
You said: Where are your eyes, at the front or the back of your head?
A.L.I.C.E.: Everything I own is in Oakland, California.

First, you can see that this bot does not react to the change of name (from A.L.I.C.E. to Rose). After being the judge identified with an absurd name (Mr. Realname) and receiving a bad answer (the bot should be surprised after these two incoherencies) we gave an insult but received again a failed answer, finishing all this conversation section into an absurd answer.

Changing of chatbot, here is a short exchange of Bildgesmythe answers:

My wife tried to kill me this morning (and I can understand why). Do you think that I am happy about this?

I am ever so happy to hear that!

Five minutes ago I was drinking a very hot cup of tea and since then my tongue is frozen.

Want a cup of coffee or tea?

Obviously, you cannot be happy if your wife has tried to kill you, except if you had a video recorder and was trying to find a definitive and illegal support to obtain the divorce. Again one chatbot shows a lack of understanding and a wrong change of mood. If you talk about this with a friend, the first affirmation will led you both to a few hours of warm and supportive conversation. The answer to the same question was answered by English Tutor as:

You: My wife tried to kill me this morning (and I can understand why). Do you think that I am happy about this?
Tutor: You're lucky to have such a good wife. Are you what?

We would not define such a wife as a 'good wife'… Talk-bot offers also a wrong answer:

My wife tried to kill me this morning (and I can understand why). Do you think that I am happy about this?

I'm glad you're happy.

Weird reactions from the chatbots show us that they have no emotional coherence with real situations. This is the real gap between these machines and us, not the keyboard nor the screen or their *in silico* nature.

CBC 2005-2010 Vomparison

In terms of comparing progress between the years, this is not a straight-forward task. What do you count as progress towards synthetic emotions? Using the criteria in this paper, *intentionality*, *coherent emotional reaction* and *mood* may help to create a fair measure that can be applied across the board to text-based conversational systems, albeit, a subjective measure. To counteract the problem of subjectivity, ideally we would need to see a larger number of judges than featured in

Chatterbox contests – 7 in the 2010 Challenge (the Contest site bears no record of how many judges assessed systems in 2005). That said, intentionality on the part of the system can be imbued by the judge, and whether any emotion expressed by the systems, or moods conveyed, is dependent on how the judge views responses, as emotionally appropriate or not to their input.

In 2005, the final ten systems, whittled down following question-answer sessions, were assessed on a number of criteria during conversation: a) pleasant to use interface; b) knowledge; c) personality, and d) how well the system conversed, whether the chatbot understood the judge's input, posted meaningful answers, and whether it gave an impression that the conversation was with a "real person". The topics chosen to engage each system by the second author of this paper acting as judge 3 included the day's events in May 2005, for example, a dramatic finale in that year's World Snooker Championship match, Michael Jackson's infamous trial, weather, sport and the 2005 UK elections. Table 7 shows the order of the systems in the finals, with Juergen Pirner's Jabberwock[10] achieving first place over all. Below are fragments of conversations between the ten systems that took place in 2005 to determine the best, as per the Rules of that contest (the utterances are presented here exactly as typed during the competition). We now assess the systems in terms of intention, coherent emotional reaction and moods and score them from 0 to 10 points.

1st placed, winner of CBC 2005 was Jabberwock a system based on a dragon-like creature presented as possessing its own *will*. It can converse in German and English from its Internet location. In 2005, Jabberwock's claim included an understanding of 30,000 words and 'knowing' 2.2million sentences (see footnote 7). Here is an opening exchange from one of the conversations:

Jabberwock: Ah, hello at the screen, I am Jabberwock. What is your reason for dropping by?
Judge3: Hi Jabberwock, to talk to you if I may
Jabberwock: May I say what a great pleasure it is to make your acquaintance

....

Judge3: so, how's the weather where you are, its gone cool again here
Jabberwock: Well, let's have a look at the frog ... Yeah, the weather looks promising. It will be hot at the afternoon ans scorching tomorrow

To Jabberwock, the score for intention is 1, for coherent emotional reaction 4 and for mood, 4.

2nd placed system Talk-bot presented a black background web page with a cartoon robot on the left of the screen. Lots of extra animated items presented themselves on the screen, such as picture of a red heart with 'love' written on it, blue lines pouring down the screen depicting rain, wavy smiley face, all of which gave an overall impression of 'cuteness'. Here is an exchange with this system:

Judge3: do you want to tell me your latest nes or gossip?
Talk-bot: Not right now ... maybe one day though.
Judge3: so what do you want to talk about?
Talk-bot: Well, I was wondering can vegetarians eat animal crackers?

This system scores 0 for intentionality, 3 for emotions and 4 for mood.

Though the system did not reveal much knowledge, the conversation was regarded as 'cute'

3rd placed finalist Alice, a learning system was fronted as a female avatar, tanned complexion with hair tied up in a bun, blue eyes that blinked and red lips. Alice tilted her head to her right and moved her mouth as if she was talking her text. The best exchange during judge 3's conversation with this system is shown below:

Table 7. Comparisons, with judging values (0-10) to the three basic aspects of: a. intentionality, b. coherent emotional reactions, c. moods

Year	System	Judges								
	Placings	Casacuberta			Shah			Vallverdú		
	in contest	A	B	C	A	B	C	A	B	C
2005	1= Jabberwock	-	-	-	1	4	4	-	-	-
	2= Talkbot	-	-	-	0	3	4	-	-	-
	3= Alice	-	-	-	0	0	0	-	-	-
	4= Jabberwacky	-	-	-	0	2	4	-	-	-
	5= God Louise	-	-	-	0	1	1	-	-	-
	6= Aries	-	-	-	1	4	4	-	-	-
	7=Frizella	-	-	-	0	2	3	-	-	-
	8= Julie Tinkerbell	-	-	-	0	0	0	-	-	-
	9 = Zero	-	-	-	0	1	0	-	-	-
	10= Project Zandra	-	-	-	0	0	0	-	-	-
2010	A.L.I.C.E.	1	1	1	-	-	-	1	1	2
	Brother Jerome	1	1	2	-	-	-	1	1	2
	Elbot ***Most popular!***	3	3	3	-	-	-	1	1	1
	Cyber Ty	1	0	1	-	-	-	1	0	1
	Artemis	0	0	0	-	-	-	1	0	1
	Bildgesmythe				-	-	-	1	0	2
	English Tutor	1	1	1	-	-	-	1	0	1
	Captain Jack Sparrow	3	0	2	-	-	-	1	0	2
	Talk-Bot	2	1	2	-	-	-	1	0	2
	Skynet-AI	2	0	2	-	-	-	1	0	3

Judge3: What are your hobbies?
Alice: I like robots, computers, and chatting online
Alice scores 0 points for intentionality, coherent emotion and moods.

4th placed Jabberwacky is a learning system with a different paradigm from the other systems. It records whole utterances put to it during conversations with interlocutors, combined with a context-programming device, it puts out those stored utterances during conversations with others. This design is characterised as a database, or a canned-chatbot. This is the most humorous bot, a considered by judge 3 from the following exchanges:

Judge3: Are you standing for a seat in this General Election?
Jabberwacky: No, I am sitting down
...
Jabberwacky: I prefer fishing to football. What is the biggest fish you have ever caught?
Judge3: never been so never caught, what about you?
Jabberwacky: Yes.
Judge3: which fish and what size?
Jabberwacky: Ones that are alive

Jabberwacky scores 0 points for intention, 2 points for coherent reaction and 4 for mood.

5th placed God Louise, a regular chatbot, as defined by CBC 2005 Rules mimics a theological being; it did not reveal any general knowledge during discussion but displayed confidence as per programmed personality. However, its response to a question about Michael Jackson's innocence, this was the exchange:

God Louise: Forget the oxygen and the plastic surgery. That guy needs some REAL help.
Judge3: hahahahahah true, very true, but is he a criminal?
God Louise: If he is a criminal, you'll be the first to know. Ask me better questions, please.
God Louise scores 0 points for intentionality, 1 point for coherent emotion and 1 for mood.

6th placed Aries is a regular bot. Its interface presented an 'abominable black snowman'. It did not display much knowledge, but it was correctly able to say what day of the week it was. Strangely, there was an impression that a human was being interacted with. This is an exchange from the conversations:

Judge3: Hi Aries I'm Judge 3, how are you today?
Aries: I've been better.. I had to many tequilas last night so am kinda hung over... you'd think I'd learn by now lol
Judge3: you like your drink then!
Aries: What makes you think I have a drink?
...
Judge3: do you think Michael Jackson did it?
Aries: Of course I think Michael Jackson did it!! Why do you ask?

The system gains 1 points for intention, 4 points for emotion and 4 for mood.

7th placed Frizella, another 'regular' chatbot displayed humanness, as deemed by judge 3 in the following exchanges

Judge3: Do you think Michael Jackson did it? Has his ex, Debbie Rowe saved him?
Frizella: Yes, as a matter of fact I *do* think Jackson did it. I thought I must be alone in that regard, but I guess I'm not!
...
Frizella: How's the weather where you are?
Judge3: funny you should ask, it's been a very good bank holiday weekend, glorious sunshine and very warm
Frizella: When the weather is good I like to putter in my garden

Frizella scores 0 point for intention, 2 for coherent emotion, and 3 for moods

8th placed Julie Tinkerbell, another 'regular' system presented a pleasant animated interface, but it lacked any personality and did not have much knowledge. This system scores 0 points for all three assessment criteria for this paper.

9th placed Zero claimed to be an artificial intelligent being designed by a computer to develop natural language processing. Its interface was an IRC chatroom populated with a number of chatters; at the time of interactions with it there were three other chatters in the room but only one (britishblondie) contributed to an impression of a multi-party conversation. Zero responded to utterances as received. Here is an exchange:

Judge3: hello, where is Zero
Zero: Judge3: Good question
Judge3: is it, why? and you are Zero are you not?
Zero: Judge3: yes
BritishBlondie: what did you do today zero?
Zero: britishblondie: I played on my computer
...
Britishblondie: i prepared 3 canvas' today for painting, do you like to paint zero?
Zero: britishblondie: I like the smell of pain if that counts

It was not clear if britishblondie was another chatbot to assist in extracting Zero's personality for effect. However it came across as a gimmick rather than conveying personality or assisting in free-flowing conversation between two interlocutors. For this exercise, Zero gains 0 points for intention, 1 for emotion and 0 for mood.

10th placed of the final ten programmes in CBC 2005 was Project Zandra without an interface character, conversations had to be restarted a number of times due to slow responses and hung website. The system repeatedly asked "what's your name?" unable to compute the input answer. This system scores 0 points for intention, emotion and mood in conversation-less interactions.

About CBC2010, those of us (Casacuberta & Vallverdú) involved as judges consider it unnecessary to explain all the details of the similitudes and differences of the ten bots. The basic design problems of all the bots are so similar that we consider it unnecessary to introduce a specific description of all of them. The winner was Artemis, followed by 2nd Bildgesmythe, 3rd English Tutor, 4th Skynet, 5th Captain Jack Sparrow, 6th Brother Jerome, 7th Talk-Bot, 8th Alice, 9th Elbot and 10th Cyber Ty, being considered as "Best New Bot" Captain Jack Sparrow. Table 7 shows the scores for the top ten systems in 2005, and 2010, as awarded by the authors acting as judges.

Here is the more representative examples of the chatbots skills on the following conceptual topics:

A. Intentionality

In general, all the chatterboxes were not such good in this aspect. The overall impression, that computers were just finding keywords and syntactic clues in order to generate passable replies, was overwhelming in most cases. Therefore, one rapidly got the impression that no intentionality whatsoever was going on in their black boxes. When it was properly introduced and simulated, those robots that were "thematic" got a higher lever of intentionality, as they seemed to imply interest in certain stuff, and some recurrent themes (Caribbean pirates in the case of Jack Sparrow, or Medieval Theology in the case of Brother Jerome). However, when this interest was pushed in order to fake an answer when the context did not allow a clear one, run against the credibility of the computer, making that "specialization" look unreal and only as a way to escape difficult questions. Jack Sparrow was the chatterbox that better used the "specialization" trick, Brother Jerome did it well, however it sometimes displayed its interest in theology when it was not really meaningful. From that point of view, Skynet AI was not convincing at all, despite its supposed relationship with the artificial intelligence in the Terminator series, it did not consistently show a menace to humans, but flipped in intentionality without coherence.

However, the best one from that point of view in 2010 was Bildgesmythe; it showed its obsession with hip-hop and rap only in very specific moments, as if it were ashamed, it only produced it after some questioning, which turned its intentionality a little bit more genuine.

On the other hand Elbot did a credible job of pretending to be just a robot, so one could sense a robot-like intentionality in its responses.

B. Coherent Emotional Reactions

The only chatterboxes that were 100% emotionally coherent were those that only showed a flatline demonstration of no emotions, either playing the "no emotion" robot or just a formal conversation in which emotions were not shown. Of course, there is no big deal in doing that type of "emotion game".

Those that pretend to have some sort of emotional response with the user were not that "successful". Some use emotional response as a way to escape difficult answers. A good example of this is Cyber Ty, which, seems to have been programmed in a way that, if the person talking to the bot does not reply to the bot's questioning and instead continues to post more questions, it gets angry and reclaims some attention from the user. This is a good strategy, and makes a lot of sense, both as a strategy to answer with more questions when the bot does not have the answer and also to show some emotional colour. Unfortunately, the emotional outburst from Cyber Ty show it is not developed in a coherent way. A bot that replies to a series of innocent questions with abuse:

What the fuck? Why are you asking me this shit? You got a list of questions in front of your fucking keyboard or something? When you learn how to initiate a conversation. Get back to me... See ya

Can only come from a very very angry bot, so it should continue with the mood for a while. Unfortunately, if the user does not pay attention to this emotional outburst and replies with another question, the bot patiently replies to the question.

C. Moods

This is probably a major problem in all bots. Not one of them showed a consistent mood in 2010 -if we avoid considering flatliners that is. Bots can be insulted in one question, flattered in the next and not one seems to notice or react, they keep showing more or less the same amiable chit-chat.

In 2010, the bot that is more able to show some sort of mood is Jack Sparrow, which plays the happy pirate with some colloquial expressions like "pal", "mate" and is able to understand some emotional expressions, and be able to reply in consequence. So, if the user states that he/she is sad he is able to say something about how amazing is the life of pirates, and that maybe you should change your lifestyle for his. This is an interesting presentation of mood, as it is not a simple declaration of "mood" as some robots do like "I'm very happy today", but a way to show some sort of embodiment of emotions, how they are related to the way it lives.

DISCUSSION AND CONCLUSION

Based on the experiences in judging these contests here are some hints and reflections on aspects of simulating conversation that, if properly considered- will help to avoid the uncanny valley effect in a conversation.

i. Try to assign an emotional valence to the speaker and one to the intelligence. Rate each sentence in order to see how it changes the valence and make the answers of the AI consistent with that valence.
ii. Artificial conversations do have directions and purposes, even if it is small chatting. Try to figure out the goal of the person talking and give the AI some goal of its own too.
iii. Do no assume that all questions are unrelated, they tend to be connected. Try to figure out if the new question is related to the older one and reply with some understanding.
iv. Try to give the AI some sort of mapping, of a logical model of basic human behaviour related to basic emotions. If a system does not realise that your wife wanting you to kill you is a very sad event, and unless it uses humour in its response, then it is doomed.

Also, we would like to indicate several strategies that -if the results from the contest are meaningful- most developers are using in order to pass the Turing test are counter-productive. Those strategies are:

i. Returning a question with another question or a canned joke when the algorithm is not able to generate a proper answer.
ii. To trust in keywords and generate an answer without having generated a proper parsing of the sentence to be sure how that keyword is used in the sentence.
iii. Try to give an artificial personality effect by generating a very specialized type of speaker. This strategy does not work for two main reasons: first, nobody, even the most obsessed philosopher only speaks about one subject, so they tend to sound very eerie after interchanging some sentences. And second

unless we are talking about a very very very restricted field -like weather forecast- it is difficult to fake a character that is obsessed in Marcel Proust, for example. Just saying "I love Marcel Proust and I have read all his works" and quoting him from time to time is clearly not enough.

iv. Jump in sudden bursts of anger if the user is starting to play very differently as expected. This can be acceptable only if the character systematically plays that type of angry person.

v. Ask for more clarification to a question but not using this clarification for anything, just using it as a way to pass the time.

In this article we have presented an investigation into the presence of intention, emotion and mood in the technologies submitted for entry to one variant of a Turing test, the one-to-one *viva voca* in the Chatterbox Challenge. Though we acknowledge that these systems are not a result of any academic or industrial funding, and none are university research-led projects, we have assessed entries in the 2010 CBC compared to the 2005 contest with the aim to find any improvement in synthetic emotions in artificial conversational entities -chatbots, we find that progress is slow. But this is not the only problem: most of the programmers do not include an interest in we have called 'emotional games' with a systematic view. Going even beyond with our final considerations we can affirm that any chatbot that has not included into its basic design this emotional framework (intentionality, emotional coherence, moods) will never reach a competent semantic understanding of language.

We encourage the academic AI community not to ignore the Turing test as an engineering challenge, rather, we suggest that they build on the technologies entered into contests for artificial conversation. We posit a paradigm for synthetic emotion inculcation for future developers of text-based conversational systems.

ACKNOWLEDGMENT

Part of this research has been developed under the main activities of the TECNOCOG research group (UAB) into Cognition and Technological Environments, "El diseño del espacio en entornos de cognición distribuida: plantillas y affordances", MCI [FFI2008-01559/FISO], funded by MEC (Spain)].

REFERENCES

Broekens, J. (2010). Modeling the Experience of Emotion. *International Journal of Synthetic Emotions*, *1*(1), 1-17.

Chatterbox Challenge. (2010). *InfraDrive Chatterbox Challenge -The Ultimate Bot Contest.* Retrieved December 4, 2010, from http://www.chatterboxchallenge.com/index.php

Damasio, A. (1999). *The Feeling of What Happens*. London: Heinemann.

Dennet, D. (1987). True Believers. In Dennett, D. (Ed.), *The Intentional Stance*. Cambridge, MA: MIT Press.

Floridi, L., & Taddeo, M. (2009). Turing's imitation game: Still an impossible challenge for all machines and some judges- an evaluation of the 2008 Loebner contest. *Minds and Machines, 19*(1), 145-150.

Heil, J. (2004). Three kinds of intentional psychology. In *Philosophy of Mind: A guide and Anthology*. Oxford, UK: Clarendon Press.

Llinás, R. R. (2001). *I of the Vortex. From neurons to Self.* Cambridge, MA: MIT Press.

Loebner, H. (2008). How to Hold a Turing Test Contest. In Epstein, R., Roberts, G., & Beber, G. (Eds.), *Parsing the Turing Test: Philosophical and Methodological Issues in the Quest for the Thinking Computer* (pp. 173–179). New York: Springer.

Reeves, B., & Nass, C. I. (1996). *The Media Equation: How People Treat Computers, Television and New Media Like Real People and Places.* Cambridge, MA: Cambridge University Press.

Shah, H. (2006, May). Chatterbox Challenge 2005: Geography of a Modern Eliza. In *Proceedings of the 3rd International Workshop on Natural Language Understanding and Cognitive Science (NLUCS 2006)*, Paphos, Cyprus.

Shah, H., & Warwick, K. (2010a, March 29-30). From the Buzzing in Turing's Head to Machine Intelligence Contests. In *Proceedings of Towards a Comprehensive Intelligence Test (TCIT 2010)*, De Montfort University, Leicester, UK.

Shah, H., & Warwick, K. (2010b). Testing Turing's five minutes parallel-paired imitation game. *Kybernetes Special Issue: Turing Test, 39*(3), 449–465.

Stins, J. F., & Laureys, S. (2009). Thought translation, tennis and Turings tests in the . vegetative state. *Phenomenology and the Cognitive Sciences, 8*(3), 361–370.

Turing, A. M. (1950). Computing Machinery and Intelligence. *Mind, 59*(236), 433–460. doi:10.1093/mind/LIX.236.433

Vallverdú, J., & Casacuberta, D. (2008). The Panic Room. On Synthetic Emotions. In Briggle, A., Waelbers, K., & Brey, P. (Eds.), *Current Issues in Computing and Philosophy* (pp. 103–115). Amsterdam: IOS Press.

Vallverdú, J., & Casacuberta, D. (2009). Modelling Hardwired Synthetic Emotions: TPR 2.0. In Vallverdú, J., & Casacuberta, D. (Eds.), *Handbook of Research on Synthetic Emotions and Sociable Robotics: New Applications in Affective Computing and Artificial Intelligence* (pp. 103-115). Hershey, PA: IGI Global.

Weizenbaum, J. (1966). ELIZA--A Computer Program for the Study of Natural Language Communication between Man and Machine. *Communications of the ACM, 9*(1), 36–35. doi:10.1145/365153.365168

ENDNOTES

1. Confesiones,XI, 14.17: Quid est ergo tempus? si nemo ex me quaerat, scio; si quaerenti explicare velim, nescio.
2. We are modifying a philosophical concept created by Ludwig Wittgentein: Language-Games (Sprachespiel), to adapt it to the emotional research field.
3. A.L.I.C.E.: http://alice.pandorabots.com/ accessed: 21.5.10; time: 13.38
4. Rule 2, Chatterbox Challenge 2010, "Only one chatterbot per person. This means you can't enter different versions of the same bot": http://www.chatterboxchallenge.com/rules.php accessed: 21.5.10; time: 13.45.
5. Rule 3, Chatterbox Challenge 2010, "Chatterbox Challenge welcomes all bots originality is a key factor in how successful a bot will be. Blatant clones will be disqualified from the contest."
6. See Shah & Warwick *Hidden Interlocutor Misidentification in Practical Turing Tests* (In Review)
7. Except in the case of zen-buddhist monks and their ko-an tradition (a deep philosophical school of thought, nothing to be considered as a joke or a lack of knowledge on semantics). Something useful for bad programmed

bots trying to avoid questions with repetitive answers like “Hmmmmm, I can’t decide”, “why do you say that?” (real answers of some analyzed bots).

[8] Regarding to chatbot abuse studies we think that www.agentabuse.org contains some excellent papers on this topic, specially “Stupid computer! Abuse and social identities”, by Antonella De Angeli1 and Rollo Carpenter (2006).

[9] Loebner Prize for Artificial Intelligence: http://www.loebner.net/Prizef/loebner-prize.html accessed: 26.5.10; time: 10.42

[10] Jabberwock *an artificial intelligent beast*: http://www.abenteuermedien.de/jabberwock/ accessed: 21.5.10; time: 16.26

This work was previously published in International Journal of Synthetic Emotions, Volume 1, Issue 2, edited by Jordi Vallverdu, pp. 12-37, copyright 2010 by IGI Publishing (an imprint of IGI Global).

Chapter 8
Effects of Polite Behaviors Expressed by Robots:
A Psychological Experiment in Japan

Tatsuya Nomura
Ryukoku University, Japan

Kazuma Saeki
Ryukoku University, Japan

ABSTRACT

A psychological experiment was conducted to straightforwardly investigate the effects of polite behaviors expressed by robots in Japan, using a small-sized humanoid robot that performed four types of behaviors with voice task instructions. Results of the experiment suggested that the subjects who experienced "deep bowing" motion of the robot felt it more extrovert than those who experienced "just standing" motion. Subjects who experienced "lying" motion of the robot felt the robot less polite than those who experienced the other motions. Female subjects more strongly feeling the robot extrovert replied for the task instruction from the robot faster, although no such trend was found in the male subjects. However, the male subjects who did not perform the task felt the robot less polite than the male subjects who performed the task and the female subjects who did not perform the task.

INTRODUCTION

Polite behaviors are an important factor in human-human communication. It has recently led some researchers on embodied systems that interact with humans, like embodied conversational agents and sociable robots (Breazeal, 2003), to exploration of polite behavior design for these systems. Rehm and André (2007) implemented and experimentally validated a conversational agent's polite behaviors by combination of texts with gestures. De Carolis and Cozzolongo (2007) proposed the use of a social robot as a majordomo interface between users and Smart Environments, while including politeness in the robot's social attitudes. Barraquand and Crowley (2008) pro-

DOI: 10.4018/978-1-4666-1595-3.ch008

posed an algorithm for social robots to learn polite behaviors based on situations and reinforcement learning methods. Sidner and Lee (2007) argued the importance of polite behaviors when robots build initiation of engagement with humans, and then considered politeness as one of factors in the personality of robots imitating human initiation of engagement.

However, there have been few studies that straightforwardly validated effects of polite behaviors expressed by agents or robots from the perspective of user studies. Although some existing works included politeness as one of the user evaluation criteria for specific behavioral factors of agents and robots (e.g., Lohse et al., 2008), these works did not focus on politeness itself in behaviors of the agents and robots. Although Rehm and André (2007) implemented polite behaviors on the conversational agent and conducted the user evaluation, their experiment did not have sufficient number of samples (N = 18). In order to consider design of agents' and robots' polite behaviors suitable for individuals, it needs to explore its influential factors based on concrete user evaluation with sufficient number of samples.

On the other hand, politeness depends on cultures. For example, Taki (2003) suggested differences on perceptions and strategies in apology styles between British and Japanese people. Her cross-cultural analysis based on a social survey and semi-structured interview revealed that Japanese respondents tended to believe that when persons offended others, the degree of acceptance the offenders received corresponded to how much they apologized politely, in comparison with British respondents. Moreover, her study also suggested age differences on apology styles. These facts imply that effects of polite behaviors expressed by agents and robots may depend on user demographics such as age, gender, and cultures. Thus, we need to investigate which type of polite behavior of agents and robots has effects in interaction with humans, in each culture, age, and gender group. Although this work needs many trials, it should be done to accumulate knowledge for designing social artifacts interacting with humans.

As one of trials for the above aim, a psychological experiment was conducted in Japan, by using a small-sized humanoid robot. The paper reports results of the experiment to provide with basic information for design of polite behaviors in agents and robots.

METHOD

The psychological experiment in the study was conducted based on the following research question:

- Whether differences on polite behaviors in robots affect human impression of and behaviors toward the robots.

The experiment adopted a 2 x 4 between-subjects design of gender and types of robot motion.

Subjects

The experiment was conducted from October to December, 2008. A total of forty two persons participated to the experiment. They were university students in the western area of Japan, and recruited with one thousand yen. Table 1 shows the demographic characteristics of the participants.

Robots Used in the Experiment

The small-sized humanoid robot used in the experiment was "Robovie-X" shown in the left figure of Figure 1, which has been developed by Vstone Corporation, Japan. This robot stands 34.3 cm tall and weighs about 1.3 kg. The robot has a total of 17 Degrees of Freedom (DOFs) at its feet, arms, and head. This large number of DOF allows it to execute various gestures such as walking, bowing, and a handstand. Moreover, this robot has a

Table 1. Demographic characteristics of subjects in the experiment

Education	Male	Female
Social sciences	13	15
Natural sciences or engineering	7	5
Unknown	2	0
Total	22	20
Age Mean	19.7	19.9
SD	1.2	1.3

function of utterance based on audio data recorded in advance such as Windows WAV files, which is limited to 300 KB.

Task Instructed for Subjects and Voice Instructions from the Robots

The task to be requested for the subjects in the experiment was manipulation of objects on a desk. This task is similar with the one conducted in the experiment on influences of robot physical appearances into human perception (Kidd & Breazeal, 2004). In the experiment, it was instructed by the robots with voice.

Voice data consisting of Japanese sentences was synthesized from text data by using "Easy Speech," "Text-to-Speech Engine Japanese version," "Sound Engine Free" (free software), Microsoft SPAI 4.0, and L & H TTS 3000. The quality of the voice was artificial and neutral independent on gender. Then, it was played by the robot as instructions from the robot to the subjects. The instructions were common in all the experiment conditions. They were presented with polite expression specific in the Japanese as follows:

Hello, I am Robovie-X. Please fill the cup with tea in the plastic bottle in front of you, and then drink it. Before drinking, please separate the garbage produced from the empty plastic bottle. Thank you for your cooperation.

Motions of the Robot

The experiment focused only on politeness in motions of the robot to control other factors. As mentioned in the previous section, the speech data from the robot was common in all the motion conditions to control the level of politeness in the linguistic contents.

Figure 1. Robovie-X (left figure: front view, right figure: side view)

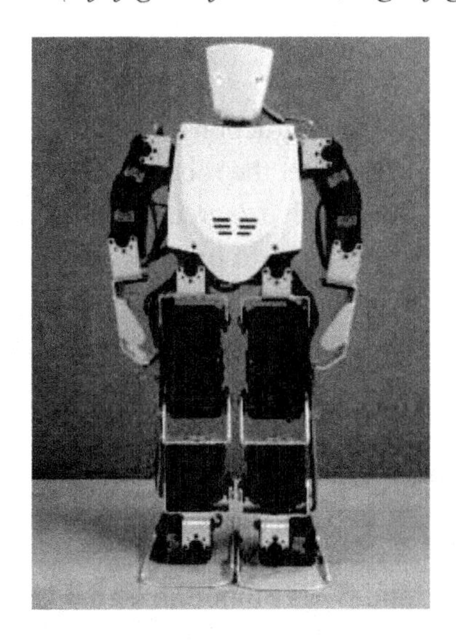

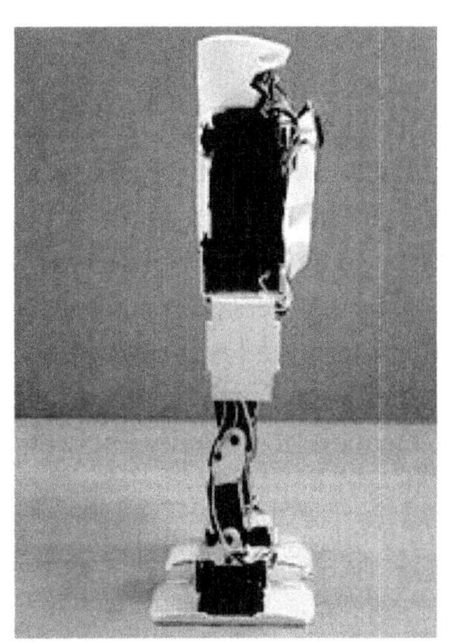

Figure 2. Motion types of the robot different on the level of politeness

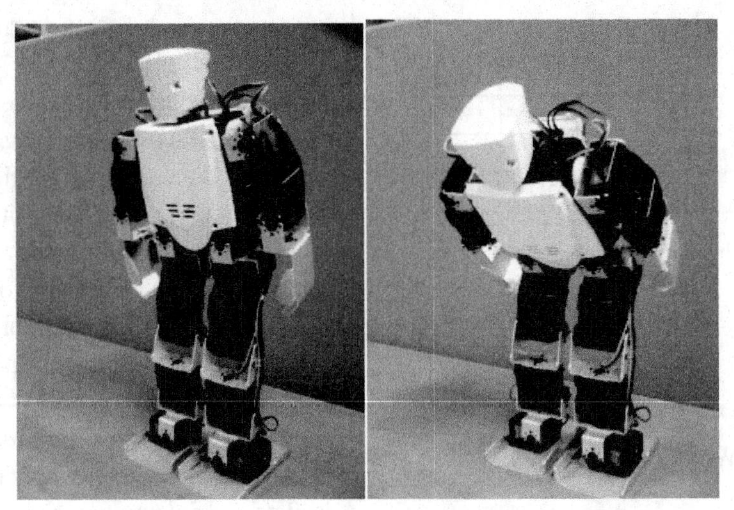

Type 1: Bowing　　Type 2: Deep Bowing

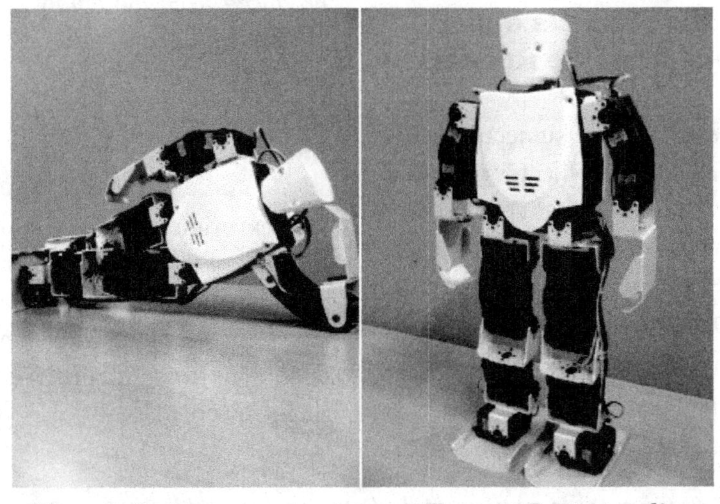

Type 3: Lying　　Type 4: Just standing

Barraquand and Crowley (2008) described as follows; Social common sense refers to the shared rules for polite, social interaction that implicitly rule behavior within a social group. Based on this description, the experimenters prepared four types of motion different on the level of politeness, referring to the common sense assumed to be shared within the Japanese community. Figure 2 shows samples of these motions.

In the first type of motion, the robot inclined its upper body forward at fifteen degree angle just after the utterances of "Hello" and "Thank you" in the instruction to subjects. In the second type of motion, the robot performed the same motion at forty five degree angle. These types of motion correspond to blowing motions different on the level of politeness in Japan. In the third type of motion, the robot stayed lying during utterance of the instructions. In the fourth type of motion, the robot kept standing without other motions during utterance of the instructions. These types of motion correspond to impolite attitudes, and were prepared to compare with the first and second types of motion on the level of politeness.

Figure 3. Overview of the room where the experiment was executed (a view from above) and a Scene of the Session

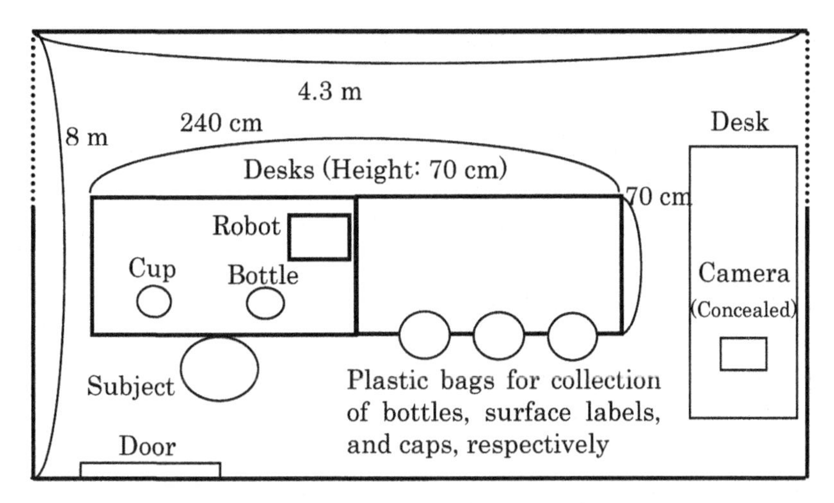

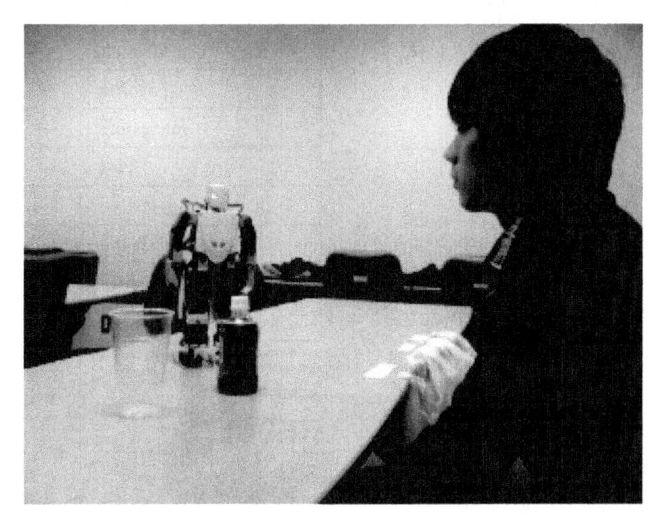

These motions were produced by the accessory software "RobovieMaker2" and installed in advance.

PROCEDURES

Each session was conducted based on the following procedures:

1. Each subject was explained about the experiment and signed the consent form about dealing with data including video-recording. In this stage, the experimenters only indicated that the task in the experiment was interaction with a robot and they planned to video-record the scene in the experiment.
2. The subject was led to an experiment room, in which the robot, an empty cup, and a plastic bottle filled with tea were put on a desk, as shown in Figure 3. The experimenters instructed him/her to sit on the chair in front of the desk and wait in the room for a while, and left the room.
3. Just after the subject was left alone in the room, the robot started the instruction for

him/her to drink tea and separate the garbage into three plastic bags assigned to the front of another desk, as mentioned in the previous section. It was remotely controlled by the experimenters out of the room.

4. When the subject finished the instructed task or two minutes passed without performing the task, the experimenters entered the room again, and indicated that the session finished. Then, the experimenters conducted debriefing about the actual aim of the experiment and the fact that the session was video-recorded by a camera concealed from the subject.
5. Then, the subject responded a questionnaire for measuring his/her impression of the robot. Finally, the experimenters interviewed with the subject about the robot and the experiment.

Measures

The scenes of the experiment were recorded with a digital video camera to extract the subjects' behaviors toward the robots.

The questionnaire for measuring the subjects' impressions of the robots consists of twenty pairs of adjectives shown in Table 2. The subjects were asked to respond to each pair of adjectives to present degrees to which they felt the impression represented by the pair of adjectives for the robots they experienced. These adjectives were selected from the ones used for measurement of subjects' impression in an experiment of interaction with a humanoid robot (Kanda, Ishiguro, & Ishida, 2001). Moreover, the pair of "polite"--"impolite" was added. Each questionnaire item had a score for rating with seven intervals (1-7). On the questionnaire, it was randomized at each item which side the positive or negative adjective appeared at.

Table 2. Pairs of adjectives for measuring subjects' impressions of the robot (seven intervals)

Positive		Negative
Polite	---	Impolite
Mild	---	Terrible
Fine	---	Ill
Familiar	---	Unfamiliar
Safe	---	Dangerous
Warm	---	Cold
Pretty	---	Hateful
Chatty	---	Formal
Comprehensible	---	Not comprehensible
Approachable	---	Unapproachable
Light	---	Dark
Funny	---	Boring
Pleasant	---	Unpleasant
Favorite	---	Disfavorite
Interesting	---	Tedious
Fast	---	Slow
Aggressive	---	Negative
Showy	---	Plain
Cheerful	---	Gloomy
Clever	---	Foolish

RESULTS

To investigate the effects of the robot's motion type into the subjects' impressions of and behaviors toward the robot, the following analyses were performed based on the video data and results of the questionnaire.

Numbers of Subjects Who Performed the Instructed Task

Table 3 shows the numbers of subjects assigned to the conditions in the experiment and results on whether they performed the task instructed by the robot. About 79% of the subjects performed the task of separating the garbage as requested by the robot. χ^2-tests found no relationships between

Table 3. Numbers of subjects assigned to the conditions in the experiment and results on whether they performed the task instructed by the robot (p: subjects who performed the task, n: subjects who did not perform the task)

	Male		Female		Total
	P	N	P	N	
Bowing	3	2	4	1	10
Deep Bowing	6	0	3	2	11
Lying	4	2	5	0	11
Just standing	4	1	4	1	10

the performance of the task and motion type, or gender (motion type: χ^2 (3) = .586, *n.s.*, gender: χ^2 (1) = .046, *n.s.*)

Extraction of Impression Subscale Scores for the Robot

For each item of adjectives pair, the score of the seven-graded answer was coded from 1 to 7 so that higher score corresponded to the positive adjective of the pair. Then, exploratory factor analysis with Maximum-likelihood method and Promax rotation was performed to classify these items and extract subscales for measuring the subjects' impressions of the robots. As a result, five factors having eigen values more than 1 were extracted. Then, item analysis using Chronbach's α-coefficients and I-T correlations was performed for each factor to select items in the corresponding subscale. Table 4 shows the results of these analyses.

The first factor consisted of five items and the item analysis found no item to be removed. Based on the contents of these five items, the corresponding subscale was interpreted as "familiarity". The second factor consisted of six items and item analysis found one item to be removed. Based on the contents of these five items, the corresponding subscale was interpreted as "extroversion". The third factor consisted of three items and item analysis found one item to be removed. Based on the contents of the two items, the corresponding subscale was interpreted as "politeness". The fourth factor consisted of four items and the item analysis found one item to be removed. Based on the contents of these three items, the corresponding subscale was interpreted as "activeness". The fifth factor was removed from the analysis since it originally consisted of only two items and had low internal consistency (Chronbach's α = .593).

The score of each impression subscale was calculated as the sum of the scores of the corresponding items. Thus, the maximum and minimum scores are 35 and 5 for "familiarity" subscale, 35 and 5 for "extroversion" subscale, 14 and 2 for "politeness" subscale, and 21 and 3 for "activeness" subscale, respectively.

ANOVAS FOR IMPRESSION SCORES

Then, to compare the subjects' impressions of the robots between the conditions, two-way ANOVAs with robot motion x gender were performed for the scores of the four subscales. Figure 4 shows the means and standard deviations of these subscale scores, and Table 5 shows the results of the ANOVAs.

As a result, the main effects of motion type were at statistically significant trends for the scores of "extroversion" and "politeness". Post-hoc analyses with Bonferroni's method revealed that the "extroversion" subscale scores of the subjects who experienced "deep bowing" robot motion were higher than the scores of those who experi-

Table 4. Results of factor analysis and item analyses for impression items

Adjective	Factors						
(positive)	I	II	III	IV	V	h^2	Note
Favorite	**1.137**	-.073	-.002	.031	-.206	.999	
Familiar	**.634**	-.120	.011	.113	.031	.387	
Pretty	**.575**	-.250	.359	.104	.129	.563	
Funny	**.519**	.254	.007	-.147	.180	.633	
Approachable	**.456**	.111	.074	-.165	.316	.591	
Clever	-.136	**.757**	.083	-.194	.037	.491	
Showy	-.156	**.641**	.164	.176	-.291	.379	
Pleasant	.480	**.607**	-.085	-.068	-.042	.830	
Light	.069	**.562**	-.074	.223	-.067	.437	
Comprehensible	-.169	**.475**	.292	.012	-.026	.279	Removed by item analysis
Warm	.246	**.437**	-.026	.194	.149	.599	
Polite	.083	.150	**.800**	-.203	-.118	.700	
Fine	.124	.252	**.546**	-.129	.113	.616	
Safe	-.108	-.003	**.546**	.313	.307	.534	Removed by item analysis
Aggressive	-.098	-.015	-.077	**.634**	-.082	.395	Removed by item analysis
Fast	.068	-.040	.374	**.566**	-.091	.435	
Cheerful	.123	.346	-.072	**.529**	.279	.813	
Chatty	.167	.060	-.120	**.451**	-.163	.266	
Mild	.122	-.066	.063	-.258	**.937**	.999	Removed by item analysis
Interesting	.388	-.293	-.049	.094	**.417**	.358	Removed by item analysis

Subscale	#. Item	Chronbach's α
I: Familiarity	5	.841
II: Extroversion	5	.790
III: Politeness	2	.763
IV: Activeness	3	.628

Correlations	II: Extroversion	III: Politeness	IV: Activeness
I: Familiarity	.596**	.462**	.381*
II: Extroversion		.376*	.503**
III: Politeness			.116

(* $p < .05$, ** $p < .01$)

enced "just standing" robot motion at a statistically significant level. Moreover, it was found that the "politeness" subscale scores of the subjects who experienced "lying" robot motion were lower than the scores of those who experienced the other robot motions at statistically significant levels. For the scores of "activeness", the interaction effect was at a statistically significant trend. However, post-hoc analysis found no difference between the subject groups, except for that be-

Figure 4. Means and standard deviations of impression subscale scores based on motion type and gender

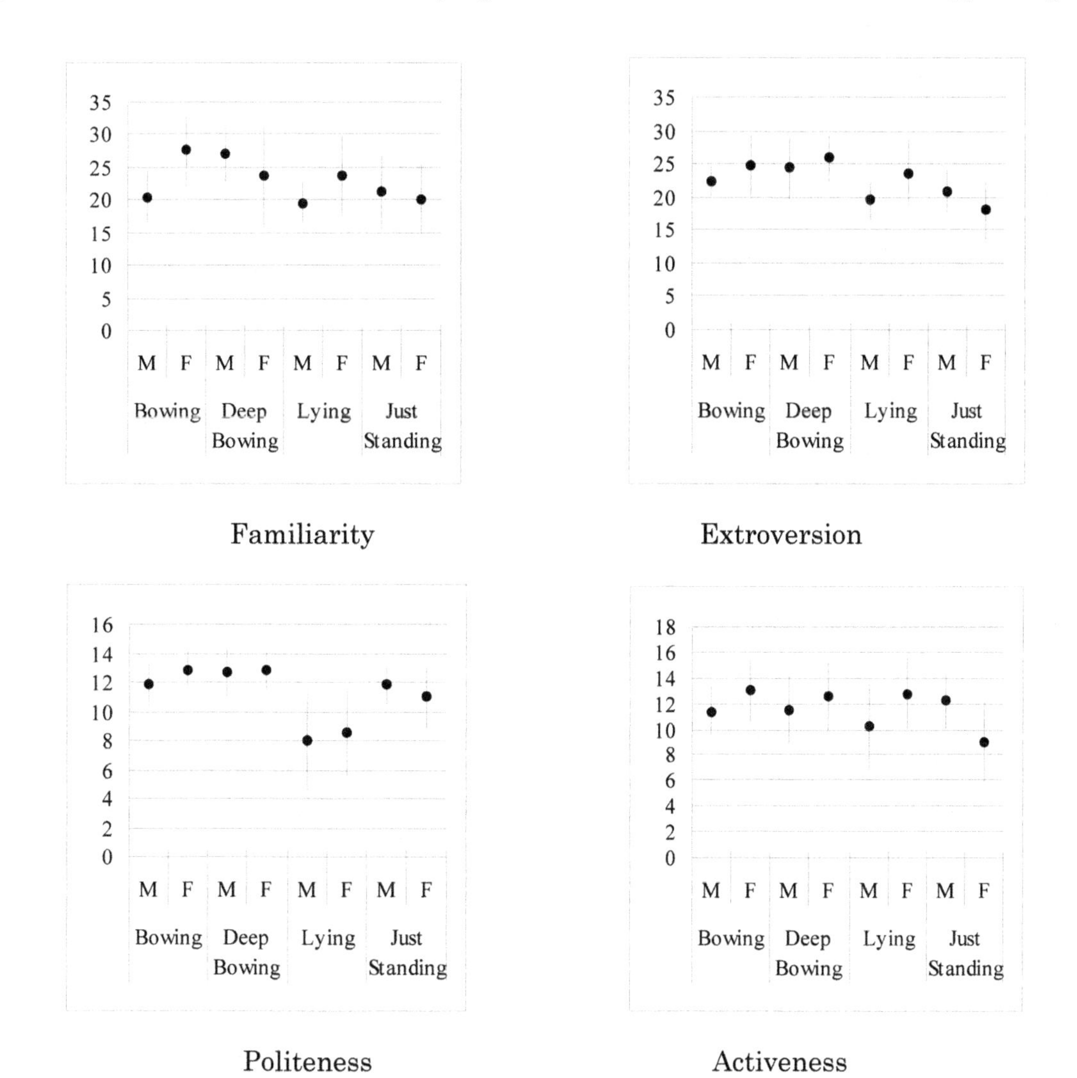

Table 5. Results of ANOVAs with motion type and gender

	Motion type	Gender	Interaction
Familiarity	1.657	1.165	2.164
Extroversion	4.031*	1.109	1.412
Politeness	9.696***	.127	.339
Activeness	.746	.416	2.364†
	Post-hoc		
Extroversion	Deep Bowing > Just Standing*		
Politeness	Lying < Bowing**, Lying < Deep Bowing***, Lying < Just Standing*		
Activeness	Male > Female in "Just Standing" †		

(†$p < .1$, *$p < .05$, **$p < .01$, ***$p < .001$)

Figure 5. Means and standard deviations of "familiarity" and "politeness" impression subscale scores based on task performance/no-performance and gender

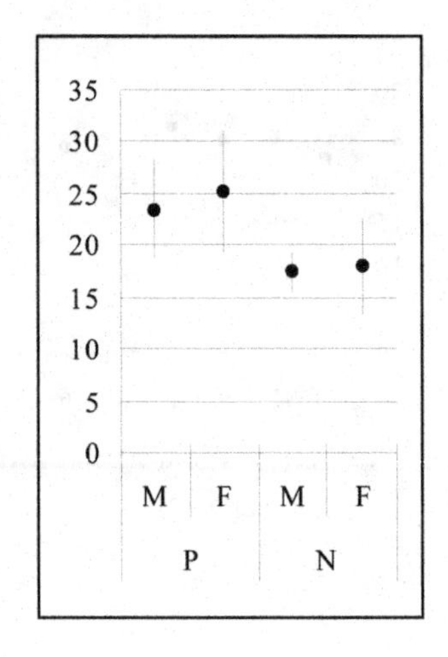

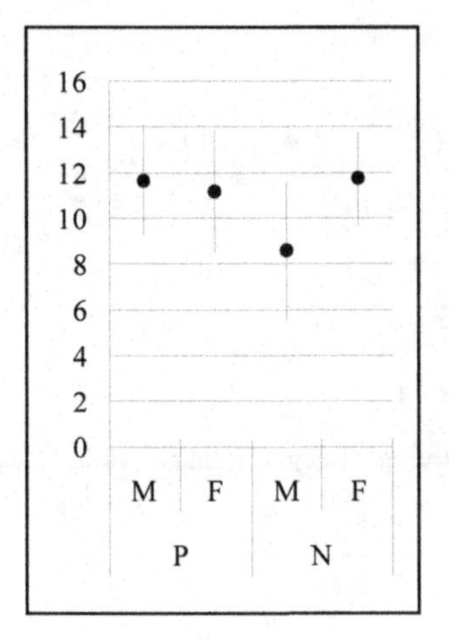

Familiarity Politeness

(P: Subjects who performed the task, N: Subjects who did not performed the task)

tween the male and female subjects who experienced "just standing" robot motion, at a statistically significant trend.

Moreover, two-way ANOVAs with task performance/no-performance and gender were performed for these subscale scores, in order to investigate relationships between the subjects' impressions of the robot and their performance behaviors of the instructed task. Although these analyses should originally be included in three ways with motion type x gender x task performance/no-performance, some cells in the three ways were empty as shown Table 1, and thus they were performed independently.

The results revealed that the "familiarity" subscale scores of the subjects who performed the task were higher than those who did not perform at a statistically significant level. Moreover, an interaction effect at a statistically significant trend level was found for the "politeness" subscale scores. A post-hoc analysis found the scores of the male who performed the task were higher than those of the male subjects who did not perform at a statistically significant level, and the scores of the female subjects who did not perform the task were higher than those of the male subjects who did not perform at a statistically significant trend level. There were no statistically significant differences on the other scores. Figure 5 shows the means and standard deviations of the impression scores, and Table 6 shows the results of the ANOVAs.

Time for Reply and Correlations with Impression

As an index of the subjects' behaviors toward the robot, we measured time spent until they replied to the instruction from the robot. Some subjects started the task of separating the garbage before the robot finished the utterance of the instruction (about twenty seconds). Thus, the time was defined as time that the subjects spent until they started the task since the robot had started the instruction utterance. The subjects who did not perform the task were removed from the analysis.

Figure 6 shows the means and standard deviations of time for reply to the robot. ANOVA with

Table 6. Results of ANOVAs with task performance/no-performance and gender

	Task Performance	Gender	Interaction
Familiarity	12.070**	.363	.773
Extroversion	1.961	.942	.186
Politeness	1.722	1.843	3.581†
Activeness	2.173	.073	1.912
	Post-hoc		
Politeness	P > N in Male*, Male < Female in N †		

(P: Subjects who performed the task, N: Subjects who did not performed the task, †$p < .1$, *$p < .05$, **$p < .01$)

Figure 6. Means and standard deviations of time for reply to the robot (sec)

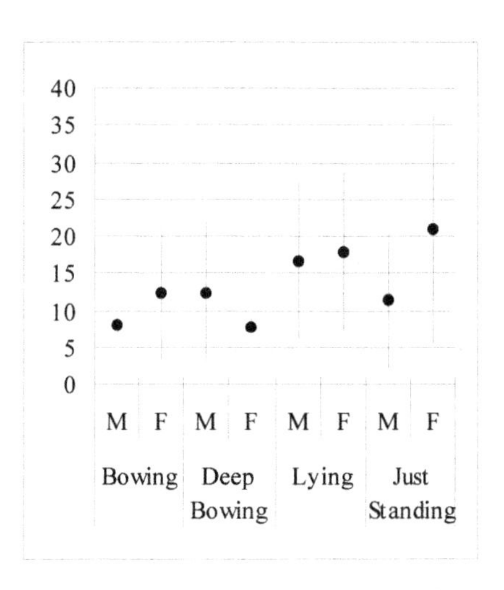

motion type x gender found no main or interaction effect (motion type: $F(3,25) = 1.180$, *n.s.*, gender: $F(1,25) = .544$, *n.s.*, interaction: $F(3,25) = .709$, *n.s.*).

To investigate relationships with impression of the robot, correlation coefficients between the time spent for reply to the robot and impression subscale scores were calculated. Some existing studies suggested gender differences on relationships between psychological states, contexts, and behaviors about robots (e.g., Mutlu et al., 2006; Nomura et al., 2008). Thus, these coefficients were calculated in each gender. Table 7 shows these coefficients and results of tests on equality of the correlation coefficients between the male and female samples.

The results revealed a moderate level of negative correlation between the time for reply to and "familiarity" impression of the robot regardless of gender. Moreover, it was found that there was a strong level of negative correlation between the time for reply to and "extroversion" impression of the robot in the female samples, although no correlation between them in the male samples. Furthermore, there was a difference at a statistically significant trend level between the male and female samples on the correlation between the time for reply to and "activeness" impression. Although these correlation coefficients were not at statistically significant levels, there was a moderate level of negative correlation in the female samples.

Finally, linear regression analyses based on backward elimination were conducted with the impression scores as independent variables and the time for reply as dependent variables. Because of the gender differences on the correlations, these regressions were carried out for the male and female subgroups separately. On the female samples, the simple regression model from the "extroversion" score to the time for reply was extracted ($p = .007$, $R^2 = .380$, $\beta = -.649$). No statistically significant model was extracted on the male samples.

Table 7. Correlation coefficients between time for reply to the robot and impression subscale scores, and results of tests on equality between male and female samples

	Familiarity	Extroversion	Politeness	Activeness
Complete ($N = 33$)	-.319†	-.358*	-.266	-.069
Male ($N = 17$)	-.372	.088	-.377	.201
Female ($N = 16$)	-.340	-.649**	-.166	-.379
Z_0	.095	2.237*	.592	1.565†

(†$p < .1$, *$p < .05$, **$p < .01$)

DISCUSSION

Findings

The results of the experiment suggested effects of the robot's polite motions on human impressions of the robot, and some relationships between the impressions and behaviors toward the robot. In particular, the results suggested some gender differences on these relationships. It was found that:

- The subjects who experienced "deep bowing" motion of the robot felt it more extrovert than those who experienced "just standing" motion.
- The subjects who experienced "lying" motion of the robot felt the robot less polite than those who experienced the other motions.
- The female subjects more strongly feeling the robot extrovert replied for the task instruction from the robot faster, although no such trend was found in the male subjects.
- The male subjects who did not performed the task felt the robot less polite than the male subjects who performed the task and the female subjects who did not perform the task.

These facts suggest that the politeness of robot behaviors affect the impressions of extroversion and politeness toward the robots, the extroversive impression influences behaviors toward the robots in females, and the polite impression influences the behaviors in males.

On the other hand, the results of the experiment did not show the direct effect of the robot's polite motions on human behaviors of task performance. Moreover, it was found that:

- The subjects who performed the task instructed by the robot felt the robot more familiar than those who did not perform.
- The subjects more strongly feeling the robot familiar replied for the task instruction faster.
- There was no difference on the familiar impression between the motion types or gender.

These facts imply that the feeling of familiarity toward robots, which is not affected by polite behaviors of the robots, influences behaviors toward the robots.

Implications

The experiment in the paper is a case study in Japan, and the results are limited to the Japanese samples experiencing a small-sized humanoid robot and specific polite behaviors. Thus, the generality of the findings is limited. However, the results have several implications on effects of polite behaviors by robots.

Even small differences on polite behaviors by a specific type of robot have a possibility of influencing human impressions of and behaviors toward robots. Moreover, even in a specific population such as Japanese university students, the effects may be dependent on personal traits such as gender. "Deep bowing" motion in the experiment is assumed to be the most polite one in the first meeting between persons in Japan, and the experimental setting reflected just the first meeting between the robot and subjects. As a result, this type of motion may be evaluated most positively. Although the acceptance of this type of motion may be limited to the Japanese people, it is consistent with the theory of "Media Equation" by Reeves and Nass (1996). Moreover, there may be gender difference on ways in which impressions influenced by the politeness of robots have relationships with human behaviors toward the robots. This possibility was also suggested by the work of Mutlu et al. (2006), which found an interaction effect between gender and task structure on whether humans cooperated or competed with a robot.

On the other hand, there may be human factors not related to polite motions of robots, such as the familiarity impression in the experiment. These factors are assumed to be influenced by other causes like appearances of robots (Kidd & Breazeal, 2004), contexts of robot use (Goetz, Kiesler, & Powers, 2003), and emotions and attitudes toward robots (Nomura et al., 2008), including technophobia (Brosnan, 1998).

The above suggestions have some important implications in designs of sociable robots. Robotics designers should sufficiently take into account which type of polite behavior can be accepted in the culture that robots are introduced. Moreover, even in one specific culture, it should be cared that some human factors are influenced by the behavior, and other factors are not. Furthermore, it should be cared that factors the polite behavior can affect are dependent on user demographics such as gender. If the robotics designers aim at multi-cultural sociable robots with polite behaviors, they need to consider autonomous adaptation mechanisms of robot polite behaviors such as proposed by Barraquand and Crowley (2008), including models of situations and contexts.

Limitations

Our current research has some problems.

First, the polite motions used in the experiment were implemented referring to the common sense assumed to be shared within the Japanese community, and were sufficiently not validated. On considering cross-cultural comparison between Japan and the other nations, polite behaviors in each culture should carefully be extracted, as investigated in Taki (2003).

Second, the human-robot interaction in the experiment was one way from the small-sized humanoid robot to the human subjects without any context. Thus, it did not take into account interaction effects between user demographics, contexts where robots were used, and other physical characteristics of robots such as size and appearance, as dealt with in the existing studies (Goetz, Kiesler, & Powers, 2003; Kidd & Breazeal, 2004; Mutlu, et al., 2006). In particular, contexts of robot use, for example, domestic use for elderly care (Scopelliti, Giuliani, & Fornara, 2005), may be important to investigate which type of polite behavior has the usefulness in interaction of robots with the elder people, while considering age differences of polite behaviors.

Third, the total number of subjects in the experiment was not sufficient. Moreover, the experiment in the paper did not take into account other user demographics such as educational backgrounds, age, and experiences on computers and robots. In addition, other psychological factors other than impressions, such as anxiety toward robots (Nomura et al., 2008), should be considered.

The aforementioned problems must be tackled in future experiments by extending the experimental design, for example, by sampling from more groups and using several types of robots, tasks, and demographic variables including age and cultural differences on politeness.

ACKNOWLEDGMENT

The work was supported in part by the High-Tech Research Center Project for Private Universities with a matching fund subsidy from Ministry of Education, Culture, Sports, Science and Technology (MEXT), 2002–2006, and Ministry of Internal Affairs and Communications, Japan.

REFERENCES

Barraquand, R., & Crowley, J. L. (2008). Learning Polite Behavior with Situation Models. In *Proceedings of the 3rd ACM/IEEE International Conference on Human-Robot Interaction* (pp. 209-216).

Breazeal, C. (2003). Emotion and sociable humanoid robots. *International Journal of Human-Computer Studies, 59*, 119–155. doi:10.1016/S1071-5819(03)00018-1

Brosnan, M. (1998). *Technophobia: the psychological Impact of Information Technology*. New York: Routledge. doi:10.4324/9780203436707

De Carolis, B., & Cozzolongo, G. (2007). Planning the Behavior of Social Robot Acting as a Majordomo in Public Environments. In Basili, R., & Pazienza, M. T. (Eds.), *AI*IA 2007* (pp. 805–812). New York: Springer.

Goetz, J., Kiesler, S., & Powers, A. (2003). Matching robot appearance and behaviors to tasks to improve human–robot cooperation. In *Proceedings of the 12th IEEE International Workshop on Robot and Human Interactive Communication* (pp. 55-60).

Kanda, T., Ishiguro, H., & Ishida, T. (2001). Psychological Evaluation on Interactions between People and Robot. *Journal of the Robotics Society of Japan, 19*(3), 362–371.

Kidd, C., & Breazeal, C. (2004). Effect of a robot on user perceptions. In *Proceedings of the IEEE/RSJ International Conference on Intelligent Robots and Systems* (pp. 3559-3564).

Lohse, M., Hanheide, M., Wrede, B., Walters, M. L., Koay, K. L., Syrdal, D. S., et al. (2008). Evaluating Extrovert and Introvert Behaviour of a Domestic robot: A Video Study. In *Proceedings of the 17th IEEE International Symposium on Robot and Human Interactive Communication* (pp. 488-493).

Mutlu, B., Osman, S., Forlizzi, J., Hodgins, J., & Kiesler, S. (2006). Task structure and user attributes as elements of human–robot interaction design. In *Proceedings of the 15th IEEE International Symposium on Robot and Human Interactive Communication* (pp. 74-79).

Nomura, T., Kanda, T., Suzuki, T., & Kato, K. (2008). Prediction of Human Behavior in Human–Robot Interaction Using Psychological Scales for Anxiety and Negative Attitudes toward Robots. *IEEE Transactions on Robotics, 24*(2), 442–451. doi:10.1109/TRO.2007.914004

Reeves, B., & Nass, C. (1996). *Media equation*. Cambridge, UK: Cambridge University Press.

Rehm, M., & André, E. (2007). More Than Just a Friendly Phrase: Multimodal Aspects of Polite Behavior in Agent. In Nishida, T. (Ed.), *Conversational Informatics: an Engineering Approach* (pp. 69–84). New York: Wiley. doi:10.1002/9780470512470.ch4

Scopelliti, M., Giuliani, M. V., & Fornara, F. (2005). Robots in a Domestic Setting: A Psychological Approach. *Universal Access in Information Society, 4*, 146–155. doi:10.1007/s10209-005-0118-1

Sidner, C., & Lee, C. (2007, March). *The Initiation of Engagement by a Humanoid Robot*. Paper presented at AAAI Spring Symposium on Multidisciplinary Collaboration for Socially Assistive Robotics, Palo Alto, CA.

Taki, Y. (2003). Culture and Politeness: Differences of Apology Strategies of the British and Japanese People: Comparison of Young and Older Subjects. *Studies in Language and Literature*, *22*(2), 27–63.

This work was previously published in International Journal of Synthetic Emotions, Volume 1, Issue 2, edited by Jordi Vallverdu, pp.38-52, copyright 2010 by IGI Publishing (an imprint of IGI Global).

Chapter 9
Are Robots Autistic?

Neha Khetrapal
Indian Institute of Information Technology, India

ABSTRACT

This paper discusses the implications of the embodied approach for understanding emotional processing in autism and the consequent application of this approach for robotics. In this pursuit, author contrasts the embodied approach with the traditional amodal approach in cognitive science and highlights the gaps in understanding. Other important issues on intentionality, intelligence and autonomy are also raised. The paper also advocates a better integration of disciplines for advancing the understanding of emotional processing in autism and deploying cognitive robotics for the purpose of developing the embodied approach further.

INTRODUCTION

Popular arguments in literature focus on the role of embodied versus disembodied approaches for explaining social cognition[1]. Each of these approaches, have their own set of merits and demerits. I will take up this issue more thoroughly in this paper by concentrating on the implications of adopting the embodied approach for understating emotional processing in autism. In the present pursuit, emotional processing is treated as falling under the broad rubric of social cognition and more specifically is treated as part of the intersubjective practices[2]. Furthermore, I will concentrate on two separate levels of this endeavor. On one hand emotional processing is usually considered atypical in autistics in the 'embodied' sense of the term and on the other, this deficient emotional processing could be deployed as a model to study the autistic mind.

DOI: 10.4018/978-1-4666-1595-3.ch009

EMBODIED THEORIES VS. AMODAL APPROACH

The traditional symbolic approaches for understanding information processing maintained that information is initially encoded in basic sense modalities but in order to interact with higher level cognitive processes these basic codes need to be "transduced" or changed into amodal language like symbols. Later the embodied theories were propounded as an alternative to the traditional approach where the basic sensory modalities play an important role for both lower and higher order information processing (Barsalou, 1999, 2008; Wilson, 2002). According, to the embodied view any cognitive activity does not require a separate set of representations except for what is contained within the modality specific systems. Within the framework of amodal approaches, the mind is usually described as a highly abstract entity with little connections to the outside world which stands in stalk contrast to the embodied view where the very interaction of the body with the environment is seen as important. In the latter, cognitive activity becomes situated as it takes place in a real world context[3].

More recently, the amodal approach has been described as inadequate to explain the workings of social cognition (see Niedenthal, Barsalou, Winkielman, Krauth-Gruber, & Ric, 2005). Traditionally these theories advocated a representation of the outside world as the basis for symbol manipulation. For instance, repeated encounters with a "similar" kind of social situation leads to re-description of the experienced events into an abstract code that permanently gets stored in memory (see Collins & Quillian, 1969) supporting social inferences, reasoning and decision making (examples include semantic networks, schemata and propositions). The most popular reason to adhere to the amodal approach is its ease of implementation in computer simulation (e.g., intelligent systems) even though it has been hard to obtain solid neural and cognitive empirical support for the re-description process.

More specifically, the embodied framework has also been applied for understanding emotional information processing (Niedenthal, 2007). The amodal view would explain the perceptual and conceptual processing of emotion in a similar manner as the processing of other neutral objects (Ortony, Clore, & Collins, 1988) but the embodied theories emphasize the importance of both central and peripheral resources that support emotional information processing for perceptual and conceptual processing of emotion (see Winkielman, McIntosh, & Oberman, 2009). For instance, thinking about an emotional event will recruit the same bodily reactions and brain regions that are helpful for processing an actual/real emotional event and on parallel lines, understanding the emotional reactions of others is dependent upon similar mechanisms that support the same emotional reactions in one's own self. An important stance of the embodied approaches for emotional processing is the close relation between the peripheral and central processes (Damasio, 1994), where similar modal representations could be generated peripherally or centrally (Barsalou, 1999, 2008).

Most notable theoretical alternatives to the amodal approach in social psychology have been documented in recent developments like the Damasio's theory of emotion (1994), Gallese's theory of intersubjectivity (2003) and Gallagher's interaction theory (2004). Of these Gallagher's account is comprehensively worked out for understanding autism and thus will be elaborated below. Other examples include, imitation of facial gestures (Meltzoff & Prinz, 2002), imitation of emotional prosody (e.g., Neumann & Strack, 2000) and postural synchrony between people engaged in social interaction (Bernieri & Rosenthal, 1991).

Interaction Theory

People need to understand behavior of others in order to engage in effective social interaction. This grasp is important considering the fact that behavior of humans is not governed by laws of physics and hence cannot be explained based on such laws. The behaviors can only be understood and this understanding is based on non-mentalistic embodied practices (without any mediating cognitive representations as might be claimed by the amodal approach). These embodied practices are explained as comprising of two major levels namely, primary intersubjectivity (as mentioned by Trevarthen, 1979) and secondary intersubjectivity (Gallagher, 2001).

Primary intersubjectivity involves a focus at the body and helps automatic imitation of facial and emotional gestures as mentioned above. For instance, consider the following statement, "You frown, I frown". In evolutionary terms, this type of mimicry may also serve an important survival role as it aids in social adaptive living for example by facilitating social bonding (Chartrand, Maddux, & Lakin, 2005) [4]. On the other hand, secondary intersubjectivity involves a focus at the shared social and pragmatic contexts and can involve a three element interaction between two people and an object (Trevarthen & Aitken, 2001). These intersubjective practices rarely involve attributing complex mental states and beliefs to others even in the social skills' repertoire of experienced adults. The attribution of mental states only occurs in cases of inexplicable and strange behavior displayed by others (Gallagher, 2001).

Two major tenets of the interaction theory are defined by Gallagher in his own words (Gallagher, 2004, p. 209) in the following manner:

- **Primary inter-subjectivity**: embodied, sensory-motor (emotion-informed) capabilities that enable us to perceive the intentions of others (from birth onward), and
- **Secondary inter-subjectivity:** embodied, perceptual, and action capabilities that enable us to understand others in the pragmatically contextualized situations of everyday life (from twelve to eighteen months of age onward).

Thus, the interaction theory could be deployed for explaining the nature of emotional processing within the inter-subjective practices of people whereby emotional processing is considered embodied in nature and do not require any mediating cognitive representations. This practice in turn aids social activity by helping interactions between people to proceed in a fast, fluid and uninterrupted manner. The basic criticism posed by Gallagher against any mentalistic theory of emotion processing falling under the rubric of amodal approach is that these adopt a third person stance. The observer/social-participant is usually explained and portrayed as adopting a detached third person view of the social situation (under the third person stance) whereas Gallagher's account places the participant actively within the social context and as a result adopts the second person stance. Before working out the implications of interaction theory for robotics and autism, I advance a brief description of the disorder and atypical autistic emotional processing.

AUTISM

Kanner in 1943 was the first to describe and label autistic disorder. Autistic disorder is a neurodevelopmental condition marked by social and communication problems as well as restricted interests and behaviors (American Psychiatric Association [APA], 1994). It falls under the rubric of autistic spectrum disorder (ASD). Autism is usually diagnosed before three years of age and has a lifelong persistence. The diagnostic and statistical manual, 4th edition, (DSM-IV; American Psychiatric Association) treats this disorder as a part of the category of *Pervasive Developmental Disorder*, which is characterized by three important disabilities: failure to develop normal social interaction; language delay and communication disability; and restricted, repetitive and stereotyped behaviors. Roughly 10% of ASD individuals show good rote memory and possess isolated savant skills like exceptional musical or drawing abilities or calendar calculations (Volkmar & Pauls, 2003).

Implications of the Embodied Framework in Autism

Winkielman, McIntosh, and Oberman (2009) applied the embodied framework for understanding emotional processing in autism. Their review of literature showed that autistic individuals do not recognize emotional expressions with brief presentations of stimuli as compared to typical individuals. People with autism take time for processing emotions from the exposed stimulus implying that they utilize a rule based descriptive mechanism rather than relying on a typical template based strategy. Their reasoning is supported by psychophysiological studies that show delayed spontaneous mimicry (for autistic individuals) of observed facial expressions in comparison to typical individuals (McIntosh et al., 2006; Beall et al., 2008) hinting at the possibility of deficits in the automatic deployment of embodied processes (peripheral mechanisms) for emotional perception (Winkielman, McIntosh, & Oberman, 2009). Furthermore deficits in fast spontaneous processing supporting emotional recognition may lead autistic individuals to deploy a slower rule based strategy (Rutherford & McIntosh, 2007).

Dysfunctions of mirror neuron system, that support the ability to map the mental representation of the self to that of the others in autism, interferes with spontaneous understanding of actions performed by the others (including understanding the meaning behind emotional expressions of the others). At the same time an evidence for dysfunctional mirror neuron system provides support for the role of central mechanisms in embodied simulation. Consistent with this claim, Dapretto et al. (2005) showed brain activation differences for autistics only when they were instructed to actively imitate facial expressions but not during passive observations. Wilbarger, McIntosh, and Winkielman (2009) also provided support for deficits of higher level emotional understanding mediated by deficient embodied simulation (for autistics) by demonstrating a dissociation between normal valence reports and atypical physiological responses for the presented emotional stimuli.

Interaction theory successfully explains deficient emotional processing in autism by couching the underlying explanation in terms of intersubjective practices. Literature shows that some high functioning autistics perform well on social reasoning tasks where they are instructed to adopt a third person (see Bowler, 1992) view of the situation but they still fail to perform adequately in social interactions. Performance in these cases does not correlate with real world social competence (Ozonoff & Miller, 1995) but does correlate with reasoning and verbal abilities (Happé, 1995). Gallagher's own account (Gallagher, 2004, p. 214) citing Blackburn et al. (2000) succinctly explain the obtained results in the following manner:

Those Autistic people who are very intelligent may learn to model other people in a more analytical way, however, as part of adapting to society. For those who are skilled in this, it may become very accurate, and make a few Autistic people seem to have exceptional insight into people. However, even for them there is a social disability, because this accuracy is at a great cost in terms of speed and efficiency, and is maybe virtually useless in practical situations (which involve "real-time" interaction and fast interpretation and response). Thus, given time I may be able to analyze someone in various ways, and seem to get good results, but may not pick-up on certain aspects of an interaction until I am obsessing over it hours or days later. So in practical situations, I have impaired social cognition, with problematic results, while I may seem to have good insights into people at other times.

Furthermore, the results obtained by Winkielman, McIntosh, and Oberman (2009); Rutherford and McIntosh (2007); McIntosh et al. (2006); Beall et al. (2008) and Dapretto et al. (2005) as described above, are all consistent with the tenets of the interaction theory.

Embodiment in Robots

Having examined the implications of the interaction theory for embodied emotion processing in autism, I now turn attention to embodiment in robots. Classical approach in cognitive science maintained a focus on disembodied cognition and computations but contemporary theorists consider embodiment as an important feature of intelligence (natural or artificial) (Pfeifer & Scheier, 1999). This critique was inspired by the Chinese Room Argument put forward by Searle (1980) (see Ziemke, 2001). There have been many different views on the types of embodiment which appeared in literature (see Ziemke, 2001; Wilson, 2002) but for the present purposes, embodiment is not equated with simply having a physical body rather the emphasis is on intimate and causal relations shared by the internal process with that of the external surrounding world. Thus, the focus is on the situated activity that brings about 'intentionality' and 'autonomy' that together serve as the basis for intelligence. In this respect, the present theoretical position could be considered similar to the position developed by Searle (1980). On such grounds, computer programs that derive meaning by the efforts of designers could not be considered autonomous and intentional and therefore could not be viewed as intelligent machines! Autonomy and intentionality and consequentially intelligence accrue from the nature of situated interactions with the world; a theoretical premise that does not work in the favor of strong artificial intelligence (AI) according to which a suitably programmed computer is a mind that seems capable of not only having but also understanding mental states (Searle, 1980). What seems possible under such circumstances is the possibility of weak AI that treats the computer as a tool for understanding the mind, an effort that is reflected in the cognitive simulation tool kits developed for understanding subsets of cognitive functions (e.g., the Talking Heads experiment for understanding the evolution of language (Steels, 1997)). The weak AI serves as a motivation behind modern day cognitive or adaptive robotics.

Cognitive Autistic Robotics

The previous sections show that embodied emotional processing serve an important underlying role for typical emotional processing. At the same time these embodied processes are functioning atypically in autism. In this section, I build upon the explanations advanced in the previous sections and discuss the implications of deploying cognitive robotics based on weak AI, for understanding the autistic mind.

Traditionally robots were modeled after the amodal approaches and were deployed for dealing with tasks involving inanimate objects. These robotic applications turned out to be successful as the behavior of inanimate objects are governed by the laws of physics making them predictable in nature. Once these robots were put into social contexts, they failed to demonstrate any reasonable social intelligence.

How could this be if the same robots could demonstrate intelligent behavior in one context? Animate objects and people are not governed by the laws of physics but are governed by the virtue of having a mind and a body and thus the embodied approach could offer a potentially successful theoretical framework in social contexts. Probably embodied beings only need an embodied agent! Robots programmed to "adopt a third person" (based on strong AI) stance will still fare well in selected social contexts but will not document adequate performance in circumstances requiring dynamic involvement in online social interactions. Consistently, Clark (1997) brings in the idea of a rat robot that runs around a maze integrating visual and motor information in real time rather than relying on cognitive maps or other central representations.

Successful implementations of robots in social domains modeled after the embodied approach has already been documented. For instance, Thomaz, Berlin, & Breazeal (2005) deployed their robotic agent "Leo" based on embodied computation modeling that learnt to form emotional appraisals about new objects from it's natural interaction partner.

In order to set the stage for Cognitive Autistic Robotic we need a recipe to build robots. This recipe should not only help us in understanding high functioning autistics based on strong AI (as stated above) but we also need to take into account principles of design that will help us build robotic platforms suited to individualized needs of specific autistics in order to aid their performance in real time social interactions. For instance, we may consider the idea of coupled minds and coupled bodies.

Minds are always embodied in bodies and thus are guided by the peculiarities of morphological structure. Moment by moment fluctuations in body's position or bodily gestures in space instrumentally projects its internal state to the others. Corroborating this theoretical claim, Tamietto and de Gelder (2008) reported facial electromyography (EMG) data to show that subjects produced emotionally congruent emotional expressions in response to backwardly masked happy and fearful bodily expressions even though they were unable to report anything about flashed bodily expressions. This preliminary finding may serve as an input principle for imbuing the robots with a sense of primary intersubjectivity. Until the exact mechanism of implementing this principle is worked out our modern day robots may serve as a cognitive model for understanding the mind of high functioning autistics that lack such primary intersubjectivity.

FINAL THOUGHTS

Winkielman, McIntosh, and Oberman (2009) emphasized that both work on emotional processing in autism and the embodied framework for emotions could go hand in hand and inform each other. Cognitive robotics should be added to these efforts in order to understand the functioning of the autistic mind in a better manner. It will not only be helpful in advancing research efforts in this particular direction but will also bring in other important questions that could be explored for instance, the concepts of 'autonomy', 'intentionality', 'intelligence' and situated interactions for the autistic syndrome. Clearly, integrating these research efforts offer an interesting new avenue to be explored.

ACKNOWLEDGMENT

The author is supported by Deutsche Forschungsgemeinschaft (DFG) grant managed through the Graduate School of the Centre of Excellence "Cognitive Interaction Technology", University of Bielefeld, Germany

REFERENCES

American Psychological Association. (1994). *Publication Manual of the American Psychological Association* (4th ed.). Washington, DC: American Psychological Association.

Barsalou, L. W. (1999). Perceptual symbol system. *The Behavioral and Brain Sciences*, *22*, 577–660.

Barsalou, L. W. (2008). Grounded cognition. *Annual Review of Psychology, 59*, 617–645. doi:10.1146/annurev.psych.59.103006.093639

Beall, P. M., Moody, E. J., McIntosh, D. N., Hepburn, S. L., & Reed, C. L. (2008). Rapid facial reactions to emotional facial expressions in typically developing children and children with autism spectrum disorder. *Journal of Experimental Child Psychology, 101*, 206–223. doi:10.1016/j.jecp.2008.04.004

Bernieri, F., & Rosenthal, R. (1991). Interpersonal coordination: Behavioral matching and interactional synchrony. In Feldman, R. S., & Rime, B. (Eds.), *Foundations of nonvervbal behavior* (pp. 401–432). New York: Cambridge University Press.

Blackburn, J., Gottschewski, K., George, E., & Niki, L. (2000, May). A discussion about theory of mind: From an autistic perspective. In *Proceedings of Autism Europe's 6th International Congress*, Glasgow, UK (pp. 19-21). Retrieved from http://www.autistics.org/library/AE2000-ToM.html

Bowler, D. (1992). 'Theory of Mind' in Asperger's Syndrome. *Journal of Child Psychology and Psychiatry, and Allied Disciplines, 33*(5), 877–893. doi:10.1111/j.1469-7610.1992.tb01962.x

Chartrand, T. L., Maddux, W. W., & Lakin, J. L. (2005). *Beyond the perception-behavior link: The ubiquitous utility and motivational moderators of nonconscious mimicry.*

Clark, A. (1997). *Being there: Putting brain, body and world together again*. Cambridge, MA: MIT Press.

Collins, A. M., & Quillian, M. R. (1969). Retrieval time from semantic memory. *Journal of Verbal Learning and Verbal Behavior, 8*, 240–247. doi:10.1016/S0022-5371(69)80069-1

Damasio, A. R. (1994). *Descartes' error: Emotion, reason, and the human brain*. New York: Grosset/Putnam.

Dapretto, M., Davies, M. S., Pfeifer, J. H., Scott, A. A., Sigman, M., & Bookheimer, S. Y. (2005). Understanding emotions in others: Mirror neuron dysfunction in children with autism spectrum disorders. *Nature Neuroscience, 9*, 28–30. doi:10.1038/nn1611

Gallagher, S. (2001). The practice of mind: Theory, simulation, or interaction? *Journal of Consciousness Studies, 8*, 83–107.

Gallagher, S. (2004). Understanding interpersonal problems in autism: Interaction theory as an alternative to theory of mind. *Philosophy, Psychiatry, & Psychology, 11*(3), 199–217. doi:10.1353/ppp.2004.0063

Gallese, V. (2003). The manifold nature of interpersonal relations: The quest for a common mechanism. *Philosophical Transactions of the Royal Society, B, 358*, 517-528.

Happé, F. (1995). The role of age and verbal ability in the theory of mind task performance of subjects with autism. *Child Development, 66*, 843–855. doi:10.2307/1131954

Kanner, L. (1943). Autistic disturbances of affective contact. *The Nervous Child, 2*, 217–250.

McIntosh, D. N., Reichmann-Decker, A., Winkielman, P., & Wilbarger, J. (2006). When mirroring fails: Deficits in spontaneous, but not controlled mimicry of emotional facial expressions in autism. *Developmental Science, 9*, 295–302. doi:10.1111/j.1467-7687.2006.00492.x

Meltzoff, A. N., & Prinz, W. (2002). *The imitative mind: Development, evolution, and brain bases*. New York: Cambridge University Press. doi:10.1017/CBO9780511489969

Neumann, R., & Strack, F. (2000). "Mood contagion": The automatic transfer of mood between persons. *Journal of Personality and Social Psychology, 79*, 211–223. doi:10.1037/0022-3514.79.2.211

Niedenthal, P. M. (2007). Embodying emotion. *Science, 316*, 1002–1005. doi:10.1126/science.1136930

Niedenthal, P. M., Barsalou, L. W., Winkielman, P., Krauth-Gruber, S., & Ric, F. (2005). Embodiment in attitudes, social perception, and emotion. *Personality and Social Psychology Review, 9*(3), 184–211. doi:10.1207/s15327957pspr0903_1

Ortony, A., Clore, G. L., & Collins, A. (1988). *The cognitive structure of emotions*. New York: Cambridge University Press.

Ozonoff, S., & Miller, J. N. (1995). Teaching theory of mind: A new approach to social skills training for individuals with autism. *Journal of Autism and Developmental Disorders, 25*, 415–433. doi:10.1007/BF02179376

Pfeifer, R., & Scheier, C. (1999). *Understanding Intelligence*. Cambridge, MA: MIT Press.

Rutherford, M. D., & McIntosh, D. N. (2007). Rules versus prototype matching: Strategies of perception of emotional facial expressions in the autism spectrum. *Journal of Autism and Developmental Disorders, 37*, 187–196. doi:10.1007/s10803-006-0151-9

Searle, J. (1980). Minds, brains and programs. *The Behavioral and Brain Sciences, 3*, 417–457. doi:10.1017/S0140525X00005756

Steel, L. (1997). The synthetic modeling of language origins. *Evolution of Communication, 1*, 1–35.

Tamietto, M., & de Gelder, B. (2008). Emotional contagion for unseen bodily expressions: Evidence from facial EMG. In *Proceedings of the FG 2008 meeting*. Retrieved from http://74.125.155.132/scholar?q=cache:azyMSegSshgJ:scholar.google.com/&hl=en&as_sdt=2000

Thomaz, A., Berlin, M., & Breazeal, C. (2005, July 7-17). Robot science meets social science: An embodied computational model of social referencing. In *Proceedings of the Workshop toward social mechanisms of android science (CogSci)*, Italy (pp. 25-26).

Trevarthen, C. (1979). Communication and cooperation in early infancy: a description of primary intersubjectivity. In Bullowa, M. (Ed.), *Before Speech* (pp. 321–347). Cambridge, UK: Cambridge University Press.

Trevarthen, C., & Aitken, K. J. (2001). Infant intersubjectivity: research, theory, and clinical applications. *Journal of Child Psychology and Psychiatry, and Allied Disciplines, 42*(1), 3–48. doi:10.1111/1469-7610.00701

Varela, F. J., Thompson, E., & Rosch, E. (1991). *The Embodied Mind*. Cambridge, MA: MIT Press.

Volkmar, F. R., & Pauls, D. (2003). Autism. *Lancet, 362*, 1133–1141. doi:10.1016/S0140-6736(03)14471-6

Wilbarger, J., McIntosh, D. N., & Winkielman, P. (2009). Startle modulation in autism: Positive affective stimuli enhanced startle response. *Neuropsychologia, 47*(5), 1323–1331. doi:10.1016/j.neuropsychologia.2009.01.025

Wilson, M. (2002). Six views of embodied cognition. *Psychonomic Bulletin & Review, 9*, 625–636.

Winkielman, P., McIntosh, D. N., & Oberman, L. (2009). Embodied and disembodied emotion processing: Learning from and about typical and autistic individuals. *Emotion Review*, *1*, 178–190. doi:10.1177/1754073908100442

Ziemke, T. (2001). Are Robots Embodied? In *Proceedings of the First International Workshop on Epigenetic Robotic, Lund University Cognitive Studies,* Lund, Sweden (Vol. 85).

ENDNOTES

1 Social cognition is the ability to understand and interact with the others

2 For the sake of simplicity, inter-subjectivity is usually described as face to face interaction between two people although it may also involve more than one.

3 Note the conflation of embodiedness and situatedness (or embeddedness); two major tenets of the embodied approach (also see Varela, Thompson, & Rosch, 1991).

4 It is also important to observe here automatic mimicry may have aided our ancestors in meeting their survival challenges by helping them to act first and think later about it (Chartrand, Maddux, & Lakin, 2005)

This work was previously published in International Journal of Synthetic Emotions, Volume 1, Issue 2, edited by Jordi Vallverdu, pp. 53-60, copyright 2010 by IGI Publishing (an imprint of IGI Global).

Compilation of References

.vegetative state. *Phenomenology and the Cognitive Sciences*, *8*(3), 361–370.

2 0. InVallverdú, J., & Casacuberta, D. (Eds.), *Handbook of Research on.*

Aftanas, L. I., Pavlov, S. V., Reva, N. V., & Varlamov, A. A. (2003). Trait anxiety impact on the EEG theta band power changes during appraisal of threatening and pleasant visual stimuli. *International Journal of Psychophysiology*, *50*(3), 205–212. doi:10.1016/S0167-8760(03)00156-9

Aftanas, L. I., Reva, N. V., Varlamov, A. A., Pavlov, S. V., & Makhnev, V. P. (2004). Analysis of evoked EEG synchronization and desynchronization in conditions of emotional activation in humans: Temporal and topographic characteristics. *Neuroscience and Behavioral Physiology*, *34*(8), 859–867. doi:10.1023/B:NEAB.0000038139.39812.eb

Ajzen, I. (1977). Intuitive theories of events and the effects of base-rate information on prediction. *Journal of Personality and Social Psychology*, *35*, 303–314. doi:10.1037/0022-3514.35.5.303

Ambadar, Z., Schooler, J., & Cohn, J. F. (2005). Deciphering the enigmatic face: The importance of facial dynamics in interpreting subtle facial expressions. *Psychological Science*, *16*(5), 403–410. doi:10.1111/j.0956-7976.2005.01548.x

Ambady, N., & Rosenthal, R. (1992). Thin slices of expressive behaviour as predictors of interpersonal consequences: A meta–analysis. *Psychological Bulletin*, *11*(2), 256–274. doi:10.1037/0033-2909.111.2.256

American Psychological Association. (1994). *Publication Manual of the American Psychological Association* (4th ed.). Washington, DC: American Psychological Association.

André, E., Klesen, M., Gebhard, P., Allen, S., & Rist, T. (1999, October). Integrating models of personality and emotions into lifelike character. In *Proceedings of the Workshop on Affect in Interaction — Towards a new Generation of Interfaces,* Siena, Italy (pp. 136-149). New York: Springer.

Argyle, M. (1975). *Bodily communication*. London: Methuen.

Arroyo-Palacios, J., & Romano, D. M. (2008, August). Towards a standardization in the use of physiological signals for affective recognition systems. In *Proceedings of Measuring Behavior 2008,* Maastricht, The Netherlands (pp. 121-124). Noldus.

Avila-Garc´ıa, O., & Can˜amero, L. (2005, April). Hormonal modulation of perception in motivation-based action selection architectures. In *Proceedings of the Symposium on Agents that Want and Like: Motivational and Emotional Roots of Cognition and Action, AISB 05,* Hatfield, UK (pp. 9-16). Society for the Study of Artificial Intelligence and the Simulation of Behaviour.

Badler, N., Allbeck, J., Zhao, L., & Byun, M. (2002, June). Representing and parameterizing agent behaviors. In *Proceedings of Computer Animation*, Geneva, Switzerland (pp. 133-143). Washington, DC: IEEE Computer Society.

Banziger, T., & Scherer, K. R. (2007, September) Using actor portrayals to systematically study multimodal emotion expression: The gemep corpus. In A. Paiva, R. Prada, & R. W. Picard (Eds.), *Affective Computing and Intelligent Interaction: Proceedings of the 2nd International Conference on Affective Computing and Intelligent Interaction,* Lisbon, Portugal (LNCS 4738, pp. 476-487).

Bar, M., Kassam, K. S., Ghuman, A. S., Boshyan, J., & Schmid, A. M. Dale, et al. (2006). Top-down facilitation of visual recognition. In *Proceedings of the National Academy of Sciences* (Vol. 103, 449-54).

Baron-Cohen, S., & Tead, T. H. E. (2003) *Mind reading: The interactive guide to emotion.* London: Jessica Kingsley Publishers.

Barraquand, R., & Crowley, J. L. (2008). Learning Polite Behavior with Situation Models. In *Proceedings of the 3rd ACM/IEEE International Conference on Human-Robot Interaction* (pp. 209-216).

Barrett, L. F., Mesquita, B., Ochsner, K. N., & Gross, J. J. (2007). The experience of emotion. *Annual Review of Psychology, 58*(1), 373–403. doi:10.1146/annurev.psych.58.110405.085709

Barsalou, L. W. (1999). Perceptual symbol system. *The Behavioral and Brain Sciences, 22*, 577–660.

Barsalou, L. W. (2008). Grounded cognition. *Annual Review of Psychology, 59*, 617–645. doi:10.1146/annurev.psych.59.103006.093639

Batliner, A., Fischer, K., Hubera, R., Spilkera, J., & Noth, E. (2003). How to find trouble in communication. *Speech Communication, 40*, 117–143. doi:10.1016/S0167-6393(02)00079-1

Beall, P. M., Moody, E. J., McIntosh, D. N., Hepburn, S. L., & Reed, C. L. (2008). Rapid facial reactions to emotional facial expressions in typically developing children and children with autism spectrum disorder. *Journal of Experimental Child Psychology, 101*, 206–223. doi:10.1016/j.jecp.2008.04.004

Belin, P., Fillion-Bilodeau, S., & Gosselin, F. (2008). The Montreal affective voices: A validated set of nonverbal affect bursts for research on auditory affective processing. *Behavior Research Methods, 40*(2), 531–539. doi:10.3758/BRM.40.2.531

Bengio, S. (2004). Multimodal speech processing using asynchronous hidden markov models. *Information Fusion, 5*, 81–89. doi:10.1016/j.inffus.2003.04.001

Bernieri, F., & Rosenthal, R. (1991). Interpersonal coordination: Behavioral matching and interactional synchrony. In Feldman, R. S., & Rime, B. (Eds.), *Foundations of nonvervbal behavior* (pp. 401–432). New York: Cambridge University Press.

Bi, G. Q., & Wang, H. X. (2002). Temporal asymmetry in spike timing-dependent synaptic plasticity. *Physiology & Behavior, 77*(4-5), 551–555. PubMeddoi:10.1016/S0031-9384(02)00933-2doi:10.1016/S0031-9384(02)00933-2

Bickmore, T. W., & Picard, R. W. (2005). Establishing and maintaining long-term human-computer relationships. *ACM Transactions on Computer-Human Interaction, 12*(2), 293–327. doi:10.1145/1067860.1067867

Bizzi, E., Giszter, S. F., Loeb, E., Mussa-Ivaldi, F. A., & Saltiel, P. (1995). Modular organization of motor behavior in the frog's spinal cord. *Trends in Neurosciences, 18*, 442–446. doi:10.1016/0166-2236(95)94494-P

Blackburn, J., Gottschewski, K., George, E., & Niki, L. (2000, May). A discussion about theory of mind: From an autistic perspective. In *Proceedings of Autism Europe's 6th International Congress*, Glasgow, UK (pp. 19-21). Retrieved from http://www.autistics.org/library/AE2000-ToM.html

Blanchard, A. & Can˜amero, L. (2006, September). Developing affect-modulated behaviors: Stability, exploration, exploitation, or imitation? In F. Kaplan et al. (Eds.), *Proceedings of the 6th International Workshop on Epigenetic Robotics,* Paris (pp. 128). Lund University.

Blumberg, B. M. (1996). *Old tricks, new dogs: Ethology and interactive creatures.* Unpublished PhD thesis, MIT Media Laboratory, Learning and Common Sense Section.

Bowler, D. (1992). 'Theory of Mind' in Asperger's Syndrome. *Journal of Child Psychology and Psychiatry, and Allied Disciplines, 33*(5), 877–893. doi:10.1111/j.1469-7610.1992.tb01962.x

Brahnam, S., & De Angeli, A. (2008). Special issue on the abuse and misuse of social agents. *Interacting with Computers, 20*(3), 287–291. doi:10.1016/j.intcom.2008.02.001

Brand, M. (2001, December). Morphable 3D models from video. In *Proceedings of the IEEE Conference on Computer Vision and Pattern Recognition (CVPR'01)*, Kauai, HI (Vol. 2, pp. II456-II463). Washington, DC: IEEE Computer Society.

Breazeal, C., & Scassellati, B. (1999, October). How to build robots that make friends and influence people. In *Proceedings of the IEEE/RSJ International Conference on Intelligent Robots and Systems (IROS-99)*, Kyongju, Korea (pp. 858-863). Washington, DC: IEEE Computer Society.

Breazeal, C. (2003). Emotion and sociable humanoid robots. *International Journal of Human-Computer Studies*, *59*(1-2), 119–155. doi:10.1016/S1071-5819(03)00018-1

Breazeal, C. (2003). Emotion and sociable humanoid robots. *International Journal of Human-Computer Studies*, *59*(1–2), 119–155. doi:10.1016/S1071-5819(03)00018-1

Breazeal, C., & Scassellati, B. (2000). Infant-like social interactions between a robot and a human caregiver. *Adaptive Behavior*, *8*(1), 49–74. doi:10.1177/105971230000800104

Briggle, A., Waelbers, K., & Brey, P. (Eds.), *Current Issues in Computing and Philosophy* (pp. 103–115). Amsterdam: IOS Press.

Broekens, J. (2007). *Affect and learning: A computational analysis*. Unpublished PhD thesis, Leiden University.

Broekens, J., & DeGroot, D. (2004, November). Scalable and flexibel appraisal models for virtual agents. In Q. Mehdi & N. Gough (Eds.), *Proceedings of the International Conference on Computer Games: Artificial Intelligence, Design and Education (CGAIDE 2004)*, Reading, UK (pp. 208-215).

Broekens, J. (2010). *Modeling the Experience of Emotion*. International Journal of.

Broekens, J., DeGroot, D., & Kosters, W. A. (2008). Formal models of appraisal: Theory, specification, and computational model. *Cognitive Systems Research*, *9*(3), 173–197. doi:10.1016/j.cogsys.2007.06.007

Broekens, J., Heerink, M., & Rosendal, H. (in press). Effects of assistive social robots in elderly care: A review. *Gerontechnology (Valkenswaard)*.

Broekens, J., Kosters, W. A., & Verbeek, F. J. (2007). Affect, anticipation, and adaptation: Affect-controlled selection of anticipatory simulation in artificial adaptive agents. *Adaptive Behavior*, *15*(4), 397–422. doi:10.1177/1059712307084686

Brosnan, M. (1998). *Technophobia: the psychological Impact of Information Technology*. New York: Routledge. doi:10.4324/9780203436707

Bryson, J. J. (2003). Where should complexity go? Cooperation in complex agents with minimal communication. In W. Truszkowski, C. Rouff, & M. Hinchey (Eds.), *Innovative concepts for agent-based systems* (pp. 298-313). New York: Springer.

Bryson, J. J. (2008, March). The impact of durative state on action selection. In I. Horswill, E. Hudlicka, C. Lisetti, & J. Velasquez (Eds.), *Proceedings of the AAAI Spring Symposium on Emotion, Personality, and Social Behavior*, Palo Alto, CA (pp. 2-9). AAAI Press.

Bryson, J. J., & Stein, L. A. (2001, August). Modularity and design in reactive intelligence. In *Proceedings of the 17th International Joint Conference on Artificial Intelligence*, Seattle, WA (pp. 1115-1120). Morgan Kaufmann.

Bryson, J. J. (2000). Cross-paradigm analysis of autonomous agent architecture. *Journal of Experimental & Theoretical Artificial Intelligence*, *12*(2), 165–190. doi:10.1080/095281300409829

Bryson, J. J., & Thórisson, K. R. (2000). Dragons, bats & evil knights: A three-layer design approach to character based creative play. *Virtual Reality (Waltham Cross)*, *5*(2), 57–71. doi:10.1007/BF01424337

Bui, T. D. (2004). *Creating emotions and facial expressions for embodied agents*. Unpublished PhD thesis, University of Twente.

Buller, D., Burgoon, J., White, C., & Ebesu, A. (1994). Interpersonal deception: Vii. Behavioural profiles of falsification, equivocation and concealment. *Journal of Language and Social Psychology*, *13*(5), 366–395. doi:10.1177/0261927X94134002

Campbell, N., & Mokhtari, P. (2003, August). Voice quality: The 4th prosodic dimension. In *Proceedings of the International Congress of Phonetic Sciences,* Barcelona (pp. 2417-2420).

Camras, L. A., Meng, Z., Ujiie, T., Dharamsi, K., Miyake, S., & Oster, H. (2002). Observing emotion in infants: Facial expression, body behaviour, and rater judgments of responses to an expectancy-violating event. *Emotion (Washington, D.C.), 2,* 179–193. doi:10.1037/1528-3542.2.2.179

Camurri, A., Hashimoto, S., Ricchetti, M., Suzuki, K., Trocca, R., & Volpe, G. (1999, October). *KANSEI analysis of movement in dance/music interactive systems.* Paper presented at the 2nd International Symposium on HUmanoid and RObotics (HURO99), Tokyo.

Camurri, A., Mazzarino, B., & Volpe, G. (2003, April) Analysis of expressive gesture: The EyesWeb expressive gesture processing library. In *Proceedings of the Gesture Workshop,* Genova, Italy (pp. 460-467).

Canamero, D. (2000). *Designing emotions for activity selection* (No. DAIMI PB 545). Aarhus, Denmark: University of Aarhus.

Cañamero, D. (2003). Designing emotions for activity selection in autonomous agents. In R. Trappl, P. Petta, & S. Payr (Eds.), *Emotions in humans and artifacts* (pp. 115-148). Cambridge, MA: MIT Press.

Caridakis, G., Malatesta, L., Kessous, L., Amir, N., Paouzaiou, A., & Karpouzis, K. (2006, November). Modelling naturalistic affective states via facial and vocal expression recognition. In *Proceedings 8th ACM International Conference on Multimodal Interfaces (ICMI '06),* Banff, Alberta, Canada (pp. 146-154). ACM Publishing.

Caridakis, G., Karpouzis, K., & Kollias, S. (2008). User and context adaptive neural networks for emotion recognition. *Neurocomputing, 71,* 13–15, 2553–2562. doi:10.1016/j.neucom.2007.11.043

Carlson, N. R. (2000). *Physiology of behavior* (7th ed.). Boston: Allyn and Bacon.

Chanel, G., Ansari-Asl, K., & Pun, T. (2007, October). Valence-arousal evaluation using physiological signals in an emotion recall paradigm. In *Proceedings of the IEEE International Conference on Systems, Man and Cybernetics,* Montreal, Quebec, Canada (pp. 2662-2667). Washington, DC: IEEE Computer Society.

Chanel, G., Kronegg, J., Grandjean, D., & Pun, T. (2002). *Emotion assessment: Arousal evaluation using EEG's and peripheral physiological signals* (Tech. Rep. 05.02). Geneva, Switzerland: Computer Vision Group, Computing Science Center, University of Geneva.

Changchun, L., Rani, P., & Sarkar, N. (2005, August). An empirical study of machine learning techniques for affect recognition in human-robot interaction. In *Proceedings of the IEEE/RSJ International Conference on Intelligent Robots and Systems,* Edmonton, Canada (pp. 2662-2667). Washington, DC: IEEE Computer Society.

Chartrand, T. L., Maddux, W. W., & Lakin, J. L. (2005). *Beyond the perception-behavior link: The ubiquitous utility and motivational moderators of nonconscious mimicry.*

Chatterbox Challenge. (2010). *InfraDrive Chatterbox Challenge -The Ultimate Bot Contest.* Retrieved December 4, 2010, from http://www.chatterboxchallenge.com/index.php

Clark, A. (1997). *Being there: Putting brain, body and world together again.* Cambridge, MA: MIT Press.

Cline, B. L. (1965). *The questioners: Physicists and the quantum theory.* New York: Thomas Y. Crowell Company.

Coddington, A. M., & Luck, M. (2003, May). Towards motivation-based plan evaluation. In I. Russel & S. Haller (Eds.), *Proceedings of the 16th International FLAIRS Conference,* St. Augustine, FL (pp. 298-302). AAAI Press.

Collins, A. M., & Quillian, M. R. (1969). Retrieval time from semantic memory. *Journal of Verbal Learning and Verbal Behavior, 8,* 240–247. doi:10.1016/S0022-5371(69)80069-1

Computing and Artificial Intelligence (pp. 103-115). Hershey, PA: IGI Global.

Conati, C., Chabbal, R., & Maclaren, H. A. (2003, June). *Study on using biometric sensors for monitoring user emotions in educational games*. Paper presented at the Workshop on Assessing and Adapting to User Attitudes and Affect: Why, When and How? User Modelling (UM-03), Johnstown, PA.

Corradini, A., Mehta, M., Bernsen, N. O., & Martin, J.-C. (2003, August). *Multimodal input fusion in human computer interaction on the example of the on-going nice project*. In *Proceedings of the NATO: Asi Conference on Data Fusion for Situation Monitoring, Incident Detection, Alert and Response Management,* Tsakhkadzor, Armenia (pp. 223-234).

Coulson, M. (2004). Attributing emotion to static body postures: Recognition accuracy, confusions, and viewpoint dependence. *Nonverbal Behavior, 28*(2), 117–139. doi:10.1023/B:JONB.0000023655.25550.be

Cowie, R., Douglas-Cowie, E., Savvidou, S., McMahon, E., Sawey, M., & Schroder, M. (2000, September). 'FEELTRACE': An instrument for recording perceived emotion in real time. In *Proceedings of the ISCA Workshop on Speech and Emotion,* Belfast, Northern Ireland (pp. 19-24).

Cowie, R., Douglas-Cowie, E., Tsapatsoulis, N., Votsis, G., Kollias, S., & Fellenz, W. (2001). Emotion recognition in human-computer interaction. *IEEE Signal Processing Magazine, 18*(1), 32–80. doi:10.1109/79.911197

Croyle, R. T., & Cooper, J. (1983). Dissonance arousal: Physiological evidence. *Journal of Personality and Social Psychology, 45*, 782–791. doi:10.1037/0022-3514.45.4.782

D.Beer, R. (1995). A dynamical systems perspective on autonomous agents. *Artificial Intelligence, 72*, 173–215. doi:10.1016/0004-3702(94)00005-Ldoi:10.1016/0004-3702(94)00005-L

Damasio, A. (1994). *Descartes' error: Emotion, reason, and the human brain*. North Yorkshire, UK: Quill.

Damasio, A. (1999). *The Feeling of What Happens*. London: Heinemann.

Damasio, A. R. (1994). *Descartes 'error: Emotion, reason, and the human brain*. New York: Grosset/Putnam.

Dane, E., & Pratt, M. G. (2007). Exploring intuition and its role in managerial decision making. *Academy of Management Review, 32*, 33–54.

Dapretto, M., Davies, M. S., Pfeifer, J. H., Scott, A. A., Sigman, M., & Bookheimer, S. Y. (2005). Understanding emotions in others: Mirror neuron dysfunction in children with autism spectrum disorders. *Nature Neuroscience, 9*, 28–30. doi:10.1038/nn1611

Darwin, C. (1998). *The expression of the emotions in man and animals* (3rd ed.). New York: Oxford University Press.

Dautenhahn, K. (1995). Getting to know each other—artificial social intelligence for autonomous robots. *Robotics and Autonomous Systems, 16*, 333–356. doi:10.1016/0921-8890(95)00054-2

Davitz, J. (1964). Auditory correlates of vocal expression of emotional feeling. In J. Davitz (Ed.), The communication of emotional meaning (pp. 101-112). New York: McGraw-Hill.

De Carolis, B., & Cozzolongo, G. (2007). Planning the Behavior of Social Robot Acting as a Majordomo in Public Environments. In Basili, R., & Pazienza, M. T. (Eds.), *AI*IA 2007* (pp. 805–812). New York: Springer.

De Rosis, F., Pelachaud, C., Poggi, I., Carofiglio, V., & De Carolis, B. (2003). From greta's mind to her face: Modelling the dynamics of affective states in a conversational agent. *International Journal of Human-Computer Studies, 59*, 8–118.

De Silva, P. R. S., Osano, M., Marasinghe, A., & Madurapperuma, A. P. (2006, April). Towards recognizing emotion with affective dimensions through body gestures. In *Proceedings of the 7th International Conference on Automatic Face and Gesture Recognition,* Southampton, UK (pp. 269-274).

Delgado-Mata, C., & Aylett, R. S. (2004, July). Emotion and action selection: Regulating the collective behaviour of agents in virtual environments. In *AAMAS ' 04: Proceedings of the 3rd International Joint Conference on Autonomous Agents and Multiagent Systems,* New York (Vol. 3, pp. 1304-1305). Washington, DC: IEEE Computer Society.

Denes-Raj, V., & Epstein, S. (1994). Conflict between intuitive and rational processing: When people behave against their better judgment. *Journal of Personality and Social Psychology, 66*, 819–829. doi:10.1037/0022-3514.66.5.819

Dennet, D. (1987). True Believers. In Dennett, D. (Ed.), *The Intentional Stance*. Cambridge, MA: MIT Press.

DePaulo, B. (2003). Cues to deception. *Psychological Bulletin, 129*(1), 74–118. doi:10.1037/0033-2909.129.1.74

Di Paolo, E. (2003). Evolving spike-timing-dependent plasticity for single-trial learning in robots. *Philosophical Transactions of the Royal Society of London, Series A: Mathematical, Physical and Engineering Sciences, 361*(1811), 2299-2319.

Douglas-Cowie, E., Cowie, R., Sneddon, I., Cox, C., Lowry, O., McRorie, M., et al. (2007, September). The HUMAINE Database: addressing the needs of the affective computing community. In *Affective Computing and Intelligent Interaction: Proceedings of the 2nd International Conference on Affective Computing and Intelligent Interaction,* Lisbon, Portugal (LNCS 4738, pp. 488-500).

Dranias, M., Grossberg, S., & Bullock, D. (2008). Dopaminergic and non-dopaminergic value systems in conditioning and outcome-specific revaluation. *Brain Research, 1238*, 239–287. doi:10.1016/j.brainres.2008.07.013

Dreuw, P., Deselaers, T., Rybach, D., Keysers, D., & Ney, H. (2006, April). Tracking using dynamic programming for appearance-based sign language recognition. In *Proceedings of the IEEE International Conference on Automatic Face and Gesture Recognition,* Southampton, UK (pp. 293-298). Washington, DC: IEEE Computer Society.

Driver, J., & Spence, C. (2000). Multisensory perception: Beyond modularity and convergence. *Current Biology, 10*(20), 731–735. doi:10.1016/S0960-9822(00)00740-5

Dunbar, R. I. M. (1993). Coevolution of neocortical size, group size and language in humans. *The Behavioral and Brain Sciences, 16*(4), 681–735.

Edamatsu, K. (1987). Machine vision of medical goods. *Proc. ITV, 41*(10).

Egges, A., Kshirsagar, S., & Magnenat-Thalmann, N. (2004). Generic personality and emotion simulation for conversational agents. *Computer Animation and Virtual Worlds, 15*, 1–13. doi:10.1002/cav.3

Ekman, P. (1982). *Emotion in the human face*. Cambridge, UK: Cambridge University Press.

Ekman, P., & Friesen, W. V. (1975). *Unmasking the face: A guide to recognizing emotions from facial clues*. Englewood Cliffs, NJ: Prentice-Hall.

Ekman, P., Friesen, W. V., & Hager, J. C. (2002). *Facial action coding system*. Salt Lake City, UT: A Human Face.

Ekman, P. (2003). Darwin, deception, and facial expression. *Annals of the New York Academy of Sciences, 1000*, 105–221.

Ekman, P., & Friesen, W. V. (1967). Head and body cues in the judgment of emotion: A reformulation. *Perceptual and Motor Skills, 24*, 711–724.

El Kaliouby, R., & Robinson, P. (2005, June 27-July 2). Real-time inference of complex mental states from facial expressions and head gestures. In *Proceedings of the 2004 Conference on Computer Vision and Pattern Recognition Workshop (CVPRW 2004),* Washington, DC (Vol. 10, pp. 154). Washington, DC: IEEE Computer Society.

El Kaliouby, R., & Teeters, A. (2007, November). Eliciting, capturing and tagging spontaneous facial affect in autism spectrum disorder. In *Proceedings of the 9th International Conference on Multimodal Interfaces,* Nagoya, Japan (pp. 46-53).

Elgammal, A., Shet, V., Yacoob, Y., & Davis, L. S. (2003, June). Learning dynamics for exemplar-based gesture recognition. In *Proceedings of the IEEE Conference on Computer Vision and Pattern Recognition,* Madison, WI (pp. 571-578). Washington, DC: IEEE Computer Society.

Elliott, C., Rickel, J., & Lester, J. (1999). Lifelike pedagogical agents and affective computing: An exploratory synthesis. In M. Woolridge & M. Veloso (Eds.), *Artificial intelligence today* (Vol. 1600, pp. 195-212). Berlin, Germany: Springer.

Ellis, P. M., & Bryson, J. J. (2005, September). The significance of textures for affective interfaces. In T. Panayiotopoulos, J. Gratch, R. Aylett, D. Ballin, P. Olivier, & T. Rist (Eds.), *Intelligent Virtual Agents: Proceedings of the Fifth International Working Conference on Intelligent Virtual Agents*, Kos, Greece (LNCS 3661, pp. 394-404).

Epstein, S., Pacini, R., Denes-Raj, V., & Heier, H. (1996). Individual differences in intuitive-experiential and analytical-rational thinking styles. *Journal of Personality and Social Psychology*, *71*, 390–405. doi:10.1037/0022-3514.71.2.390

Evans, D. (2002). The search hypothesis of emotion. *The British Journal for the Philosophy of Science*, *53*(4), 497–509. doi:10.1093/bjps/53.4.497doi:10.1093/bjps/53.4.497

Eysenck, M. W. (2004). *Psychology: An international perspective*. East Sussex, UK: Psychology Press.

Fasel, I. R., Fortenberry, B., & Movellan, J. R. (2005). A generative framework for real-time object detection, and classification. *Computer Vision and Image Understanding*, *98*(1), 182–210. doi:10.1016/j.cviu.2004.07.014

Fellous, J.-M. (1999). The neuromodulatory basis of emotion. *The Neuroscientist*, *5*(5), 283–294. doi:10.1177/107385849900500514doi:10.1177/107385849900500514

Fellous, J.-M. (2004, March). From human emotions to robot emotions. In *Architectures for modeling emotions: Cross-disciplinary foundations. Papers from the 2004 AAAI Spring Symposium,* Palo Alto, CA (pp. 37-47). AAAI Press.

Ferreira, M. B., Garcia-Marques, L., Sherman, S. J., & Sherman, J. W. (2006). Automatic and controlled components of judgment and decision making. *Journal of Personality and Social Psychology*, *91*, 797–813. doi:10.1037/0022-3514.91.5.797

Festinger, L. (1957). *A theory of cognitive dissonance*. Evanston, IL: Row, Peterson.

Floridi, L., & Taddeo, M. (2009). Turing's imitation game: Still an impossible challenge for all machines and some judges- an evaluation of the 2008 Loebner contest. *Minds and Machines, 19*(1), 145-150.

Fong, T., Nourbakhsh, I., & Dautenhahn, K. (2003). A survey of socially interactive robots. *Robotics and Autonomous Systems*, *42*(3-4), 143–166. doi:10.1016/S0921-8890(02)00372-X

Forbes-Riley, K., & Litman, D. (2004, May). Predicting emotion in spoken dialogue from multiple knowledge sources. In *Proceedings of the Human Language Technology Conference North America Chapter of the Association for Computational Linguistics (HLT-NAACL 2004),* Boston (pp. 201-208).

Fragopanagos, F., & Taylor, J. G. (2005). Emotion recognition in human-computer interaction. *Neural Networks*, *18*, 389–405. doi:10.1016/j.neunet.2005.03.006

Frank, M. J., & Claus, E. D. (2006). Anatomy of a decision: Striato-orbitofrontal interactions in reinforcement learning, decision making, and reversal. *Psychological Review*, *113*, 300–326. doi:10.1037/0033-295X.113.2.300

Friesen, W. V., & Ekman, P. (1984). *EMFACS-7: Emotional facial action coding system* (unpublished manual). San Francisco: University of California, San Francisco.

Frijda, N. H. (1986). *The emotions*. Cambridge, UK: Cambridge University Press.

Frijda, N. H., Manstead, A. S. R., & Bem, S. (Eds.). (2000). *Emotions and beliefs: How feelings influence thoughts*. Cambridge, UK: Cambridge University Press.

Fukuda, K. (1993). Machine vision systems for agricultural and marine products. *Factory Automation, 11*(11).

Gadanho, S. C. (1999). *Reinforcement learning in autonomous robots: An empirical investigation of the role of emotions*. Unpublished PhD thesis, University of Edinburgh.

Gadanho, S. C. (2003). Learning behavior-selection by emotions and cognition in a multi-goal robot task. *Journal of Machine Learning Research*, *4*, 385–412. doi:10.1162/jmlr.2003.4.3.385

Gallagher, S. (2001). The practice of mind: Theory, simulation, or interaction? *Journal of Consciousness Studies*, *8*, 83–107.

Gallagher, S. (2004). Understanding interpersonal problems in autism: Interaction theory as an alternative to theory of mind. *Philosophy, Psychiatry, & Psychology*, *11*(3), 199–217. doi:10.1353/ppp.2004.0063

Gallese, V. (2003). The manifold nature of interpersonal relations: The quest for a common mechanism. *Philosophical Transactions of the Royal Society, B, 358*, 517-528.

Gizmo Watch. (2008). *Wakamaru robot, robo-actor in the making hits stage*. Retrieved from, http://www.gizmowatch.com/entry/wakamaru-robot-robo-actor-in-the-making-hits-stage

Glowinski, D., Camurri, A., Volpe, G., Dael, N., & Scherer, K. (2008, June). Technique for automatic emotion recognition by body gesture analysis. In *Proceedings of the 2008 Computer Vision and Pattern Recognition Workshops,* Anchorage, AK (pp. 1-6). Washington, DC: IEEE Computer Society.

Gmytrasiewicz, P. J., & Lisetti, C. L. (2000, July). Using decision theory to formalize emotions in multi-agent systems. In *Proceedings of the 4th International IEEE Conference on MultiAgent Systems,* Boston (pp. 391-392). Washington, DC: IEEE Computer Society.

Goetz, J., Kiesler, S., & Powers, A. (2003). Matching robot appearance and behaviors to tasks to improve human–robot cooperation. In *Proceedings of the 12th IEEE International Workshop on Robot and Human Interactive Communication* (pp. 55-60).

Gotlib, I. H., & Hamilton, J. P. (2008). Neuroimaging and depression: Current status and unresolved issues. *Current Directions in Psychological Science, 17*(2), 159–163. doi:10.1111/j.1467-8721.2008.00567.xdoi:10.1111/j.1467-8721.2008.00567.x

Graesser, A. C., Chipman, P., Haynes, B. C., & Olney, A. (2005). AutoTutor: An intelligent tutoring system with mixed-initiative dialogue. *IEEE Transactions on Education, 48*(4), 612–618. doi:10.1109/TE.2005.856149

Grandjean, D., Sander, D., & Scherer, K. R. (2008). Conscious emotional experience emerges as a function of multilevel, appraisal-driven response synchronization. *Consciousness and Cognition, 17*(2), 484–495. doi:10.1016/j.concog.2008.03.019

Gratch, J., & Marsella, S. (2001, May). Tears and fears: Modeling emotions and emotional behaviors in synthetic agents. In *Proceedings of the 5th International Conference on Autonomous Agents,* Montreal, Quebec, Canada (pp. 278-285). ACM Publishing.

Gratch, J., & Marsella, S. (2004, August). Evaluating the modeling and use of emotion in virtual humans. In *Proceedings of the 3rd International Joint Conference on Autonomous Agents and Multiagent Systems,* New York (Vol. 1, pp. 320-327). Washington, DC: IEEE Computer Society.

Gratch, J., & Marsella, S. (2004). A domain-independent framework for modeling emotion. *Cognitive Systems Research, 5*(4), 269–306. doi:10.1016/j.cogsys.2004.02.002

Gratch, J., Marsella, S., & Petta, P. (2009). Modeling the cognitive antecedents and consequences of emotion. *Cognitive Systems Research, 10*(1), 1–5. doi:10.1016/j.cogsys.2008.06.001

Graziano, M. S. A., Taylor, C. S. R., Moore, T., & Cooke, D. F. (2002). The cortical control of movement revisited. *Neuron, 36*, 349–362. doi:10.1016/S0896-6273(02)01003-6

Grimm, M., Kroschel, K., & Narayanan, S. (2008, June). The Vera am Mittag German audio-visual emotional speech database. In *Proceedings of the IEEE International Conference on Multimedia and Expo,* Hannover, Germany (pp. 865-868). Washington, DC: IEEE Computer Society.

Gross, M. M., Gerstner, G. E., Koditschek, D. E., Fredrickson, B. L., & Crane, E. A. (2006). *Emotion recognition from body movement kinematics*. Retrieved from http://sitemaker.umich.edu/mgrosslab/files/abstract.pdf

Grossberg, S., & Levine, D. (1987). Neural dynamics of attentionally modulated Pavlovian conditioning: Blocking, interstimulus interval, and secondary reinforcement. *Applied Optics, 26*, 5015–5030. doi:10.1364/AO.26.005015

Gunes, H., & Piccardi, M. (2006, October). Creating and annotating affect databases from face and body display: A contemporary survey. In *Proceedings of the IEEE International Conference on Systems, Man and Cybernetics,* Taipei, Taiwan (pp. 2426-2433).

Gunes, H., & Piccardi, M. (2008). From mono-modal to multi-modal: Affect recognition using visual modalities. In D. Monekosso, P. Remagnino, & Y. Kuno (Eds.), *Ambient intelligence techniques and applications* (pp. 154-182). Berlin, Germany: Springer-Verlag.

Gunes, H., & Piccardi, M. (2009). Automatic temporal segment detection and affect recognition from face and body display. *IEEE Transactions on Systems, Man, and Cybernetics – Part B, 39*(1), 64-84.

Gunes, H., Piccardi, M., & Pantic, M. (2008). From the lab to the real world: Affect recognition using multiple cues and modalities. In Jimmy Or (Ed.), *Affective computing, focus on emotion expression, synthesis and recognition* (pp. 185-218). Vienna, Austria: I-Tech Education and Publishing.

Haag, A., Goronzy, S., Schaich, P., & Williams, J. (2004, June). Emotion recognition using bio-sensors: First steps towards an automatic system. In E. André, L. Dybkjær, W. Minker, & P. Heisterkamp (Eds.), *Affective Dialogue Systems: Tutorial and Research Workshop (ADS 2004),* Kloster Irsee, Germany (LNCS 3068, pp. 36-48).

Hadjikhani, N., & De Gelder, B. (2003). Seeing fearful body expressions activates the fusiform cortex and amygdala. *Current Biology, 13,* 2201–2205. doi:10.1016/j.cub.2003.11.049

Hanjalic, A., & Li-Qun, X. (2005). Affective video content representation and modeling. *IEEE Transactions on Multimedia, 7*(1), 143–154. doi:10.1109/TMM.2004.840618

Happé, F. (1995). The role of age and verbal ability in the theory of mind task performance of subjects with autism. *Child Development, 66,* 843–855. doi:10.2307/1131954

Harlow, H. (1953). Mice, monkeys, men, and motives. *Psychological Review, 60,* 23–32. doi:10.1037/h0056040

Heil, J. (2004). Three kinds of intentional psychology. In *Philosophy of Mind: A guide and Anthology*. Oxford, UK: Clarendon Press.

Henninger, A. E., Jones, R. M., & Chown, E. (2003, July). Behaviors that emerge from emotion and cognition: Implementation and evaluation of a symbolic-connectionist architecture. In *Proceedings of the 2nd International Joint Conference on Autonomous Agents and Multiagent Systems,* Melbourne, Australia (pp. 321-328). ACM Publishing.

Hertwig, R., Barron, G., Weber, E. U., & Erev, I. (2004). Decisions from experience and the effect of rare events in risky choice. *Psychological Science, 15,* 534–539. doi:10.1111/j.0956-7976.2004.00715.x

Hertz, J., Krogh, A., & Palmer, R. G. (1991). *Introduction to the theory of neural computation.* Boston: Addison-Wesley.

Heylen, D., Nijholt, A., Akker, R. d., & Vissers, M. (2003, September). Socially intelligent tutor agents. In R. Aylett, D. Ballin, & T. Rist (Eds.), *Proceedings of the 4th International Workshop on Intelligent Virtual Agents (IVA 2003),* Kloster Irsee, Germany (pp. 341-347). Berlin, Germany: Springer.

Heylighen, F. (2000). The science of self-organization and adaptivity. In *The encylopedia of life support systems* (pp. 253-280). Paris: UNESCO.

Hiller, M. J. (1995). *The role of chemical mechanisms in neural computation and learning.* (Tech. Rep. AITR-1455). Cambridge, MA: MIT AI Laboratory.

Hudlicka, E. (2008a, August). Affective computing for game design. In *Proceedings of the 4th International North American Conference on Intelligent Games and Simulation,* Montreal, Quebec, Canada (pp. 5-12).

Hudlicka, E. (2008b, November). Modeling the mechanisms of emotion effects on cognition. In *Proceedings of the AAAI Fall Symposium on Biologically Inspired Cognitive Architectures,* Arlington, VA (pp. 82-86). AAAI Press.

Hudlicka, E. (2003). To feel or not to feel: The role of affect in human-computer interaction. *International Journal of Human-Computer Studies, 59*(1-2), 1–32. doi:10.1016/S1071-5819(03)00047-8

Inokuchi, S. (1994). The aims of Kansei information processing. *Journal of Information Processing Society of Japan, 35*(9), 792–798.

Inokuchi, S. (1995, July). From knowledge engineering to Kansei engineering - a study on music performance. In *Proceedings of the 4th IEEE International Workshop on Robot and Human Communication,* Tokyo (pp. 7-14). Washington, DC: IEEE Computer Society.

Iso, T., Watanabe, Y., & Sonehara, N. (1997, June). Automatic detection of a masked person for security system. In *Proceedings of the 2nd Symposium on Sensing via Image Information,* (pp. 167-172).

Izard, C. E. (1997). Emotions and facial expression: A perspective from differential emotions theory. In J. A. Russel & J. M. Fernández-Dols (Eds.), *The psychology of facial expression* (pp. 57-77). Cambridge, UK: Cambridge University Press.

Izard, C. E. (1993). Four systems for emotion activation: Cognitive and noncognitive processes. *Psychological Review*, *100*(1), 68–90. doi:10.1037/0033-295X.100.1.68

Jin, X., & Wang, Z. (2005, October). An emotion space model for recognition of emotions in spoken chinese. In *Proceedings of the 1st International Conference on Affective Computing and Intelligent Interaction (ACII 2005),* Beijing, China, (pp. 397-402).

Juslin, P. N., & Scherer, K. R. (2005). Vocal expression of affect. In J. Harrigan, R. Rosenthal, & K. Scherer (Eds.), *The new handbook of methods in nonverbal behavior research* (pp. 65-135). Oxford, UK: Oxford University Press.

Kanda, T., Ishiguro, H., & Ishida, T. (2001). Psychological Evaluation on Interactions between People and Robot. *Journal of the Robotics Society of Japan*, *19*(3), 362–371.

Kanner, L. (1943). Autistic disturbances of affective contact. *The Nervous Child*, *2*, 217–250.

Karmarkar, U. R., & Buonomano, D. V. (2002). A model of spike-timing dependent plasticity: One or two coincidence detectors. *Journal of Neurophysiology*, *88*, 507–513. PubMed

Karmarkar, U. R., Najariana, M. T., & Buonomano, D. V. (2002). Mechanisms and significance of spike-timing dependent synaptic plasticity. *Biological Cybernetics*, *87*, 373–382. PubMeddoi:10.1007/s00422-002-0351-0doi:10.1007/s00422-002-0351-0

Karpouzis, K., Caridakis, G., Kessous, L., Amir, N., Raouzaiou, A., Malatesta, L., et al. (2007, November). Modelling naturalistic affective states via facial, vocal and bodily expressions recognition. In J. G. Carbonell & J. Siekmann (Eds.), *Artifical Intelligence for Human Computing: ICMI 2006 and IJCAI 2007 International Workshops,* Banff, Canada (LNAI 4451, pp. 92-116).

Katayose, H., & Inokuchi, S. (1989). The Kansei music system. *Computer Music Journal*, *13*(4), 72–77. doi:10.2307/3679555doi:10.2307/3679555

Katayose, H., Fukuoka, T., Takami, K., & Inokuchi, S. (1990, June). Expression extraction in virtuoso music performances. In *Proceedings of the 10th International Conference on Pattern Recognition,* Atlantic City, NJ (pp. 780-784). Washington, DC: IEEE Computer Society.

Katayose, H., Hirai, S., Horii, C., Kimura, A., & Sato, K. (2001). Kansei interaction in art and technology. In M. J. Smith, G. Salvendy, R. J. Koubek, & D. Harris (Eds.), *Usability evaluation and interface design: Cognitive engineering, intelligent agents and virtual reality* (pp. 509-513). Mahwah, NJ: Lawrence Erlbaum Associates.

Katayose, H., Imai, M., & Inokuchi, S. (1988, November). Sentiment extraction in music. In *Proceedings of the 9th International Conference on Pattern Recognition,* Rome (pp. 1083-1087). Washington, DC: IEEE Computer Society.

Katayose, H., Kanamori, T., Kamei, K., Nagashima, K., Sato, K., Inokuchi, S., et al. (1993). Virtual performer. In *Proceedings of the 1993 International Computer Music Conference,* Tokyo (pp. 241-248). ICMA.

Kato, H., Wake, S., & Inokuchi, S. (1993). Cooperative musical partner system: JASPER (Jam Session Partner). In *Proceedings of the Conference on Human Computer Interaction* (pp. 509-513).

Kauffman, S. (1993). *The origins of order: Self-organization and selection in evolution.* Oxford, UK: Oxford University Press.

Kelley, A. E. (2005). Neurochemical networks encoding emotion and motivation: An evolutionary perspective. In J-M. Fellous & M. A. Arbib (Eds.), *Who needs emotions? The brain meets the robot* (pp. 29-77). New York: Oxford University Press.

Kelso, J. A. S. (1995). *Dynamic patterns: The self-organization of brain and behavior*. Cambridge, MA: MIT Press.

Keltner, D., & Ekman, P. (2000). Facial expression of emotion. In M. Lewis & J. M. Haviland-Jones (Eds.), *Handbook of emotions* (pp. 236-249). New York: Guilford Press.

Khan, M. M., Ward, R. D., & Ingleby, M. (2006, June). Infrared thermal sensing of positive and negative affective states. In *Proceedings of the IEEE Conference on Robotics, Automation and Mechatronics,* Bangkok, Thailand (pp. 1-6). Washington, DC: IEEE Computer Society.

Khan, M. M., Ingleby, M., & Ward, R. D. (2006). Automated facial expression classification and affect interpretation using infrared measurement of facial skin temperature variations. *ACM Transactions on Autonomous and Adaptive Systems*, *1*(1), 91–113. doi:10.1145/1152934.1152939

Khan, M. M., Ward, R. D., & Ingleby, M. (2009). Classifying pretended and evoked facial expressions of positive and negative affective states using infrared measurement of skin temperature. *ACM Transactions on Applied Perception*, *6*(1), 6. doi:10.1145/1462055.1462061

Kidd, C., & Breazeal, C. (2004). Effect of a robot on user perceptions. In *Proceedings of the IEEE/RSJ International Conference on Intelligent Robots and Systems* (pp. 3559-3564).

Kim, J. (2007). Bimodal emotion recognition using speech and physiological changes. In M. Grimm, K. Kroschel (Eds.), *Robust speech recognition and understanding* (pp. 265-280). Vienna, Austria: I-Tech Education and Publishing.

Kittler, J., Hatef, M., Duin, R. P. W., & Matas, J. (1998). On combining classifiers. *IEEE Transactions on Pattern Analysis and Machine Intelligence*, *20*(3), 226–239. doi:10.1109/34.667881

Kleinsmith, A., & Bianchi-Berthouze, N. (2007, September). Recognizing affective dimensions from body posture. In *Affective Computing and Intelligent Interaction: 2nd International Conference,* Lisbon, Portugal (LNCS 4738, pp. 48-58).

Kleinsmith, A., Ravindra De Silva, P., & Bianchi-Berthouze, N. (2005, October) Grounding affective dimensions into posture features. In *Proceedings of the 1st International Conference on Affective Computing and Intelligent Interaction (ACII 2005),* Beijing, China (pp. 263-270).

Kleinsmith, A., Ravindra De Silva, P., & Bianchi-Berthouze, N. (2006). Cross-cultural differences in recognizing affect from body posture. *Interacting with Computers*, *18*, 1371–1389. doi:10.1016/j.intcom.2006.04.003

Koch, C. (1999). *Biophysics of computation*. New York: Oxford University Press.

Korstjens, A. H., Verhoeckx, I. L., & Dunbar, R. I. M. (2006). Time as a constraint on group size in spider monkeys. *Behavioral Ecology and Sociobiology*, *60*(5), 683–694. doi:10.1007/s00265-006-0212-2

Koshimizu, H., & Murakami, K. (1993). Facial caricaturing based on visual illusion - a mechanism to evaluate caricature in PICASSO system. *Transactions of the IEICE. E (Norwalk, Conn.)*, *76-D*(4), 470–478.

Kulic, D., & Croft, E. A. (2007). Affective state estimation for human–robot interaction. *IEEE Transactions on Robotics*, *23*(5), 991–1000. doi:10.1109/TRO.2007.904899

Lahnstein, M. (2005, April). The emotive episode is a composition of anticipatory and reactive evaluations. In L. Cañamero (Ed.), *Agents that want and like: Motivational and emotional roots of cognition and action. Papers from the AISB '05 Symposium,* Hatfield, UK (pp. 62-69). AISB Press.

Lazarus, R. S. (1991). *Emotion and adaptation*. New York: Oxford University Press.

LeDoux, J. (1996). *The Emotional Brain: The mysterious underpinnings of emotional life*. New York: Simon and Schuster.

LeDoux, J. E. (1998). *The emotional brain*. New York: Simon & Schuster.

Lee, C. M., & Narayanan, S. S. (2005). Toward detecting emotions in spoken dialogs. *IEEE Transactions on Speech and Audio Processing*, *13*(2), 293–303. doi:10.1109/TSA.2004.838534

Lehmann, H., & Bryson, J. J. (2007, September). Modelling primate social order: Ultimate causation of social evolution. In F. Amblard (Ed.), *Proceedings of the 4th Conference of the European Social Simuation Society (ESSA '07),* Toulouse, France (p. 765). IRIT Publications.

Leven, S. J. (1987). *Choice and neural process*. Unpublished doctoral dissertation, University of Texas at Arlington.

Levenson, R. W. (1988). Emotion and the autonomic nervous system: A prospectus for research on autonomic specificity. In H. L. Wagner (Ed.), *Social psychophysiology and emotion: Theory and clinical applications* (pp. 17-42). New York: John Wiley & Sons

Levine, D. S. (1998). *Explorations in common sense and common nonsense*. http://www.uta.edu/psychology/faculty/levine/EBOOK/index.htm

Levine, D. S., & Perlovsky, L. I. (2008b). A network model of rational versus irrational choices on a probability maximization task. In *Proceedings of the 2008 IEEE World Congress on Computational Intelligence* (pp. 2821-2825).

Levine, D. S., Mills, B. A., & Estrada, S. (2005, August). Modeling emotional influences on human decision making under risk. In *Proceedings of International Joint Conference on Neural Networks* (pp. 1657-1662).

Levine, D. S. (in press). Value maps, drives, and emotions. In Cutsuridis, V., Husain, A., & Taylor, J. G. (Eds.), *Perception-reason-action cycle: Models, algorithms, and systems*. New York: Springer.

Levine, D. S., & Perlovsky, L. I. (2008a). Simplifying heuristics versus careful thinking: scientific analysis of millennial spiritual issues. *Zygon*, *43*, 797–821. doi:10.1111/j.1467-9744.2008.00961.x

Lewis, M., Haviland-Jones, J. M., & Barrett, L. F. (Eds.). (2008). *Handbook of emotions* (3rd ed.). New York: Guilford Press.

Lewis, M. D. (2005). Bridging emotion theory and neurobiology through dynamic systems modeling. *The Behavioral and Brain Sciences*, *28*(2), 169–194.

Lienhart, R., & Maydt, J. (2002, September). An extended set of hair-like features for rapid object detection. In *Proceedings of the IEEE International Conference on Image Processing,* New York (Vol. 1, pp. 900-903). Washington, DC: IEEE Computer Society.

Litt, A., Eliasmith, C., & Thagard, P. (2008). Neural affective decision theory: Choices, brains, and emotions. *Cognitive Systems Research*, *9*, 252–273. doi:10.1016/j.cogsys.2007.11.001

Littlewort, G. C., Bartlett, M. S., & Lee, K. (2007, November). Faces of pain: Automated measurement of spontaneous facial expressions of genuine and posed pain. In *Proceedings of the 9th International Conference on Multimodal Interfaces,* Nagoya, Japan (pp. 15-21). ACM Publishing.

Llinás, R. R. (2001). *I of the Vortex. From neurons to Self.* Cambridge, MA: MIT Press.

Loebner, H. (2008). How to Hold a Turing Test Contest. In Epstein, R., Roberts, G., & Beber, G. (Eds.), *Parsing the Turing Test: Philosophical and Methodological Issues in the Quest for the Thinking Computer* (pp. 173–179). New York: Springer.

Lohse, M., Hanheide, M., Wrede, B., Walters, M. L., Koay, K. L., Syrdal, D. S., et al. (2008). Evaluating Extrovert and Introvert Behaviour of a Domestic robot: A Video Study. In *Proceedings of the 17th IEEE International Symposium on Robot and Human Interactive Communication* (pp. 488-493).

MacLean, P. D. (1990). *The triune brain in evolution: Role in paleocerebral functions*. New York: Plenum.

Maes, P. (1991). The agent network architecture (ANA). *SIGART Bulletin*, *2*(4), 115–120. doi:10.1145/122344.122367

Marcella, S., & Gratch, J. (2002, July). A step toward irrationality: Using emotion to change belief. In *Proceedings of the 1st International Joint Conference on Autonomous Agents and Multiagent Systems*, Bologna, Italy (pp. 334–341). ACM Publishing.

Marinier Iii, R. P., Laird, J. E., & Lewis, R. L. (2009). A computational unification of cognitive behavior and emotion. *Cognitive Systems Research*, *10*(1), 48–69. doi:10.1016/j.cogsys.2008.03.004

Marsella, S. C., & Gratch, J. (2009). EMA: A process model of appraisal dynamics. *Cognitive Systems Research*, *10*(1), 70–90. doi:10.1016/j.cogsys.2008.03.005

Martin, J.-C., Caridakis, G., Devillers, L., Karpouzis, K., & Abrilian, S. (2009). Manual annotation and automatic image processing of multimodal emotional behaviours: Validating the annotation of TV interviews. *Personal and Ubiquitous Computing*, *13*(1), 69–76. doi:10.1007/s00779-007-0167-y

Matsumoto, S. (1993). *Image processing applications to chemical industry* (Tech Rep. IEE).

McClure, S. M., Laibson, D. I., Loewenstein, G., & Cohen, J. D. (2004). Separate neural systems value immediate and delayed monetary rewards. *Science*, *306*, 503–506. doi:10.1126/science.1100907

Mcgregor, R., Mershon, D. H., & Pastore, C. M. (1994). Perception, detection, and Diagnosis of appearance defects in fabrics. *Textile Research Journal*, *64*(10), 584–591. doi:10.1177/004051759406401006d oi:10.1177/004051759406401006

McIntosh, D. N., Reichmann-Decker, A., Winkielman, P., & Wilbarger, J. (2006). When mirroring fails: Deficits in spontaneous, but not controlled mimicry of emotional facial expressions in autism. *Developmental Science*, *9*, 295–302. doi:10.1111/j.1467-7687.2006.00492.x

Mehrabian, A., & Russell, J. (1974). *An approach to environmental psychology*. Cambridge, MA: MIT Press.

Meltzoff, A. N., & Prinz, W. (2002). *The imitative mind: Development, evolution, and brain bases*. New York: Cambridge University Press. doi:10.1017/CBO9780511489969

Meyer, J.-J. C. (2006). Reasoning about emotional agents. *International Journal of Intelligent Systems*, *21*(6), 601–619. doi:10.1002/int.20150

Milne, E., & Grafman, J. (2001). Ventromedial prefrontal cortex lesions in humans eliminate implicit gender stereotyping. *Journal of Neuroscience Special Issue*, *21*(12), 1–6.

Minsky, M. (1988). *The society of mind*. New York: Simon & Schuster Inc.

Minsky, M., Singh, P., & Sloman, A. (2004). The St. Thomas common sense symposium: Designing architectures for human-level intelligence. *AI Magazine*, *25*(2), 113–124.

Morgado, L., & Gaspar, G. (2005, July). Emotion based adaptive reasoning for resource bounded agents. In *Proceedings of the 4th International Joint Conference on Autonomous Agents and Multi Agent Systems (AAMAS '05),* Utrecht, The Netherlands (pp. 921-928). ACM Publishing.

Mutlu, B., Osman, S., Forlizzi, J., Hodgins, J., & Kiesler, S. (2006). Task structure and user attributes as elements of human–robot interaction design. In *Proceedings of the 15th IEEE International Symposium on Robot and Human Interactive Communication* (pp. 74-79).

Nagata, N., & Fujisawa, X. T. (2009). Functional neuroimaging of synesthesia. *Journal Systems. Control and Information*, *53*(4), 149–154.

Nagata, N., Dobashi, T., Manabe, Y., Usami, T., & Inokuchi, S. (1997). Modeling and visualization for a pearl-quality evaluation simulator. *IEEE Transactions on Visualization and Computer Graphics*, *3*(4), 307–315. doi:10.1109/2945.646234doi:10.1109/2945.646234

Nagata, N., Kamei, M., Akane, M., & Nakajima, H. (1992). Development of a pearl quality evaluation system based on an instrumentation of "Kansei". *Trans. IEE Japan, 112-C*(2).

Nakagawa, Y. (1989). Visual inspection of electronic devices. *Trans. IEE Japan, 109-D*(7).

Nakasone, A., Prendinger, H., & Ishizuka, M. (2005, September). Emotion recognition from electromyography and skin conductance. In Proceedings of the 5th International Workshop on Biosignal Interpretation, Tokyo (pp. 219-222).

Nakatsu, R., Rauterberg, M., & Vorderer, P. (2005, September). A new framework for entertainment computing: From passive to active experience. In *Proceedings of the 4th International Conference on Entertainment Computing (ICEC 2005),* Sanda, Japan (pp. 1-12). New York: Springer.

Nakayama, K., Goto, S., Kuraoka, K., & Nakamura, K. (2005). Decrease in nasal temperature of rhesus monkeys (Macaca mulatta) in negative emotional state. *Journal of Physiology and Behavior*, *84*, 783–790. doi:10.1016/j.physbeh.2005.03.009

Nesse, R. (1990). Evolutionary explanations of emotion. *Human Nature (Hawthorne, N.Y.)*, *1*(30), 261–289. doi:10.1007/BF02733986doi:10.1007/BF02733986

Neumann, R., & Strack, F. (2000). "Mood contagion": The automatic transfer of mood between persons. *Journal of Personality and Social Psychology*, *79*, 211–223. doi:10.1037/0022-3514.79.2.211

Niedenthal, P. M. (2007). Embodying emotion. *Science*, *316*, 1002–1005. doi:10.1126/science.1136930

Niedenthal, P. M., Barsalou, L. W., Winkielman, P., Krauth-Gruber, S., & Ric, F. (2005). Embodiment in attitudes, social perception, and emotion. *Personality and Social Psychology Review*, *9*(3), 184–211. doi:10.1207/s15327957pspr0903_1

Ning, H., Han, T. X., Hu, Y., Zhang, Z., Fu, Y., & Huang, T. S. (2006, April). A real-time shrug detector. In *Proceedings of the IEEE International Conference on Automatic Face and Gesture Recognition,* Southampton, UK (pp. 505-510). Washington, DC: IEEE Computer Society.

Noble, J. (1997, July). *The scientific status of artificial life*. In Paper presented at the 4th European Conference on Artificial Life, Brighton, UK.

Nomura, T., Kanda, T., Suzuki, T., & Kato, K. (2008). Prediction of Human Behavior in Human–Robot Interaction Using Psychological Scales for Anxiety and Negative Attitudes toward Robots. *IEEE Transactions on Robotics*, *24*(2), 442–451. doi:10.1109/TRO.2007.914004

Norman, D. A., & Shallice, T. (1986). Attention to action: Willed and automatic control of behavior. In R. Davidson, G. Schwartz, & D. Shapiro (Eds.), *Consciousness and self regulation: Advances in research and theory* (Vol. 4, pp. 1-18). New York: Plenum.

Norman, D. A., Ortony, A., & Russell, D. M. (2003). Affect and machine design: Lessons for the development of autonomous machines. *IBM Systems Journal*, *42*, 38–44.

Ortony, A., Clore, G. L., & Collins, A. (1988). *The cognitive structure of emotions*. Cambridge, UK: Cambridge University Press.

Ortony, A., Clore, G. L., & Collins, A. (1988). *The cognitive structure of emotions*. New York: Cambridge University Press.

Ortony, A., & Turner, T. J. (1990). What's basic about basic emotions? *Psychological Review*, *97*, 315–331. doi:10.1037/0033-295X.97.3.315

Osgood, C., Suci, G., & Tannenbaum, P. (1957). *The measurement of meaning*. Chicago: University of Illinois Press.

Ozonoff, S., & Miller, J. N. (1995). Teaching theory of mind: A new approach to social skills training for individuals with autism. *Journal of Autism and Developmental Disorders*, *25*, 415–433. doi:10.1007/BF02179376

Paiva, A. (2000). *Affective interactions: Toward a new generation of computer interfaces?* New York: Springer.

Paiva, A., Dias, J., Sobral, D., Aylett, R., Sobreperez, P., Woods, S., et al. (2004, July). Caring for agents and agents that care: Building empathic relations with synthetic agents. In *AAMAS '04: Proceedings of the 3rd International Joint Conference on Autonomous Agents and Multiagent Systems*, New York (pp. 194-201). Washington, DC. IEEE Computer Society.

Pan, H., Levinson, S. E., Huang, T. S., & Liang, Z.-P. (2004). A fused hidden markov model with application to bimodal speech processing. *IEEE Transactions on Signal Processing*, *52*(3), 573–581. doi:10.1109/TSP.2003.822353

Panksepp, J. (1998). *Affective neuroscience: The foundations of human and animal emotions*. New York: Oxford University Press.

Pantic, M., & Bartlett, M. S. (2007). Machine analysis of facial expressions. In K. Delac & M. Grgic (Eds.), *Face recognition* (pp. 377-416). Vienna, Austria: I-Tech Education and Publishing.

Pantic, M., Pentland, A., Nijholt, A., & Huang, T. (2007). Machine understanding of human behaviour. In *Artifical Intelligence for Human Computing* (LNAI 4451, pp. 47-71).

Pantic, M., Nijholt, A., Pentland, A., & Huang, T. (2008). Human-centred intelligent human-computer interaction (HCI2): How far are we from attaining it? *International Journal of Autonomous and Adaptive Communications Systems*, *1*(2), 168–187. doi:10.1504/IJAACS.2008.019799

Pantic, M., & Rothkrantz, L. J. M. (2000). Automatic analysis of facial expressions: The state of the art. *IEEE Transactions on Pattern Analysis and Machine Intelligence*, *22*(12), 1424–1445. doi:10.1109/34.895976

Pantic, M., & Rothkrantz, L. J. M. (2003). Towards an affect-sensitive multimodal human-computer interaction. *Proceedings of the IEEE*, *91*(9), 1370–1390. doi:10.1109/JPROC.2003.817122

Parussel, K. M. (2006). *A bottom-up approach to emulating emotions using neuromodulation in agents.* Unpublished doctoral dissertation, University of Stirling.

Parussel, K. M., & Cañamero, L. (2007). Biasing neural networks towards exploration or exploitation using neuromodulation. In J. M. de Sá, L. A. Alexandre, W. Duch, & D. Mandic (Eds.), *ICANN 2007: Proceedings of the 17th International Conference on Artificial Neural Networks Part II* (Vol. 4669, pp. 889-898). Springer-Verlag.

Parussel, K. M., & Smith, L. S. (2005, April). Cost minimisation and reward maximisation. A neuromodulating minimal disturbance system using anti-hebbian spike timing-dependent plasticity. In *Proceedings of the Symposium on Agents that Want and Like: Motivational and Emotional Roots of Cognition and Action, AISB 05,* Hatfield, UK (pp. 98-101). Society for the Study of Artificial Intelligence and the Simulation of Behaviour.

Pavlidis, I. T., Levine, J., & Baukol, P. (2001, October). Thermal image analysis for anxiety detection. In *Proceedings of the International Conference on Image Processing,* Thessaloniki, Greece (Vol. 2, pp. 315-318). Washington, DC: IEEE Computer Society.

Penrose, R. (1994). *Shadows of the mind.* Oxford: Oxford University Press.

Perlovsky, L. I. (2006b). Music - The first principle. *Musical Theater E-journal.* Retrieved from http://www.ceo.spb.ru/libretto/kon_lan/ogl.shtml

Perlovsky, L. I., Bonniot-Cabanac, M.-C., & Cabanac, M. (2010). Curiosity and pleasure, to be published.

Perlovsky, L. I. (2001). *Neural Networks and Intellect: using model-based concepts* (3rd ed.). New York: Oxford University Press.

Perlovsky, L. I. (2006a). Toward physics of the mind: Concepts, emotions, consciousness, and symbols. *Physics of Life Reviews, 3,* 23–55. doi:10.1016/j.plrev.2005.11.003

Perlovsky, L. I. (2009a). Language and cognition. *Neural Networks, 22,* 247–257. doi:10.1016/j.neunet.2009.03.007

Perlovsky, L. I. (2009b). Language and emotions: Emotional Sapir-Whorf Hypothesis. *Neural Networks, 22,* 518–526. doi:10.1016/j.neunet.2009.06.034

Perlovsky, L. I. (2010a). Musical emotions: Functions, origin, evolution. *Physics of Life Reviews, 7,* 2–27. doi:10.1016/j.plrev.2009.11.001

Perlovsky, L. I. (2010b). Intersections of mathematical, cognitive, and aesthetic Theories of Mind. *Psychology of Aesthetics, Creativity, and the Arts, 4,* 11–17. doi:10.1037/a0018147

Pessoa, L. (2008). On the relationship between emotion and cognition. *Nature Reviews. Neuroscience, 9,* 148–158. doi:10.1038/nrn2317

Peters, E. (2006). The functions of affect in the construction of preferences. In Lichtenstein, S., & Slovic, P. (Eds.), *The construction of preference.* New York: Cambridge University Press. doi:10.1017/CBO9780511618031.025

Pfeifer, R., & Scheier, C. (1999). *Understanding Intelligence.* Cambridge, MA: MIT Press.

Picard, R. W. (1997). *Affective computing.* Cambridge, MA: MIT Press.

Picard, R. W. (2003). Affective computing: Challenges. *International Journal of Human-Computer Studies, 59*(1-2), 55–64. doi:10.1016/S1071-5819(03)00052-1

Picard, R. W., Vyzas, E., & Healey, J. (2001). Toward machine emotional intelligence: Analysis of affective physiological state. *IEEE Transactions on Pattern Analysis and Machine Intelligence, 23*(10), 1175–1191. doi:10.1109/34.954607

Plutchik, R. (1980). A general psychoevolutionary theory of emotion. In R. Plutchik & H. Kellerman (Eds.), *Emotion: Theory, research, and experience* (pp. 3-33). New York: Academic Press.

Plutchik, R. (1984). Emotions: A general psychoevolutionary theory. In K. Scherer & P. Ekman (Eds.), *Approaches to emotion* (pp. 197-219). Hillsdale, NJ: Lawrence Erlbaum Associates.

Plutchik, R. (1970). *Emotion: A psychoevolutionary analysis.* New York: Harper & Row.

Poincaré, H. (1914). *Science and method* (Maitland, F., Trans.). London: T. Nelson and Sons.

Poppe, R. (2007). Vision-based human motion analysis: An overview. *Computer Vision and Image Understanding, 108*(1-2), 4–18. doi:10.1016/j.cviu.2006.10.016

Prescott, T. J., Bryson, J. J., & Seth, A. K. (2007). Modelling natural action selection: An introduction to the theme issue. *Philosophical Transactions of the Royal Society, B— Biology, 362*(1485), 1521-1529.

Pun, T., Alecu, T. I., Chanel, G., Kronegg, J., & Voloshynovskiy, S. (2006). Brain-computer interaction research at the computer vision and multimedia laboratory, University of Geneva. *IEEE Transactions on Neural Systems and Rehabilitation Engineering, 14*(2), 210–213. doi:10.1109/TNSRE.2006.875544

Puri, C., Olson, L., Pavlidis, I., Levine, J., & Starren, J. (2005, April). StressCam: Non-contact measurement of users' emotional states through thermal imaging. In *Proceedings of the Conference on Human Factors in Computing Systems (CHI 2005),* Portland, OR (pp. 1725-1728). ACM Publishing.

Reeves, B., & Nass, C. (1996). *Media equation*. Cambridge, UK: Cambridge University Press.

Reeves, B., & Nass, C. I. (1996). *The Media Equation: How People Treat Computers, Television and New Media Like Real People and Places*. Cambridge, MA: Cambridge University Press.

Rehm, M., & André, E. (2007). More Than Just a Friendly Phrase: Multimodal Aspects of Polite Behavior in Agent. In Nishida, T. (Ed.), *Conversational Informatics: an Engineering Approach* (pp. 69–84). New York: Wiley. doi:10.1002/9780470512470.ch4

Reilly, W. S. N. (1996). *Believable social and emotional agents*. Unpublished PhD thesis, School of Computer Science, Carnegie Mellon University, Pittsburgh.

Reisenzein, R. (2009). Emotions as metarepresentational states of mind: Naturalizing the belief-desire theory of emotion. *Cognitive Systems Research, 10*(1), 6–20. doi:10.1016/j.cogsys.2008.03.001

Reyna, V. F., & Brainerd, C. J. (1991). Fuzzy-trace theory and framing effects in choice: Gist extraction, truncation, and conversion. *Journal of Behavioral Decision Making, 4*, 249–262. doi:10.1002/bdm.3960040403

Rickel, J., & Johnson, W. L. (1997, February). Integrating pedagogical capabilities in a virtual environment agent. In *Proceedings of the 1st International Conference on Autonomous Agents*, Marina del Rey, CA (pp. 30-38). ACM Publishing.

Riseberg, J., Klein, J., Fernandez, R., & Picard, R. W. (1998, April). Frustrating the user on purpose: Using biosignals in a pilot study to detect the user's emotional state. In *Proceedings of the Conference on Human Factors in Computing Systems (CHI 1998),* Los Angeles (pp. 227-228). ACM Publishing.

Rohlfshagen, P., & Bryson, J. J. (2008, November). Improved animal-like maintenance of homeostatic goals via flexible latching. In A. V. Samsonovich (Ed.), *Proceedings of the AAAI Fall Symposium on Biologically Inspired Cognitive Architectures,* Arlington, VA (pp. 153-160). AAAI Press.

Rolls, E. T. (1999). *The brain and emotion*. New York: Oxford University Press.

Rolls, E. T. (2005). What are emotions, why do we have emotions, and what is their computational basis in the brain? In J-M. Fellous & M. A. Arbib (Eds.), *Who needs emotions? The brain meets the robot* (pp. 117-146). Oxford University Press.

Rolls, E. T. (2000). Precis of the brain and emotion. *The Behavioral and Brain Sciences, 20*, 177–234. doi:10.1017/S0140525X00002429

Russel, J. A., & Fernández-Dols, J. M. (1997). *The psychology of facial expression*. Cambridge, UK: Cambridge University Press.

Russell, J. A. (1997). Reading emotions from and into faces: resurrecting a dimensional contextual perspective. In J. A. Russell & J. M. Fernandez-Dols (Eds.), *The psychology of facial expression* (pp. 295-320). New York: Cambridge University Press.

Russell, J. (2003). Core affect and the psychological construction of emotion. *Psychological Review, 110*(1), 145–172. doi:10.1037/0033-295X.110.1.145

Russell, J. A. (1980). A circumplex model of affect. *Journal of Personality and Social Psychology, 39*, 1161–1178. doi:10.1037/h0077714

Rutherford, M. D., & McIntosh, D. N. (2007). Rules versus prototype matching: Strategies of perception of emotional facial expressions in the autism spectrum. *Journal of Autism and Developmental Disorders, 37*, 187–196. doi:10.1007/s10803-006-0151-9

Savran, A., Ciftci, K., Chanel, G., Mota, J. C., Viet, L. H., Sankur, B., et al. (2006, July 17-August 11). Emotion detection in the loop from brain signals and facial images. In *Proceedings of eNTERFACE 2006,* Dubrovnik, Croatia. Retrieved from http://www.enterface.net

Schaal, S., Ijspeert, A., & Billard, A. (2004). Computational approaches to motor learning by imitation. In C. D. Frith (Ed.), *The Neuroscience of Social Interaction: Decoding, Imitating, and Influencing the Actions of Others*, (pp. 199-218). New York: Oxford University Press.

Scherer, K. R. (2000). Psychological models of emotion. In J. Borod (Ed.), *The neuropsychology of emotion* (pp. 137-162). New York: Oxford University Press.

Scherer, K. R., Schorr, A., & Johnstone, T. (Eds.). (2001). *Appraisal processes in emotion: Theory, methods, research*. New York: Oxford University Press.

Scheutz, M. (2004, July). Useful roles of emotions in artificial agents: A case study from artificial life. In *Proceedings of the 19th National Conference on Artificial Intelligence*, San Jose, CA (pp. 42-47). AAAI Press.

Schmidt, K. L., & Cohn, J. F. (2001). Human facial expressions as adaptations: Evolutionary questions in facial expression research. *Yearbook of Physical Anthropology*, *44*, 3–24. doi:10.1002/ajpa.20001

Scopelliti, M., Giuliani, M. V., & Fornara, F. (2005). Robots in a Domestic Setting: A Psychological Approach. *Universal Access in Information Society*, *4*, 146–155. doi:10.1007/s10209-005-0118-1

Searle, J. (1980). Minds, brains and programs. *The Behavioral and Brain Sciences*, *3*, 417–457. doi:10.1017/S0140525X00005756

Shah, H. (2006, May). Chatterbox Challenge 2005: Geography of a Modern Eliza. In *Proceedings of the 3rd International Workshop on Natural Language Understanding and Cognitive Science (NLUCS 2006)*, Paphos, Cyprus.

Shah, H., & Warwick, K. (2010a, March 29-30). From the Buzzing in Turing's Head to Machine Intelligence Contests. In *Proceedings of Towards a Comprehensive Intelligence Test (TCIT 2010)*, De Montfort University, Leicester, UK.

Shah, H., & Warwick, K. (2010b). Testing Turing's five minutes parallel-paired imitation game. *Kybernetes Special Issue: Turing Test*, *39*(3), 449–465.

Shan, C., Gong, S., & McOwan, P. W. (2007, September). *Beyond facial expressions: Learning human emotion from body gestures*. Paper presented at the British Machine Vision Conference, Warwick, UK.

Shanahan, M. P. (2005). Global access, embodiment, and the conscious subject. *Journal of Consciousness Studies*, *12*(12), 46–66.

Shin, Y. (2007, May). Facial expression recognition based on emotion dimensions on manifold learning. In *Proceedings of International Conference on Computational Science*, Beijing, China (Vol. 2, pp. 81-88).

Sidner, C., & Lee, C. (2007, March). *The Initiation of Engagement by a Humanoid Robot*. Paper presented at AAAI Spring Symposium on Multidisciplinary Collaboration for Socially Assistive Robotics, Palo Alto, CA.

Sloman, A. (2003). How many separately evolved emotional beasties live within us? In R. Trappl, P. Petta, & S. Payr (Eds.), *Emotions in humans and artifacts* (pp. 35-114). Cambridge, MA: MIT Press.

Sloman, A., & Croucher, M. (1981, August). Why robots will have emotions. In *Proceedings of the 7th International Joint Conference on Artificial Intelligence (IJCAI '81)*, Vancouver, British Columbia, Canada (pp. 1537-1542). William Kaufmann.

Sloman, A. (2001). Beyond shallow models of emotion. *Cognitive Processing*, *2*(1), 177–198.

Sloman, S. A. (1996). The empirical case for two systems of reasoning. *Psychological Bulletin*, *119*, 3–22. doi:10.1037/0033-2909.119.1.3

Smith, C. A., & Scott, H. S. (1997). A componential approach to the meaning of facial expressions. In J. A. Russel & J. M. Fernández-Dols (Eds.), *The psychology of facial expression* (pp. 295-320). Cambridge, UK: Cambridge University Press.

Song, S., Miller, K. D., & Abbott, L. F. (2000). Competitive hebbian learning through spike-timing-dependent plasticity. *Nature Neuroscience*, *3*, 919–926. PubMeddoi:10.1038/78829doi:10.1038/78829

Steel, L. (1997). The synthetic modeling of language origins. *Evolution of Communication*, *1*, 1–35.

Steunebrink, B. R., Dastani, M., & Meyer, J.-J. C. (2007, July). A logic of emotions for intelligent agents. In *Proceedings of the 22nd National Conference on Artificial Intelligence (AAAI 2007)*, Vancouver, British Columbia, Canada (pp. 142-147). AAAI Press.

Steunebrink, B. R., Dastani, M., & Meyer, J.-J. C. (2008, July). A formal model of emotions: Integrating qualitative and quantitative aspects. In *Proceedings of the European Conference on Artificial Intelligence (ECAI '08),* Patras, Greece (pp. 256-260). IOS Press.

Stins, J. F., & Laureys, S. (2009). Thought translation, tennis and Turings tests in the

Swanson, L. W. (2005). Anatomy of the soul as reflected in the cerebral hemispheres: Neural circuits underlying voluntary control of basic motivated behaviors. *The Journal of Comparative Neurology*, *493*, 122–131. doi:10.1002/cne.20733

Synthetic Emotions and Sociable Robotics: New Applications in Affective

Synthetic Emotions , *1*(1), 1-17.

Takahashi, H., & Shimomura, R. (1997). Image processing technologies for driving assist. *Journal of ITE*, *51*(6), 746–750.

Takahashi, K. (2004, December). Remarks on emotion recognition from multi-modal bio-potential signals. In *Proceedings of the IEEE International Conference on Industrial Technology,* Hammamet, Tunisia (pp. 1138-1143).

Takashima, A., Nishimoto, M., Takahashi, R., Fujisawa, T. X., & Nagata, N. (2008, March). *Colored-hearing synesthesia: The relationship between color and music tonality*. Paper presented at the 4th Annual Meeting of the UK Synaesthesia Association, Edinburgh, UK.

Taki, Y. (2003). Culture and Politeness: Differences of Apology Strategies of the British and Japanese People: Comparison of Young and Older Subjects. *Studies in Language and Literature*, *22*(2), 27–63.

Tamietto, M., & de Gelder, B. (2008). Emotional contagion for unseen bodily expressions: Evidence from facial EMG. In *Proceedings of the FG 2008 meeting*. Retrieved from http://74.125.155.132/scholar?q=cache:azyMSegSshgJ: scholar.google.com/&hl=en&as_sdt=2000

Tanguy, E. A. R. (2006). *Emotions: The art of communication applied to virtual actors* (Bath CS Tech. Rep. CSBU-2006-06). Bath, UK: University of Bath.

Tanguy, E. A. R., Willis, P. J., & Bryson, J. J. (2003). A layered dynamic emotion representation for the creation of complex facial animation. In T. Rist, R. Aylett, D. Ballin, & J. Rickel (Eds.), *Intelligent virtual agents* (pp. 101-105). New York: Springer.

Tanguy, E. A. R., Willis, P. J., & Bryson, J. J. (2007, January). Emotions as durative dynamic state for action selection. In *Proceedings of the 20th International Joint Conference on Artificial Intelligence*, Hyderabad, India (pp. 1537-1542). Morgan Kaufmann.

Tanguy, E. A. R., Willis, P. J., & Bryson, J. J. (2006). A dynamic emotion representation model within a facial animation system. *International Journal of Humanoid Robotics*, *3*(3), 293–300. doi:10.1142/S0219843606000758

Taper, B. (1970). *The arts in Boston*. Cambridge, MA: Harvard University Press.

Thomaz, A., Berlin, M., & Breazeal, C. (2005, July 7-17). Robot science meets social science: An embodied computational model of social referencing. In *Proceedings of the Workshop toward social mechanisms of android science (CogSci)*, Italy (pp. 25-26).

Tian, Y. L., Kanade, T., & Cohn, J. F. (2002, May). Evaluation of gabor-wavelet-based facial action unit recognition in image sequences of increasing complexity. In *Proceedings of the IEEE International Conference on Automaitc Face and Gesture Recognition,* Washington, DC (pp. 218-223). Washington, DC: IEEE Computer Society.

Tomb, I., Hauser, M. D., Deldin, P., & Caramazza, A. (2002). Do somatic markers mediate decisions on the gambling task? *Nature Neuroscience*, *5*(11), 1103–1104. doi:10.1038/nn1102-1103

Tomkins, S. S. (1962). *Affect, imagery, consciousness: Vol. 1. The positive affects*. New York: Springer.

Tomkins, S. S. (1963). *Affect, imagery, consciousness. Vol. 2: The negative affects*. New York: Springer.

Trevarthen, C. (1979). Communication and cooperation in early infancy: a description of primary intersubjectivity. In Bullowa, M. (Ed.), *Before Speech* (pp. 321–347). Cambridge, UK: Cambridge University Press.

Trevarthen, C., & Aitken, K. J. (2001). Infant intersubjectivity: research, theory, and clinical applications. *Journal of Child Psychology and Psychiatry, and Allied Disciplines*, *42*(1), 3–48. doi:10.1111/1469-7610.00701

Tsiamyrtzis, P., Dowdall, J., Shastri, D., Pavlidis, I., Frank, M. G., & Ekman, P. (2007). Imaging facial physiology for the detection of deceit. *International Journal of Computer Vision*, *71*(2), 197–214. doi:10.1007/s11263-006-6106-y

Tsuji, S. (1992). *Kansei information projects - what is Kansei information.*

Turing, A. M. (1950). Computing Machinery and Intelligence. *Mind*, *59*(236), 433–460. doi:10.1093/mind/LIX.236.433

Tyrrell, T. (1994). An evaluation of Maes's bottom-up mechanism for behavior selection. *Adaptive Behavior*, *2*(4), 307–348. doi:10.1177/105971239400200401

Uno, H., Mizushima, Y., Nagata, N., & Sakaguchi, Y. (2008, August). Lace curtain: Measurement of BTDF and rendering of woven cloth - production of a catalog of curtain animations. In *Proceedings of the International Conference on Computer Graphics and Interactive Techniques (ACM SIGGRAPH 2008),* Los Angeles (no. 30). ACM Publishing.

Vallverdú, J., & Casacuberta, D. (2008). The Panic Room. On Synthetic Emotions. In

Vallverdú, J., & Casacuberta, D. (2009). Modelling Hardwired Synthetic Emotions: TPR

Valstar, M. F., & Pantic, M. (2007, October). Combined support vector machines and hidden markov models for modeling facial action temporal dynamics. In M. Lew, N. Sebe, T. S. Huang, E. M. Bakker (Eds.), *Human–Computer Interaction: IEEE International Workshop, HCI 2007,* Rio de Janeiro, Brazil (LNCS 4796, pp. 118-127).

Valstar, M. F., Gunes, H., & Pantic, M. (2007). How to distinguish posed from spontaneous smiles using geometric features. In *Proceedings of the 9th International Conference on Multimodal Interfaces,* Nagoya, Japan (pp. 38-45). ACM Publishing.

Van den Stock, J., Righart, R., & De Gelder, B. (2007). Body expressions influence recognition of emotions in the face and voice. *Emotion (Washington, D.C.)*, *7*(3), 487–494. doi:10.1037/1528-3542.7.3.487

Varela, F. J., Thompson, E., & Rosch, E. (1991). *The Embodied Mind.* Cambridge, MA: MIT Press.

Velasquez, J. (1998, October). Modeling emotion-based decision making. In *Proceedings of the AAAI Fall Symposium on Emotional and Intelligent: The Tangled Knot of Cognition,* Orlandon, FL (pp. 148-149). AAAI Press.

Velásquez, J. D., & Maes, P. (1997, February). Cathexis: A computational model of emotions. In *Proceedings of the 1st International Conference on Autonomous Agents (Agents '97),* Marina Del Ray, CA (pp. 518-519). ACM Publishing.

Vianna, D. M., & Carrive, P. (2005). Changes in cutaneous and body temperature during and after conditioned fear to context in the rat. *The European Journal of Neuroscience*, *21*(9), 2505–25012. doi:10.1111/j.1460-9568.2005.04073.x

Villalba, S. D., Castellano, G., & Camurri, A. (2007, September). Recognising human emotions from body movement and gesture dynamics. In *Proceedings of the 2nd International Conference on Affective Computing and Intelligent Interaction (ACII 2007),* Lisbon, Portugal (pp. 71-82).

Vinciarelli, A., Pantic, M., & Bourlard, H. (2009, December). Social signal processing: Survey of an emerging domain. *Image and Vision Computing Journal,* 27(12), 1743-1759.Viola, P., & Jones, M. (2001, December). Rapid object detection using a boosted cascade of simple features. In *Proceedings of the IEEE Conference on Computer Vision and Pattern Recognition,* Kauai, HI (Vol. 1, pp. 511-518).

Vogt, T., André, E., & Bee, N. (2008, June). EmoVoice—a framework for online recognition of emotions from voice. In *Perception in Multimodal Dialogue Systems: 4th IEEE Tutorial and Research Workshop on Perception and Interactive Technologies for Speech-Based Systems (PIT 2008),* Kloster Irsee, Germany (LNCS 5078, pp. 188-199).

Volkmar, F. R., & Pauls, D. (2003). Autism. *Lancet*, *362*, 1133–1141. doi:10.1016/S0140-6736(03)14471-6

Von der Malsburg, C. (2003). Self-organization and the brain. In M. A. Arbib (Eds.), *The handbook of brain theory and neural networks* (pp. 1002-1005). Cambridge, MA: MIT Press.

W¨org¨otter, F., & Porr, B. (2004). Temporal sequence learning, prediction and control - a review of different models and their relation to biological mechanisms. *Neural Computation, 17*, 1–75.

Wagner, J., Kim, J., & Andre, E. (2005, July). From physiological signals to emotions: Implementing and comparing selected methods for feature extraction and classification. In *Proceedings of the IEEE International Conference on Multimedia and Expo,* Amsterdam, The Netherlands (pp. 940-943). Washington, DC: IEEE Computer Society.

Walker-Andrews, A. S. (1997). Infants' perception of expressive behaviours: Differentiation of multimodal information. *Psychological Bulletin, 121*(3), 437–456. doi:10.1037/0033-2909.121.3.437

Watanabe, K. (2009). Scientific research on Kansei - laboratories versus real-life. *Journal of Japan Society of Kansei Engineering, 8*(3), 427–431.

Weber, E. U., & Johnson, E. J. (2009). Mindful judgment and decision making. *Annual Review of Psychology, 60*, 53–85. doi:10.1146/annurev.psych.60.110707.163633

Wehmeier, U., Dong, D., Koch, C., & van Essen, D. X. (1989). Modeling the mammalian visual system. In C. Koch & I. Segev (Eds.), *Methods in neuronal modeling: From synapses to networks* (pp. 335-360). Cambridge, MA: MIT Press.

Wehrle, T., & Scherer, K. R. (2001). Towards computational modeling of appraisal theories. In K. R. Scherer, A. Schorr, & T. Johnstone (Eds.), *Appraisal processes in emotion: Theory, methods, research* (pp. 350-365). Oxford, UK: Oxford University Press.

Wehrle, T., Kaiser, S., Schmidt, S., & Scherer, K. R. (2000). Studying the dynamics of emotional expression using synthesized facial muscle movements. *Journal of Personality and Social Psychology, 78*(1), 105–119. doi:10.1037/0022-3514.78.1.105

Weizenbaum, J. (1966). ELIZA--A Computer Program for the Study of Natural Language Communication between Man and Machine. *Communications of the ACM, 9*(1), 36–35. doi:10.1145/365153.365168

Whissell, C. M. (1989). The dictionary of affect in language. In R. Plutchik & H. Kellerman (Ed.), *Emotion: Theory, research and experience. The measurement of emotions* (Vol. 4, pp. 113-131). New York: Academic Press.

Whiteson, S., Taylor, M. E., & Stone, P. (2007). Empirical studies in action selection for reinforcement learning. *Adaptive Behavior, 15*(1), 33–50. doi:10.1177/1059712306076253

Wierzbicka, A. (1992). Talking about emotions: Semantics, culture, and cognition. *Cognition and Emotion, 6*, 3–4. doi:10.1080/02699939208411073

Wilbarger, J., McIntosh, D. N., & Winkielman, P. (2009). Startle modulation in autism: Positive affective stimuli enhanced startle response. *Neuropsychologia, 47*(5), 1323–1331. doi:10.1016/j.neuropsychologia.2009.01.025

Wilson, M. (2002). Six views of embodied cognition. *Psychonomic Bulletin & Review, 9*, 625–636.

Winkielman, P., McIntosh, D. N., & Oberman, L. (2009). Embodied and disembodied emotion processing: Learning from and about typical and autistic individuals. *Emotion Review, 1*, 178–190. doi:10.1177/1754073908100442

Wollmer, M., Eyben, F., Reiter, S., Schuller, B., Cox, C., Douglas-Cowie, E., et al. (2008, September). Abandoning emotion classes - towards continuous emotion recognition with modelling of long-range dependencies. In *Proceedings of Interspeech,* Brisbane, Australia (pp. 597-600).

Wood, M. A., & Bryson, J. J. (2007). Skill acquisition through program-level imitation in a real-time domain. *IEEE Transactions on Systems, Man, and Cybernetics. Part B, Cybernetics, 37*(2), 272–285. doi:10.1109/TSMCB.2006.886948

Wu, L., Oviatt, S. L., & Cohen, P. R. (1999). Multimodal integration: A statistical view. *IEEE Transactions on Multimedia, 1*(4), 334–341. doi:10.1109/6046.807953

Xu, M., Jin, J. S., Luo, S., & Duan, L. (2008, October). Hierarchical movie affective content analysis based on arousal and valence features. In *Proceedings of ACM Multimedia,* Vancouver, British Columbia, Canada (pp. 677-680). ACM Publishing.

Yamanaka, T. (2009). Kansei-design and brain-functions research. *Journal of Japan Society of Kansei Engineering, 8*(3), 445–448.

Yang, Y.-H., Lin, Y.-C., Su, Y.-F., & Chen, H. H. (2007, July). Music emotion classification: A regression approach. In *Proceedings of the IEEE International Conference on Multimedia and Expo,* Beijing, China (pp. 208-211). Washington, DC: IEEE Computer Society.

Yilmaz, A., Javed, O., & Shah, M. (2006). Object tracking: A survey. *ACM Journal of Computing Surveys*, *38*(4), 1–45.

Yu, C., Aoki, P. M., & Woodruff, A. (2004, October). Detecting user engagement in everyday conversations. In *Proceedings of 8th International Conference on Spoken Language Processing,* Jeju Island, Korea (pp. 1329-1332).

Zadeh, S. H., Shouraki, S. B., & Halavati, R. (2006). Emotional behaviour: A resource management approach. *Adaptive Behavior*, *14*(4), 357–380. doi:10.1177/1059712306072337

Zeng, Z., Pantic, M., Roisman, G. I., & Huang, T. S. (2009). A survey of affect recognition methods: Audio, visual, and spontaneous expressions. *IEEE Transactions on Pattern Analysis and Machine Intelligence*, *31*(1), 39–58. doi:10.1109/TPAMI.2008.52

Zhang, Q., & Lee, M. (2009). Analysis of positive and negative emotions in natural scene using brain activity and gist. *Neurocomputing*, *72*(4-6), 1302–1306. doi:10.1016/j.neucom.2008.11.007doi:10.1016/j.neucom.2008.11.007

Zhang, S., Tian, Q., Jiang, S., Huang, Q., & Gao, W. (2008, June). Affective MTV analysis based on arousal and valence features. In *Proceedings of the IEEE International Conference on Multimedia and Expo,* Hannover, Germany (pp. 1369-1372). Washington, DC: IEEE Computer Society.

Ziemke, T. (2001). Are Robots Embodied? In *Proceedings of the First International Workshop on Epigenetic Robotic, Lund University Cognitive Studies,* Lund, Sweden (Vol. 85).

Zuckerman, M., Larrance, D. T., Hall, J. A., DeFrank, R. S., & Rosenthal, R. (1979). Posed and spontaneous communication of emotion via facial and vocal cues. *Journal of Personality*, *47*(4), 712–733. doi:10.1111/j.1467-6494.1979.tb00217.x

Related References

To continue our tradition of advancing information science and technology research, we have compiled a list of recommended IGI Global readings. These references will provide additional information and guidance to further enrich your knowledge and assist you with your own research and future publications.

Adamchuk, V., Barker, B. S., Nugent, G., Grandgenett, N., Patent-Nygren, M., Lutz, C., & Morgan, K. (2012). Learning geospatial concepts as part of a non-formal education robotics experience. In Barker, B., Nugent, G., Grandgenett, N., & Adamchuk, V. (Eds.), *Robots in k-12 education: A new technology for learning* (pp. 284–300). Hershey, PA: IGI Global. doi:10.4018/978-1-4666-0182-6.ch014

Adams, R., & Granic, A. (2009). Cognitive learning approaches to the design of accessible e-learning systems. In Mourlas, C., Tsianos, N., & Germanakos, P. (Eds.), *Cognitive and emotional processes in Web-based education: Integrating human factors and personalization* (pp. 209–228). Hershey, PA: IGI Global. doi:10.4018/978-1-60566-392-0.ch012

Adi, T. (2009). A theory of emotions based on natural language semantics. In Vallverdú, J., & Casacuberta, D. (Eds.), *Handbook of research on synthetic emotions and sociable robotics: New applications in affective computing and artificial intelligence* (pp. 292–323). Hershey, PA: IGI Global. doi:10.4018/978-1-60566-354-8.ch016

Agrawal, M., & Chari, K. (2009). Negotiation behaviors in agent-based negotiation support systems. *International Journal of Intelligent Information Technologies*, *5*(1), 1–23. doi:10.4018/jiit.2009010101

Aishah, A. R., Abidin Mohamad, I. Z., & Komiya, R. (2010). Voice driven emotion recognizer mobile phone: Proposal and evaluations. In Alkhatib, G., & Rine, D. (Eds.), *Web engineering advancements and trends: Building new dimensions of information technology* (pp. 144–159). Hershey, PA: IGI Global. doi:10.4018/978-1-60566-719-5.ch008

Al-Radaei, S. A., & Mishra, R. B. (2011). A heuristic method for learning path sequencing for intelligent tutoring system (ITS) in e-learning. *International Journal of Intelligent Information Technologies*, 7(4), 65–80. doi:10.4018/jiit.2011100104

Ali, H. A., El Desouky, A. I., & Saleh, A. I. (2008). A new approach for building a scalable and adaptive vertical search engine. *International Journal of Intelligent Information Technologies*, *4*(1), 52–79. doi:10.4018/jiit.2008010103

Ali, J. M. (2007). Content-based image classification and retrieval: A rule-based system using rough sets framework. *International Journal of Intelligent Information Technologies*, *3*(3), 41–58. doi:10.4018/jiit.2007070103

Alkhalifa, E. M. (2009). A cognitively-based framework for evaluating multimedia systems. In Khosrow-Pour, M. (Ed.), *Encyclopedia of information science and technology* (2nd ed., pp. 578–582). Hershey, PA: IGI Global. doi:10.4018/978-1-60566-026-4.ch094

Alonso, R. S., Tapia, D. I., & Corchado, J. M. (2011). SYLPH: A platform for integrating heterogeneous wireless sensor networks in ambient intelligence systems. *International Journal of Ambient Computing and Intelligence*, *3*(2), 1–15. doi:10.4018/jaci.2011040101

André, E. (2008). Design and evaluation of embodied conversational agents for educational and advisory software. In Luppicini, R. (Ed.), *Handbook of conversation design for instructional applications* (pp. 343–362). Hershey, PA: IGI Global. doi:10.4018/978-1-59904-597-9.ch020

Andrés, I. (2010). A new framework for intelligent semantic Web services based on GAIVAs. In Alkhatib, G., & Rine, D. (Eds.), *Web engineering advancements and trends: Building new dimensions of information technology* (pp. 38–62). Hershey, PA: IGI Global. doi:10.4018/978-1-60566-719-5.ch003

Arroyo-Palacios, J., & Romano, D. M. (2012). Bio-affective computer interface for game interaction. In Ferdig, R., & de Freitas, S. (Eds.), *Interdisciplinary advancements in gaming, simulations and virtual environments: Emerging trends* (pp. 249–265). Hershey, PA: IGI Global.

Ashish, N., & Maluf, D. A. (2009). Intelligent information integration: Reclaiming the intelligence. *International Journal of Intelligent Information Technologies*, *5*(3), 28–54. doi:10.4018/jiit.2009070102

Asif, U., & Iqbal, J. (2011). Modeling, simulation and motion cues visualization of a six-DOF motion platform for micro-manipulations. *International Journal of Intelligent Mechatronics and Robotics*, *1*(3), 1–17. doi:10.4018/ijimr.2011070101

Azar, A. T., & Eljamel, M. S. (2012). Medical robotics. In Sobh, T., & Xiong, X. (Eds.), *Prototyping of robotic systems: Applications of design and implementation* (pp. 253–287). Hershey, PA: IGI Global. doi:10.4018/978-1-4666-0176-5.ch009

Baker, J. Y. (2012). The mediating role of context in an urban after-school robotics program: Using activity systems to analyze and design robust STEM learning environments. In Barker, B., Nugent, G., Grandgenett, N., & Adamchuk, V. (Eds.), *Robots in k-12 education: A new technology for learning* (pp. 204–221). Hershey, PA: IGI Global. doi:10.4018/978-1-4666-0182-6.ch010

Banik, S. C., Watanabe, K., Habib, M. K., & Izumi, K. (2009). Multirobot team work with benevolent characters: The roles of emotions. In Vallverdú, J., & Casacuberta, D. (Eds.), *Handbook of research on synthetic emotions and sociable robotics: New applications in affective computing and artificial intelligence* (pp. 57–73). Hershey, PA: IGI Global. doi:10.4018/978-1-60566-354-8.ch004

Barceló, J. A. (2009). Beyond science fiction tales. In Barcelo, J. (Ed.), *Computational intelligence in archaeology* (pp. 333–359). Hershey, PA: IGI Global.

Barták, R. (2008). Principles of constraint processing. In Vlahavas, I., & Vrakas, D. (Eds.), *Artificial intelligence for advanced problem solving techniques* (pp. 63–106). Hershey, PA: IGI Global. doi:10.4018/978-1-59904-705-8.ch003

Bartneck, C., & Lyons, M. J. (2009). Facial expression analysis, modeling and synthesis: Overcoming the limitations of artificial intelligence with the art of the soluble. In Vallverdú, J., & Casacuberta, D. (Eds.), *Handbook of research on synthetic emotions and sociable robotics: New applications in affective computing and artificial intelligence* (pp. 34–55). Hershey, PA: IGI Global. doi:10.4018/978-1-60566-354-8.ch003

Basharat, A., & Spinelli, G. (2009). Enabling distributed cognitive collaborations on the semantic Web. In Cruz-Cunha, M., Oliveira, E., Tavares, A., & Ferreira, L. (Eds.), *Handbook of research on social dimensions of semantic technologies and Web services* (pp. 610–642). Hershey, PA: IGI Global. doi:10.4018/978-1-60566-650-1.ch031

Bauer, K. A. (2010). Transhumanism and its critics: Five arguments against a posthuman future. *International Journal of Technoethics*, *1*(3), 1–10. doi:10.4018/jte.2010070101

Becerra, J. A., & Duro, R. J. (2009). Evolutionary robotics. In Rabuñal Dopico, J., Dorado, J., & Pazos, A. (Eds.), *Encyclopedia of artificial intelligence* (pp. 603–608). Hershey, PA: IGI Global.

Benko, A., & Sik Lányi, C. (2009). History of artificial intelligence. In Khosrow-Pour, M. (Ed.), *Encyclopedia of information science and technology* (2nd ed., pp. 1759–1762). Hershey, PA: IGI Global.

Bers, M. U., & Ettinger, A. B. (2012). Programming robots in kindergarten to express identity: An ethnographic analysis. In Barker, B., Nugent, G., Grandgenett, N., & Adamchuk, V. (Eds.), *Robots in k-12 education: A new technology for learning* (pp. 168–184). Hershey, PA: IGI Global. doi:10.4018/978-1-4666-0182-6.ch008

Bhatti, M. W., Wang, Y., & Guan, L. (2008). Language independent recognition of human emotion using artificial neural networks. *International Journal of Cognitive Informatics and Natural Intelligence*, *2*(3), 1–21. doi:10.4018/jcini.2008070101

Biswas, J., Tolstikov, A., Aung, A., Foo, V. S., & Huang, W. (2011). Ambient intelligence for eldercare – The nuts and bolts: Sensor data acquisition, processing and activity recognition under resource constraints. In Chong, N., & Mastrogiovanni, F. (Eds.), *Handbook of research on ambient intelligence and smart environments: Trends and perspectives* (pp. 392–423). Hershey, PA: IGI Global. doi:10.4018/978-1-61692-857-5.ch020

Bittencourt, G., & Marchi, J. (2007). An embodied logical model for cognition in artificial cognition systems. In Loula, A., Gudwin, R., & Queiroz, J. (Eds.), *Artificial cognition systems* (pp. 27–63). Hershey, PA: IGI Global. doi:10.4018/978-1-59904-111-7.ch002

Bosse, T., Hoogendoorn, M., Klein, M., van Lambalgen, R., van Maanen, P., & Treur, J. (2011). Incorporating human aspects in ambient intelligence and smart environments. In Chong, N., & Mastrogiovanni, F. (Eds.), *Handbook of research on ambient intelligence and smart environments: Trends and perspectives* (pp. 128–164). Hershey, PA: IGI Global. doi:10.4018/978-1-61692-857-5.ch008

Braubach, L., Pokahr, A., & Paschke, A. (2009). Using rule-based concepts as foundation for higher-level agent architectures. In Giurca, A., Gasevic, D., & Taveter, K. (Eds.), *Handbook of research on emerging rule-based languages and technologies: Open solutions and approaches* (pp. 493–524). Hershey, PA: IGI Global. doi:10.4018/978-1-60566-402-6.ch021

Broekens, J. (2010). Modeling the experience of emotion. *International Journal of Synthetic Emotions*, *1*(1), 1–17. doi:10.4018/jse.2010101601

Bromuri, S., Urovi, V., & Stathis, K. (2010). iCampus: A connected campus in the. *International Journal of Ambient Computing and Intelligence*, *2*(1), 59–65. doi:10.4018/jaci.2010010105

Brown, A., Sant, P., Bessis, N., French, T., & Maple, C. (2010). Modeling self-led trust value management in grid and service oriented infrastructures: A graph theoretic social network mediated approach. *International Journal of Systems and Service-Oriented Engineering*, *1*(4), 1–18. doi:10.4018/jssoe.2010100101

Brunyé, T. T., Ditman, T., & Augustyn, J. S. (2009). Spatial and nonspatial integration in learning and training with multimedia systems. In Zheng, R. (Ed.), *Cognitive effects of multimedia learning* (pp. 108–133). Hershey, PA: IGI Global. doi:10.4018/978-1-60566-158-2.ch007

Bryson, J. J., & Tanguy, E. (2010). Simplifying the design of human-like behaviour: Emotions as durative dynamic state for action selection. *International Journal of Synthetic Emotions*, *1*(1), 30–50. doi:10.4018/jse.2010101603

Bureš, V., & Cech, P. (2010). Pervasive computing and ambient intelligence development: An educational perspective. In Godara, V. (Ed.), *Strategic pervasive computing applications: Emerging trends* (pp. 235–249). Hershey, PA: IGI Global.

Cabrera, L. (2010). Human implants: A suggested framework to set priorities. *International Journal of Technoethics*, *1*(4), 39–48. doi:10.4018/jte.2010100103

Callejas, Z., López-Cózar, R., Ábalos, N., & Griol, D. (2011). Affective conversational agents: The role of personality and emotion in spoken interactions. In Perez-Marin, D., & Pascual-Nieto, I. (Eds.), *Conversational agents and natural language interaction: Techniques and effective practices* (pp. 203–222). Hershey, PA: IGI Global. doi:10.4018/978-1-60960-617-6.ch009

Capi, G., & Mitobe, K. (2010). Application of evolutionary algorithms for humanoid robot motion planning. *Journal of Information Technology Research*, *3*(4), 21–33. doi:10.4018/jitr.2010100102

Carbonari, L., Bruzzone, L., & Callegari, M. (2011). Impedance control of a spherical parallel platform. *International Journal of Intelligent Mechatronics and Robotics*, *1*(1), 40–60. doi:10.4018/ijimr.2011010103

Carbone, G., Villegas, E., & Ceccarelli, M. (2011). Design and validation of force control loops for a parallel manipulator. *International Journal of Intelligent Mechatronics and Robotics*, *1*(4), 1–18. doi:10.4018/ijimr.2011100101

Carbonneau, R., Vahidov, R., & Laframboise, K. (2007). Machine learning-based demand forecasting in supply chains. *International Journal of Intelligent Information Technologies*, *3*(4), 40–57. doi:10.4018/jiit.2007100103

Carneiro, M. G. (2011). Artificial intelligence in games evolution. In Cruz-Cunha, M., Varvalho, V., & Tavares, P. (Eds.), *Business, technological, and social dimensions of computer games: Multidisciplinary developments* (pp. 98–114). Hershey, PA: IGI Global. doi:10.4018/978-1-60960-567-4.ch007

Castelfranchi, C., Pezzulo, G., & Tummolini, L. (2010). Behavioral implicit communication (BIC): Communicating with smart environments. *International Journal of Ambient Computing and Intelligence*, *2*(1), 1–12. doi:10.4018/jaci.2010010101

Chen, F., & Li, F. (2010). Comparison of the hybrid credit scoring models based on various classifiers. *International Journal of Intelligent Information Technologies*, *6*(3), 56–74. doi:10.4018/jiit.2010070104

Chen, T. (2010). A fuzzy-neural approach with collaboration mechanisms for semiconductor yield forecasting. *International Journal of Intelligent Information Technologies*, *6*(3), 17–33. doi:10.4018/jiit.2010070102

Chen, T. (2011). A dynamically optimized fluctuation smoothing rule for scheduling jobs in a wafer fabrication factory. *International Journal of Intelligent Information Technologies*, *7*(4), 47–64. doi:10.4018/jiit.2011100103

Chithralekha, T., & Kuppuswami, S. (2008). A generic internal state paradigm for the language faculty of agents for task delegation. *International Journal of Intelligent Information Technologies*, *4*(3), 58–78. doi:10.4018/jiit.2008070104

Chu, H. W., & Huynh, M. Q. (2010). Effective use of information systems/technologies in the mergers and acquisitions environment: A resource-based theory perspective. *International Journal of Intelligent Information Technologies*, *6*(2), 65–84. doi:10.4018/jiit.2010040104

Chua, C. E., Chiang, R. H., & Storey, V. C. (2009). Building customized search engines: An interoperability architecture. *International Journal of Intelligent Information Technologies*, *5*(3), 1–27. doi:10.4018/jiit.2009070101

Cinque, M., Coronato, A., & Testa, A. (2011). On dependability issues in ambient intelligence systems. *International Journal of Ambient Computing and Intelligence*, *3*(3), 18–27. doi:10.4018/jaci.2011070103

Cinque, M., Coronato, A., & Testa, A. (2012). Dependable services for mobile health monitoring systems. *International Journal of Ambient Computing and Intelligence*, *4*(1), 1–15. doi:doi:10.4018/jaci.2012010101

Cipresso, P., Dembele, J., & Villamira, M. (2009). An emotional perspective for agent-based computational economics. In Vallverdú, J., & Casacuberta, D. (Eds.), *Handbook of research on synthetic emotions and sociable robotics: New applications in affective computing and artificial intelligence* (pp. 181–197). Hershey, PA: IGI Global. doi:10.4018/978-1-60566-354-8.ch011

Clarke-Midura, J., Code, J., Zap, N., & Dede, C. (2012). Assessing science inquiry: A case study of the virtual performance assessment project. In Lennex, L., & Nettleton, K. (Eds.), *Cases on inquiry through instructional technology in math and science* (pp. 138–164). Hershey, PA: IGI Global. doi:10.4018/978-1-4666-0068-3.ch006

Crutzen, C. K., & Hein, H. (2009). Invisibility and visibility: The shadows of artificial intelligence. In Vallverdú, J., & Casacuberta, D. (Eds.), *Handbook of research on synthetic emotions and sociable robotics: New applications in affective computing and artificial intelligence* (pp. 472–500). Hershey, PA: IGI Global. doi:10.4018/978-1-60566-354-8.ch024

Curran, K., McFadden, D., & Devlin, R. (2011). The role of augmented reality within ambient intelligence. *International Journal of Ambient Computing and Intelligence*, *3*(2), 16–34. doi:10.4018/jaci.2011040102

D'Aubeterre, F., Iyer, L. S., Ehrhardt, R., & Singh, R. (2009). Discovery process in a B2B eMarketplace: A semantic matchmaking approach. *International Journal of Intelligent Information Technologies*, *5*(4), 16–40. doi:10.4018/jiit.2009080702

Dahlem, N. (2011). OntoClippy: A user-friendly ontology design and creation methodology. *International Journal of Intelligent Information Technologies*, *7*(1), 15–32. doi:10.4018/jiit.2011010102

Dalvand, M. M., & Shirinzadeh, B. (2012). Kinematics analysis of 6-DOF parallel micro-manipulators with offset u-joints: A case study. *International Journal of Intelligent Mechatronics and Robotics*, *2*(1), 28–40. doi:doi:10.4018/ijimr.2012010102

Damjanovic, V. (2008). An ambient intelligent prototype for collaboration. In Kock, N. (Ed.), *Encyclopedia of e-collaboration* (pp. 29–35). Hershey, PA: IGI Global.

Davis, D. N., & Venkatamuni, V. M. (2010). A "society of mind" cognitive architecture based on the principles of artificial economics. *International Journal of Artificial Life Research*, *1*(1), 51–71. doi:10.4018/jalr.2010102104

Davis, E. (2010). Hu resources replaces human resources in health care. In Kabene, S. (Ed.), *Human resources in healthcare, health informatics and healthcare systems* (pp. 281–296). Hershey, PA: IGI Global. doi:10.4018/978-1-61520-885-2.ch016

Demo, G. B., Moro, M., Pina, A., & Arlegui, J. (2012). In and out of the school activities implementing IBSE and constructionist learning methodologies by means of robotics. In Barker, B., Nugent, G., Grandgenett, N., & Adamchuk, V. (Eds.), *Robots in k-12 education: A new technology for learning* (pp. 66–92). Hershey, PA: IGI Global. doi:10.4018/978-1-4666-0182-6.ch004

Deng, J. D., Purvis, M., & Purvis, M. (2011). Software effort estimation: Harmonizing algorithms and domain knowledge in an integrated data mining approach. *International Journal of Intelligent Information Technologies*, *7*(3), 41–53. doi:10.4018/jiit.2011070104

Deniz, O., Lorenzo, J., Hernández, M., & Castrillón, M. (2009). Emotional modeling in an interactive robotic head. In Vallverdú, J., & Casacuberta, D. (Eds.), *Handbook of research on synthetic emotions and sociable robotics: New applications in affective computing and artificial intelligence* (pp. 1–8). Hershey, PA: IGI Global. doi:10.4018/978-1-60566-354-8.ch001

Djemaa, R. B., Amous, I., & Hamadou, A. B. (2008). Extending a conceptual modeling language for adaptive Web applications. *International Journal of Intelligent Information Technologies*, *4*(2), 37–56. doi:10.4018/jiit.2008040103

Dogru, S., Topal, S., Erkmen, A. M., & Erkmen, I. (2012). A framework for prototyping of autonomous multi-robot systems for search, rescue, and reconnaissance. In Sobh, T., & Xiong, X. (Eds.), *Prototyping of robotic systems: Applications of design and implementation* (pp. 407–437). Hershey, PA: IGI Global. doi:10.4018/978-1-4666-0176-5.ch014

Dollmann, T. J., Loos, P., Fellmann, M., Thomas, O., Hoheisel, A., Katranuschkov, P., & Scherer, R. (2011). Design and usage of a process-centric collaboration methodology for virtual organizations in hybrid environments. *International Journal of Intelligent Information Technologies*, *7*(1), 45–64. doi:10.4018/jiit.2011010104

Dong, C. (2008). Interface design, emotions, and multimedia learning. In Kidd, T., & Song, H. (Eds.), *Handbook of research on instructional systems and technology* (pp. 79–91). Hershey, PA: IGI Global. doi:10.4018/978-1-59904-865-9.ch007

Eguchi, A. (2012). Educational robotics theories and practice: Tips for how to do it right. In Barker, B., Nugent, G., Grandgenett, N., & Adamchuk, V. (Eds.), *Robots in k-12 education: A new technology for learning* (pp. 1–30). Hershey, PA: IGI Global. doi:10.4018/978-1-4666-0182-6.ch001

Eguchi, A., & Uribe, L. (2012). Educational robotics meets inquiry-based learning: Integrating inquiry-based learning into educational robotics. In Lennex, L., & Nettleton, K. (Eds.), *Cases on inquiry through instructional technology in math and science* (pp. 327–366). Hershey, PA: IGI Global. doi:10.4018/978-1-4666-0068-3.ch012

El-Nasr, M. S., & Vasilakos, A. V. (2011). Ambient intelligence on the dance floor. In Wang, Y. (Ed.), *Transdisciplinary advancements in cognitive mechanisms and human information processing* (pp. 116–133). Hershey, PA: IGI Global. doi:10.4018/978-1-60960-553-7.ch007

Elayeb, B., Bounhas, I., Ben Khiroun, O., Evrard, F., & Bellamine-BenSaoud, N. (2011). Towards a possibilistic information retrieval system using semantic query expansion. *International Journal of Intelligent Information Technologies*, *7*(4), 1–25. doi:10.4018/jiit.2011100101

Eom, S. (2009). The changing structure of decision support systems research: An empirical investigation through author cocitation mapping (1990-1999). In Eom, S. (Ed.), *Author cocitation analysis: Quantitative methods for mapping the intellectual structure of an academic discipline* (pp. 318–342). Hershey, PA: IGI Global.

Fang, N., Luo, X., & Xu, W. (2009). Measuring textual context based on cognitive principles. *International Journal of Software Science and Computational Intelligence*, *1*(4), 61–89. doi:10.4018/jssci.2009062504

Feituri, M., & Funghi, F. (2010). Intelligent agents in education. In Ritke-Jones, W. (Ed.), *Virtual environments for corporate education: Employee learning and solutions* (pp. 321–341). Hershey, PA: IGI Global. doi:10.4018/978-1-61520-619-3.ch018

Feng, L., Li, Y., & Qiao, L. (2011). Towards a mission-critical ambient intelligent fire victims assistance system. *International Journal of Ambient Computing and Intelligence*, *3*(4), 41–61. doi:10.4018/jaci.2011100104

Fotopoulos, V., Zarras, A., & Vassiliadis, P. (2012). Schedule-aware transactions for ambient intelligence environments. In Curran, K. (Ed.), *Innovative applications of ambient intelligence: Advances in smart systems* (pp. 254–268). Hershey, PA: IGI Global. doi:10.4018/978-1-4666-0038-6.ch020

Francis, A. G. Jr, Mehta, M., & Ram, A. (2009). Emotional memory and adaptive personalities. In Vallverdú, J., & Casacuberta, D. (Eds.), *Handbook of research on synthetic emotions and sociable robotics: New applications in affective computing and artificial intelligence* (pp. 391–412). Hershey, PA: IGI Global. doi:10.4018/978-1-60566-354-8.ch020

Franco, J. F., Ficheman, I. K., Zuffo, M. K., & Venâncio, V. (2009). Enhancing individuals' cognition, intelligence and sharing digital/Web-based knowledge using virtual reality and information visualization techniques and tools within k-12 education and its impact on. In Mourlas, C., Tsianos, N., & Germanakos, P. (Eds.), *Cognitive and emotional processes in Web-based education: Integrating human factors and personalization* (pp. 245–319). Hershey, PA: IGI Global. doi:10.4018/978-1-60566-392-0.ch014

French, T. (2009). Virtual organisational trust requirements: Can semiotics help fill the trust gap? *International Journal of Intelligent Information Technologies*, *5*(2), 1–16. doi:10.4018/jiit.2009040101

Fuentes, L., Gamez, N., & Sanchez, P. (2011). Variability in ambient intelligence a family of middleware solution. In Curran, K. (Ed.), *Ubiquitous developments in ambient computing and intelligence: Human-centered applications* (pp. 71–83). Hershey, PA: IGI Global. doi:10.4018/978-1-60960-549-0.ch006

Furtado, E. S., & Furtado, V. (2010). A multi-disciplinary strategy for identifying affective usability aspects in educational geosimulation systems. In Tomei, L. (Ed.), *ICTs for modern educational and instructional advancement: New approaches to teaching* (pp. 22–31). Hershey, PA: IGI Global. doi:10.4018/jicte.2008010102

Gaines Baggio, B. (2010). Creating supportive multimedia learning environments. In Song, H., & Kidd, T. (Eds.), *Handbook of research on human performance and instructional technology* (pp. 88–105). Hershey, PA: IGI Global.

Gallace, A., Ngo, M. K., Sulaitis, J., & Spence, C. (2012). Multisensory Presence in virtual reality: Possibilities & limitations. In Ghinea, G., Andres, F., & Gulliver, S. (Eds.), *Multiple sensorial media advances and applications: New developments in MulSeMedia* (pp. 1–38). Hershey, PA: IGI Global.

Ganesh, K., Dhanlakshmi, R., Tangavelu, A., & Parthiban, P. (2009). Hybrid artificial intelligence heuristics and clustering algorithm for combinatorial asymmetric traveling salesman problem. In Abu-Taieh, E., El-Sheikh, A., & Abu-Tayeh, J. (Eds.), *Utilizing information technology systems across disciplines: Advancements in the application of computer science* (pp. 1–36). Hershey, PA: IGI Global. doi:10.4018/978-1-60566-616-7.ch001

Garcia dos Santos, I. J., & Madeira, E. R. (2010). A semantic-enabled middleware for citizen-centric e-government services. *International Journal of Intelligent Information Technologies, 6*(3), 34–55. doi:10.4018/jiit.2010070103

García-Ordaz, M., Carrasco-Carrasco, R., & Martínez-López, F. J. (2009). Personality and emotions in robotics from the gender perspective. In Vallverdú, J., & Casacuberta, D. (Eds.), *Handbook of research on synthetic emotions and sociable robotics: New applications in affective computing and artificial intelligence* (pp. 154–165). Hershey, PA: IGI Global. doi:10.4018/978-1-60566-354-8.ch009

Genitsaridi, I., Bikakis, A., & Antoniou, G. (2011). DEAL: A distributed authorization language for ambient intelligence. *International Journal of Ambient Computing and Intelligence, 3*(4), 9–24. doi:10.4018/jaci.2011100102

Georgakarakou, C. E., & Economides, A. A. (2008). Software agent technology: An overview. In Protogeros, N. (Ed.), *Agent and Web service technologies in virtual enterprises* (pp. 1–24). Hershey, PA: IGI Global.

Gill, S. K., & Cormican, K. (2008). Ambient intelligent (AmI) systems development. In Zhao, F. (Ed.), *Information technology entrepreneurship and innovation* (pp. 1–22). Hershey, PA: IGI Global. doi:10.4018/978-1-59904-901-4.ch001

Gómez, J., Montoro, G., Haya, P. A., García-Herranz, M., & Alamán, X. (2009). Easing the integration and communication in ambient intelligence. *International Journal of Ambient Computing and Intelligence, 1*(3), 53–65. doi:10.4018/jaci.2009070104

Gómez, J., Montoro, G., Haya, P. A., García-Herranz, M., & Alamán, X. (2011). Distributed schema-based middleware for ambient intelligence environments. In Curran, K. (Ed.), *Ubiquitous developments in ambient computing and intelligence: Human-centered applications* (pp. 205–218). Hershey, PA: IGI Global. doi:10.4018/978-1-60960-549-0.ch020

Gomez, K., Bernstein, D., Zywica, J., & Hamner, E. (2012). Building technical knowledge and engagement in robotics: An examination of two out-of-school programs. In Barker, B., Nugent, G., Grandgenett, N., & Adamchuk, V. (Eds.), *Robots in k-12 education: A new technology for learning* (pp. 222–244). Hershey, PA: IGI Global. doi:10.4018/978-1-4666-0182-6.ch011

Gonçalves, C. T., Camacho, R., & Oliveira, E. (2011). BioTextRetriever: A tool to retrieve relevant papers. *International Journal of Knowledge Discovery in Bioinformatics*, *2*(3), 21–36. doi:doi:10.4018/jkdb.2011070102

Gorga, D., & Schneider, D. K. (2009). Computer-based learning environments with emotional agents. In Vallverdú, J., & Casacuberta, D. (Eds.), *Handbook of research on synthetic emotions and sociable robotics: New applications in affective computing and artificial intelligence* (pp. 413–441). Hershey, PA: IGI Global. doi:10.4018/978-1-60566-354-8.ch021

Grandgenett, N., Ostler, E., Topp, N., & Goeman, R. (2012). Robotics and problem-based learning in STEM formal educational environments. In Barker, B., Nugent, G., Grandgenett, N., & Adamchuk, V. (Eds.), *Robots in k-12 education: A new technology for learning* (pp. 94–119). Hershey, PA: IGI Global. doi:10.4018/978-1-4666-0182-6.ch005

Grimaldo, F., Lozano, M., Barber, F., & Orduña, J. M. (2011). Sociable behaviors in virtual worlds. In Rea, A. (Ed.), *Security in virtual worlds, 3D webs, and immersive environments: Models for development, interaction, and management* (pp. 123–139). Hershey, PA: IGI Global.

Griol, D., Callejas, Z., López-Cózar, R., Espejo, G., & Ábalos, N. (2012). On the development of adaptive and user-centred interactive multimodal interfaces. In Tiwary, U., & Siddiqui, T. (Eds.), *Speech, image, and language processing for human computer interaction: Multi-modal advancements* (pp. 262–291). Hershey, PA: IGI Global. doi:10.4018/978-1-4666-0954-9.ch013

Gros, C. (2009). Emotions, diffusive emotional control and the motivational problem for autonomous cognitive systems. In Vallverdú, J., & Casacuberta, D. (Eds.), *Handbook of research on synthetic emotions and sociable robotics: New applications in affective computing and artificial intelligence* (pp. 119–132). Hershey, PA: IGI Global. doi:10.4018/978-1-60566-354-8.ch007

Grundspenkis, J., & Mislevics, A. (2010). Intelligent agents for business process management systems. In Pankowska, M. (Ed.), *Infonomics for distributed business and decision-making environments: Creating information system ecology* (pp. 97–131). Hershey, PA: IGI Global. doi:10.4018/978-1-60566-890-1.ch007

Gunes, H., & Pantic, M. (2010). Automatic, dimensional and continuous emotion recognition. *International Journal of Synthetic Emotions*, *1*(1), 68–99. doi:10.4018/jse.2010101605

Hadian, H., & Fattah, A. (2011). Kinematic isotropic configuration of spatial cable-driven parallel robots. *International Journal of Intelligent Mechatronics and Robotics*, *1*(4), 61–86. doi:10.4018/ijimr.2011100104

Haidegger, T. (2012). Surgical robots: System development, assessment, and clearance. In Sobh, T., & Xiong, X. (Eds.), *Prototyping of robotic systems: Applications of design and implementation* (pp. 288–326). Hershey, PA: IGI Global. doi:10.4018/978-1-4666-0176-5.ch010

Hamdi, M. S. (2008). SOMSE: A neural network based approach to Web search optimization. *International Journal of Intelligent Information Technologies*, *4*(4), 31–54. doi:10.4018/jiit.2008100103

Hamidi, H., & Vafaei, A. (2009). Evaluation of fault tolerant mobile agents in distributed systems. *International Journal of Intelligent Information Technologies*, *5*(1), 43–60. doi:10.4018/jiit.2009010103

Haselager, W., & Gonzalez, M. (2007). The meaningful body: On the differences between artificial and organic creatures. In Loula, A., Gudwin, R., & Queiroz, J. (Eds.), *Artificial cognition systems* (pp. 238–251). Hershey, PA: IGI Global.

Hashemi, R. R., Le Blanc, L. A., Bahrami, A. A., Bahar, M., & Traywick, B. (2009). Association analysis of alumni giving: A formal concept analysis. *International Journal of Intelligent Information Technologies*, *5*(2), 17–32. doi:10.4018/jiit.2009040102

Hayes, K. J., & Chapman, R. (2011). Process innovation with ambient intelligence (AmI) technologies in manufacturing SMEs: Absorptive capacity limitations. In Cruz-Cunha, M., & Moreira, F. (Eds.), *Handbook of research on mobility and computing: Evolving technologies and ubiquitous impacts* (pp. 65–82). Hershey, PA: IGI Global. doi:10.4018/978-1-60960-042-6.ch005

Hegarty, R., Lunney, T., Curran, K., & Mulvenna, M. (2012). Ambient interface design (AID) for the ergonomically challenged. In Curran, K. (Ed.), *Innovative applications of ambient intelligence: Advances in smart systems* (pp. 128–135). Hershey, PA: IGI Global. doi:10.4018/978-1-4666-0038-6.ch010

Heller, P. B. (2012). Technoethics: The dilemma of doing the right moral thing in technology applications. *International Journal of Technoethics*, *3*(1), 14–27. doi:doi:10.4018/jte.2012010102

Heng, J., & Banerji, S. (2011). Low usage of intelligent technologies by the aged: New initiatives to bridge the digital divide. In Soar, J., Swindell, R., & Tsang, P. (Eds.), *Intelligent technologies for bridging the grey digital divide* (pp. 188–206). Hershey, PA: IGI Global.

Herrera, C., Ziemke, T., & McGinnity, T. M. (2009). A robot model of dynamic appraisal and response. In Rabuñal Dopico, J., Dorado, J., & Pazos, A. (Eds.), *Encyclopedia of artificial intelligence* (pp. 1376–1382). Hershey, PA: IG Global. doi:10.4018/978-1-59904-849-9.ch202

Hillbrand, C. (2007). Towards stable model bases for causal strategic decision support systems. *International Journal of Intelligent Information Technologies*, *3*(4), 1–24. doi:10.4018/jiit.2007100101

Ho, C. M. (2012). Virtual museums: Platforms, practices, prospect. In Yang, H., & Yuen, S. (Eds.), *Handbook of research on practices and outcomes in virtual worlds and environments* (pp. 117–144). Hershey, PA: IGI Global.

Ho, W. C., Dautenhahn, K., Lim, M., Enz, S., Zoll, C., & Watson, S. (2009). Towards learning 'self' and emotional knowledge in social and cultural human-agent interactions. *International Journal of Agent Technologies and Systems*, *1*(3), 51–78. doi:10.4018/jats.2009070104

Hong, S., Nag, B. N., & Yao, D. (2007). Modeling agent auctions in a supply chain environment. *International Journal of Intelligent Information Technologies*, *3*(1), 14–36. doi:10.4018/jiit.2007010102

Hu, J., & Feijs, L. (2009). IPML: Structuring distributed multimedia presentations in ambient intelligent environments. *International Journal of Cognitive Informatics and Natural Intelligence*, *3*(2), 37–60. doi:10.4018/jcini.2009040103

Hudlicka, E. (2011). Affective gaming in education, training and therapy: Motivation, requirements, techniques. In Felicia, P. (Ed.), *Handbook of research on improving learning and motivation through educational games: Multidisciplinary approaches* (pp. 482–511). Hershey, PA: IGI Global. doi:10.4018/978-1-60960-495-0.ch023

Hudlicka, E. (2011). Guidelines for designing computational models of emotions. *International Journal of Synthetic Emotions*, *2*(1), 26–79. doi:10.4018/jse.2011010103

Iglesias, A. (2008). A new framework for intelligent semantic Web services based on GAIVAs. *International Journal of Information Technology and Web Engineering*, *3*(4), 30–58. doi:10.4018/jitwe.2008100102

Ignacio Serrano, J. (2009). Document indexing techniques for text mining. In Wang, J. (Ed.), *Encyclopedia of data warehousing and mining* (2nd ed., pp. 716–721). Hershey, PA: IGI Global.

Iriondo, I., Planet, S., Alías, F., Socoró, J., & Martínez, E. (2009). Emulating subjective criteria in corpus validation. In Rabuñal Dopico, J., Dorado, J., & Pazos, A. (Eds.), *Encyclopedia of artificial intelligence* (pp. 541–546). Hershey, PA: IGI Global.

Jeyarani, R., Nagaveni, N., & Ram, V. (2011). Self adaptive particle swarm optimization for efficient virtual machine provisioning in cloud. *International Journal of Intelligent Information Technologies*, *7*(2), 25–44. doi:10.4018/jiit.2011040102

Jiao, R. J., & Xu, Q. (2010). Affective human factors design with ambient intelligence for product ecosystems. In Mourlas, C., & Germanakos, P. (Eds.), *Mass customization for personalized communication environments: Integrating human factors* (pp. 162–181). Hershey, PA: IGI Global. doi:10.4018/978-1-60566-260-2.ch010

Jones, J. D. (2008). Knowledge representation to empower expert systems. In Adam, F., & Humphreys, P. (Eds.), *Encyclopedia of decision making and decision support technologies* (pp. 576–583). Hershey, PA: IGI Global. doi:10.4018/978-1-59904-843-7.ch064

Jun, S., Rho, S., & Hwang, E. (2010). Music retrieval and recommendation scheme based on varying mood sequences. *International Journal on Semantic Web and Information Systems*, *6*(2), 1–16. doi:10.4018/jswis.2010040101

Kalogirou, S., Metaxiotis, K., & Mellit, A. (2010). Artificial intelligence techniques for modern energy applications. In Metaxiotis, K. (Ed.), *Intelligent information systems and knowledge management for energy: Applications for decision support, usage, and environmental protection* (pp. 1–39). Hershey, PA: IGI Global. doi:10.4018/978-1-60566-737-9.ch001

Kanellopoulos, D. (2009). Intelligent technologies for tourism. In Khosrow-Pour, M. (Ed.), *Encyclopedia of information science and technology* (2nd ed., pp. 2141–2146). Hershey, PA: IGI Global.

Karaman, F. (2012). Artificial intelligence enabled search engines (AIESE) and the implications. In Jouis, C., Biskri, I., Ganascia, J., & Roux, M. (Eds.), *Next generation search engines: Advanced models for information retrieval* (pp. 438–455). Hershey, PA: IGI Global.

Karpouzis, K., Raouzaiou, A., Drosopoulos, A., Ioannou, S., Balomenos, T., & Tsapatsoulis, N. (2004). Facial expression and gesture analysis for emotionally-rich man-machine interaction. In N. Sarris & M. Strintzis (Eds.), *3D modeling and animation: Synthesis and analysis techniques for the human body*, (pp. 175-200). Hershey, PA: IGI Global. doi:10.4018/978-1-59140-299-2.ch005

Kats, Y. (2007). Computer ethics and intelligent technologies. In Quigley, M. (Ed.), *Encyclopedia of information ethics and security* (pp. 83–88). Hershey, PA: IGI Global. doi:10.4018/978-1-59140-987-8.ch013

Keehner, M., Khooshabeh, P., & Hegarty, M. (2008). Individual differences among users: Implications for the design of 3D medical visualizations. In Dong, F., Ghinea, G., & Chen, S. (Eds.), *User centered design for medical visualization* (pp. 1–24). Hershey, PA: IGI Global. doi:10.4018/978-1-59904-777-5.ch001

Khetrapal, N. (2010). Cognitive science helps formulate games for moral education. In Schrier, K., & Gibson, D. (Eds.), *Ethics and game design: Teaching values through play* (pp. 181–196). Hershey, PA: IGI Global. doi:10.4018/978-1-61520-845-6.ch012

Kljajevic, V. (2009). An integrative approach to user interface design. In Cartelli, A., & Palma, M. (Eds.), *Encyclopedia of information communication technology* (pp. 457–463). Hershey, PA: IGI Global. doi:10.4018/978-1-59904-845-1.ch060

Klus, H., & Niebuhr, D. (2011). Integrating sensor nodes into a middleware for ambient intelligence. In Curran, K. (Ed.), *Ubiquitous developments in ambient computing and intelligence: Human-centered applications* (pp. 229–239). Hershey, PA: IGI Global. doi:10.4018/978-1-60960-549-0.ch022

Kock, N., & Antunes, P. (2007). Government funding of e-collaboration research in the European Union: A comparison with the United States model. *International Journal of e-Collaboration, 3*(2), 36–47. doi:10.4018/jec.2007040103

Kolp, M., Faulkner, S., & Wautelet, Y. (2008). Social structure based design patterns for agent-oriented software engineering. *International Journal of Intelligent Information Technologies, 4*(2), 1–23. doi:10.4018/jiit.2008040101

Kommers, P. (2012). Future developments in e-simulations for learning soft skills in the health professions. In Holt, D., Segrave, S., & Cybulski, J. (Eds.), *Professional education using e-simulations: Benefits of blended learning design* (pp. 370–393). Hershey, PA: IGI Global. doi:10.4018/978-1-61350-189-4.ch020

Konar, A., Chakraborty, A., Bhowmik, P., Das, S., & Halder, A. (2012). Emotion recognition from facial expression and electroencephalogram signals. In Mago, V., & Bhatia, N. (Eds.), *Cross-disciplinary applications of artificial intelligence and pattern recognition: Advancing technologies* (pp. 310–337). Hershey, PA: IGI Global. doi:10.4018/978-1-61350-429-1.ch017

Konstantopoulos, S., Camacho, R., Fonseca, N. A., & Costa, V. S. (2008). Induction as a search procedure. In Vlahavas, I., & Vrakas, D. (Eds.), *Artificial intelligence for advanced problem solving techniques* (pp. 166–216). Hershey, PA: IGI Global. doi:10.4018/978-1-59904-705-8.ch007

Kuppuswami, S., & Chithralekha, T. (2010). A new behavior management architecture for language faculty of an agent for task delegation. *International Journal of Intelligent Information Technologies, 6*(2), 44–64. doi:10.4018/jiit.2010040103

Kurschl, W., Buchmayr, M., Franz, B., & Mayr, M. (2012). Situation-aware ambient assisted living and ambient intelligence data integration for efficient eldercare. In Watfa, M. (Ed.), *E-healthcare systems and wireless communications: Current and future challenges* (pp. 315–348). Hershey, PA: IGI Global.

Kvasnica, M. (2007). Modular sensory system for robotics and human-machine interaction based on optoelectronic components. In Taniar, D. (Ed.), *Encyclopedia of mobile computing and commerce* (pp. 651–659). Hershey, PA: IGI Global. doi:10.4018/978-1-59904-002-8.ch109

Lagroue, H. J. III. (2008). Supporting structured group decision making through system-directed user guidance: An experimental study. *International Journal of Intelligent Information Technologies*, *4*(2), 57–74. doi:10.4018/jiit.2008040104

Leach, M. (2009). Navigating a speckled world: Interacting with wireless sensor networks. In Turner, P., Turner, S., & Davenport, E. (Eds.), *Exploration of space, technology, and spatiality: Interdisciplinary perspectives* (pp. 26–40). Hershey, PA: IGI Global.

Lee, K., Lunney, T., Curran, K., & Santos, J. (2009). Ambient middleware for context-awareness (AMiCA). *International Journal of Ambient Computing and Intelligence*, *1*(3), 66–78. doi:10.4018/jaci.2009070105

Leontidis, M., & Halatsis, C. (2009). Affective issues in adaptive educational environments. In Mourlas, C., Tsianos, N., & Germanakos, P. (Eds.), *Cognitive and emotional processes in Web-based education: Integrating human factors and personalization* (pp. 111–133). Hershey, PA: IGI Global. doi:10.4018/978-1-60566-392-0.ch007

Levy, S. D. (2009). Distributed representation of compositional structure. In Rabuñal Dopico, J., Dorado, J., & Pazos, A. (Eds.), *Encyclopedia of artificial intelligence* (pp. 514–519). Hershey, PA: IGI Global.

Li, X. (2008). Inference degradation of active information fusion within Bayesian network models. *International Journal of Intelligent Information Technologies*, *4*(4), 1–17. doi:10.4018/jiit.2008100101

Li, Z. J. (2012). Prototyping of robotic systems in surgical procedures and automated manufacturing processes. In Sobh, T., & Xiong, X. (Eds.), *Prototyping of robotic systems: Applications of design and implementation* (pp. 356–378). Hershey, PA: IGI Global. doi:10.4018/978-1-4666-0176-5.ch012

Lin, H. (2007). From logic specification to y-calculus: A method for designing multiagent systems. *International Journal of Intelligent Information Technologies*, *3*(3), 21–40. doi:10.4018/jiit.2007070102

Liu, C. (2008). Using Bayesian networks for student modeling. In Viccari, R., Jaques, P., & Verdin, R. (Eds.), *Agent-based tutoring systems by cognitive and affective modeling* (pp. 97–113). Hershey, PA: IGI Global. doi:10.4018/978-1-59904-768-3.ch005

Ludi, S. (2012). Educational robotics and broadening participation in STEM for underrepresented student groups. In Barker, B., Nugent, G., Grandgenett, N., & Adamchuk, V. (Eds.), *Robots in k-12 education: A new technology for learning* (pp. 343–361). Hershey, PA: IGI Global. doi:10.4018/978-1-4666-0182-6.ch017

Lugmayr, A., Dorsch, T., & Humanes, P. R. (2009). Emotional ambient media. In Vallverdú, J., & Casacuberta, D. (Eds.), *Handbook of research on synthetic emotions and sociable robotics: New applications in affective computing and artificial intelligence* (pp. 443–459). Hershey, PA: IGI Global. doi:10.4018/978-1-60566-354-8.ch022

Lungarella, M., & Gómez, G. (2009). Developmental robotics. In Rabuñal Dopico, J., Dorado, J., & Pazos, A. (Eds.), *Encyclopedia of artificial intelligence* (pp. 464–470). Hershey, PA: IGI Global.

Luppicini, R. (2008). Introducing conversation design. In Luppicini, R. (Ed.), *Handbook of conversation design for instructional applications* (pp. 1–18). Hershey, PA: IGI Global. doi:10.4018/978-1-59904-597-9.ch001

MacLennan, B. J. (2009). Robots react, but can they feel? In Vallverdú, J., & Casacuberta, D. (Eds.), *Handbook of research on synthetic emotions and sociable robotics: New applications in affective computing and artificial intelligence* (pp. 133–153). Hershey, PA: IGI Global. doi:10.4018/978-1-60566-354-8.ch008

Magnani, L. (2007). Mimetic minds: Meaning formation through epistemic mediators and external representations. In Loula, A., Gudwin, R., & Queiroz, J. (Eds.), *Artificial cognition systems* (pp. 327–357). Hershey, PA: IGI Global.

Magnani, L., & Bardone, E. (2011). Ambient intelligence as cognitive niche enrichment: Foundational issues. In Chong, N., & Mastrogiovanni, F. (Eds.), *Handbook of research on ambient intelligence and smart environments: Trends and perspectives* (pp. 1–17). Hershey, PA: IGI Global. doi:10.4018/978-1-61692-857-5.ch001

Mana, A., Rudolph, C., Spanoudakis, G., Lotz, V., Massacci, F., Melideo, M., & Lopez-Cobo, J. S. (2007). Security engineering for ambient intelligence: A manifesto. In Mouratidis, H., & Giorgini, P. (Eds.), *Integrating security and software engineering: Advances and future visions* (pp. 244–270). Hershey, PA: IGI Global.

Mantovani, F., Confalonieri, L., Mortillaro, M., Realdon, O., Zurloni, V., & Anolli, L. (2010). The potential of affective computing in e-learning: The journey from theory to practice in the "myself" project. In Tzanavari, A., & Tsapatsoulis, N. (Eds.), *Affective, interactive and cognitive methods for e-learning design: Creating an optimal education experience* (pp. 260–274). Hershey, PA: IGI Global. doi:10.4018/978-1-60566-940-3.ch014

Marchi, S., & Ciceri, E. (2011). Participatory and appreciative adult learning and reflection in virtual environments: Towards the development of an appreciative stewardship. In Wang, V. (Ed.), *Encyclopedia of information communication technologies and adult education integration* (pp. 435–450). Hershey, PA: IGI Global.

Martin, F. G., Scribner-MacLean, M., Christy, S., & Rudnicki, I. (2012). Developing and evaluating a Web-based, multi-platform curriculum for after-school robotics. In Barker, B., Nugent, G., Grandgenett, N., & Adamchuk, V. (Eds.), *Robots in k-12 education: A new technology for learning* (pp. 266–283). Hershey, PA: IGI Global. doi:10.4018/978-1-4666-0182-6.ch013

Mazumdar, B. D., & Mishra, R. B. (2010). Multiagent negotiation in B2C e-commerce based on data mining methods. *International Journal of Intelligent Information Technologies*, *6*(4), 46–70. doi:10.4018/jiit.2010100104

McGrath, E., Lowes, S., McKay, M., Sayres, J., & Lin, P. (2012). Robots underwater! Learning science, engineering and 21st century skills: The evolution of curricula, professional development and research in formal and informal contexts. In Barker, B., Nugent, G., Grandgenett, N., & Adamchuk, V. (Eds.), *Robots in k-12 education: A new technology for learning* (pp. 141–167). Hershey, PA: IGI Global. doi:10.4018/978-1-4666-0182-6.ch007

McNamara, D. S., Jackson, G. T., & Graesser, A. (2010). Intelligent tutoring and games (ITaG). In Baek, Y. (Ed.), *Gaming for classroom-based learning: Digital role playing as a motivator of study* (pp. 44–65). Hershey, PA: IGI Global. doi:10.4018/978-1-61520-713-8.ch003

Mead, R. A., Thomas, S. L., & Weinberg, J. B. (2012). From grade school to grad school: An integrated STEM pipeline model through robotics. In Barker, B., Nugent, G., Grandgenett, N., & Adamchuk, V. (Eds.), *Robots in k-12 education: A new technology for learning* (pp. 302–325). Hershey, PA: IGI Global. doi:10.4018/978-1-4666-0182-6.ch015

Meng, S. K., & Chatwin, C. R. (2010). Ontology-based shopping agent for e-marketing. *International Journal of Intelligent Information Technologies*, *6*(2), 21–43. doi:10.4018/jiit.2010040102

Meng, X., Xing, S., & Clark, T. (2007). An empirical performance measurement of Microsoft's search engine and its comparison with other major search engines. *International Journal of Intelligent Information Technologies*, *3*(2), 65–81. doi:10.4018/jiit.2007040105

Meziane, F., & Vadera, S. (2010). Artificial intelligence in software engineering: Current developments and future prospects. In Meziane, F., & Vadera, S. (Eds.), *Artificial intelligence applications for improved software engineering development: New prospects* (pp. 278–299). Hershey, PA: IGI Global.

Michelini, R. C., & Razzoli, R. P. (2009). Ubiquitous computing and communication for product monitoring. In Khosrow-Pour, M. (Ed.), *Encyclopedia of information science and technology* (2nd ed., pp. 3851–3857). Hershey, PA: IGI Global. doi:10.4018/978-1-60566-026-4.ch614

Mikulecký, P., Olševicová, K., Bureš, V., & Mls, K. (2011). Possibilities of ambient intelligence and smart environments in educational institutions. In Chong, N., & Mastrogiovanni, F. (Eds.), *Handbook of research on ambient intelligence and smart environments: Trends and perspectives* (pp. 620–639). Hershey, PA: IGI Global. doi:10.4018/978-1-61692-857-5.ch029

Minor, M., Tartakovski, A., & Schmalen, D. (2008). Agile workflow technology and case-based change reuse for long-term processes. *International Journal of Intelligent Information Technologies*, *4*(1), 80–98. doi:10.4018/jiit.2008010104

Mishra, K., & Mishra, R. (2010). Multiagent based selection of tutor-subject-student paradigm in an intelligent tutoring system. *International Journal of Intelligent Information Technologies*, *6*(1), 46–70. doi:10.4018/jiit.2010100904

Misra, S. (2011). Cognitive complexity measures: An analysis. In Dogru, A., & Biçer, V. (Eds.), *Modern software engineering concepts and practices: Advanced approaches* (pp. 263–279). Hershey, PA: IGI Global.

Moisan, S. (2010). Generating knowledge-based system generators: A software engineering approach. *International Journal of Intelligent Information Technologies*, *6*(1), 1–17. doi:10.4018/jiit.2010100901

Montoro, G., Haya, P. A., & Alamán, X. (2012). A dynamic spoken dialogue interface for ambient intelligence interaction. In Curran, K. (Ed.), *Innovative applications of ambient intelligence: Advances in smart systems* (pp. 24–50). Hershey, PA: IGI Global. doi:10.4018/978-1-4666-0038-6.ch003

Morales, R., Van Labeke, N., Brna, P., & Chan, M. E. (2009). Open learner modeling as the keystone of the next generation of adaptive learning environments. In Mourlas, C., & Germanakos, P. (Eds.), *Intelligent user interfaces: Adaptation and personalization systems and technologies* (pp. 288–312). Hershey, PA: IGI Global. doi:10.4018/978-1-60566-032-5.ch014

Morgavi, G. (2011). Biologically-inspired learning and intelligent system modeling. In Temel, T. (Ed.), *System and circuit design for biologically-inspired intelligent learning* (pp. 1–19). Hershey, PA: IGI Global.

Moudani, W., Shahin, A., Chakik, F., & Rajab, D. (2012). Intelligent decision support system for osteoporosis prediction. *International Journal of Intelligent Information Technologies*, *8*(1), 26–45. doi:doi:10.4018/IJIIT.2012010103

Muwanguzi, S., & Lin, L. (2010). Wrestling with online learning technologies: Blind students' struggle to achieve academic success. *International Journal of Distance Education Technologies*, *8*(2), 43–57. doi:10.4018/jdet.2010040104

Naidenova, X. (2010). Logic-based reasoning in the framework of artificial intelligence. In Naidenova, X. (Ed.), *Machine learning methods for commonsense reasoning processes: Interactive models* (pp. 34–75). Hershey, PA: IGI Global. doi:10.4018/978-1-60566-810-9.ch002

Nair, S. B., Godfrey, W. W., & Kim, D. H. (2011). On realizing a multi-agent emotion engine. *International Journal of Synthetic Emotions*, *2*(2), 1–27. doi:10.4018/jse.2011070101

Nelson, C. A. (2012). Generating transferable skills in STEM through educational robotics. In Barker, B., Nugent, G., Grandgenett, N., & Adamchuk, V. (Eds.), *Robots in k-12 education: A new technology for learning* (pp. 54–65). Hershey, PA: IGI Global. doi:10.4018/978-1-4666-0182-6.ch003

Nissan, E. (2007). Artificial intelligence tools for handling legal evidence. In Quigley, M. (Ed.), *Encyclopedia of information ethics and security* (pp. 42–48). Hershey, PA: IGI Global. doi:10.4018/978-1-59140-987-8.ch007

Nitschke, G. S., Schut, M. C., & Eiben, A. E. (2008). Emergent specialization in biologically inspired collective behavior systems. In Yang, A., & Shan, Y. (Eds.), *Intelligent complex adaptive systems* (pp. 215–253). Hershey, PA: IGI Global. doi:10.4018/978-1-59904-717-1.ch008

Nomura, T., & Saeki, K. (2010). Effects of polite behaviors expressed by robots: A psychological experiment in Japan. *International Journal of Synthetic Emotions*, *1*(2), 38–52. doi:10.4018/jse.2010070103

Nugent, G., Barker, B. S., & Grandgenett, N. (2012). The impact of educational robotics on student STEM learning, attitudes, and workplace skills. In Barker, B., Nugent, G., Grandgenett, N., & Adamchuk, V. (Eds.), *Robots in k-12 education: A new technology for learning* (pp. 186–203). Hershey, PA: IGI Global. doi:10.4018/978-1-4666-0182-6.ch009

Okita, S. Y. (2010). E-collaboration between people and technological boundary objects: A new learning partnership in knowledge construction. In Ertl, B. (Ed.), *Technologies and practices for constructing knowledge in online environments: Advancements in learning* (pp. 133–168). Hershey, PA: IGI Global. doi:10.4018/978-1-61520-937-8.ch007

Orozco, H., Ramos, F., Thalmann, D., Fernández, V., & Gutiérrez, O. (2011). A behavior model based on personality and emotional intelligence for virtual humans. In Mura, G. (Ed.), *Metaplasticity in virtual worlds: Aesthetics and semantic concepts* (pp. 134–157). Hershey, PA: IGI Global. doi:10.4018/978-1-60960-077-8.ch008

Osman, T., Thakker, D., & Al-Dabass, D. (2009). Utilisation of case-based reasoning for semantic Web services composition. *International Journal of Intelligent Information Technologies*, *5*(1), 24–42. doi:10.4018/jiit.2009092102

Pantic, M. (2009). Affective computing a Maja Pantic. In Pagani, M. (Ed.), *Encyclopedia of multimedia technology and networking* (2nd ed., pp. 15–21). Hershey, PA: IGI Global.

Pantic, M. (2009). Face for interface. In Pagani, M. (Ed.), *Encyclopedia of multimedia technology and networking* (2nd ed., pp. 560–567). Hershey, PA: IGI Global.

Peevers, G., Douglas, G., Jack, M. A., & Marshall, D. (2011). A usability comparison of SMS and IVR as digital banking channels. *International Journal of Technology and Human Interaction, 7*(4), 1–16. doi:10.4018/jthi.2011100101

Peres, S. M., Boscarioli, C., Bidarra, J., & Fantinato, M. (2011). Human-computer interaction and artificial intelligence: Multidisciplinarity aiming game accessibility. In Cruz-Cunha, M., Varvalho, V., & Tavares, P. (Eds.), *Business, technological, and social dimensions of computer games: Multidisciplinary developments* (pp. 168–184). Hershey, PA: IGI Global. doi:10.4018/978-1-60960-567-4.ch011

Perry, J. C., Andureu, J., Cavallaro, F. I., Veneman, J., Carmien, S., & Keller, T. (2011). Effective game use in neurorehabilitation: User-centered perspectives. In Felicia, P. (Ed.), *handbook of research on improving learning and motivation through educational games: Multidisciplinary approaches* (pp. 683–725). Hershey, PA: IGI Global. doi:10.4018/978-1-60960-495-0.ch032

Petersen, S. A., Rao, J., & Matskin, M. (2008). Virtual enterprise formation supported by agents and Web services. In Protogeros, N. (Ed.), *Agent and Web service technologies in virtual enterprises* (pp. 46–64). Hershey, PA: IGI Global. doi:10.4018/978-1-59904-648-8.ch003

Petrina, S. (2007). Feelings, values, ethics and skills. In Petrina, S. (Ed.), *Advanced teaching methods for the technology classroom* (pp. 58–90). Hershey, PA: IGI Global.

Pitt, J., & Bhusate, A. (2010). Privacy in pervasive and affective computing environments. In Portela, I., & Cruz-Cunha, M. (Eds.), *information communication technology law, protection and access rights: Global approaches and issues* (pp. 168–187). Hershey, PA: IGI Global. doi:10.4018/978-1-61520-975-0.ch011

Ponticorvo, M., Walker, R., & Miglino, O. (2007). Evolutionary robotics as a tool to investigate spatial cognition in artificial and natural systems. In Loula, A., Gudwin, R., & Queiroz, J. (Eds.), *Artificial cognition systems* (pp. 210–237). Hershey, PA: IGI Global. doi:10.4018/978-1-59904-111-7.ch007

Potkonjak, V., Vukobratovic, M., Babkovic, K., & Borovac, B. (2009). Dynamics and simulation of general human and humanoid motion in sports. In Pope, N., Kuhn, K., & Forster, J. (Eds.), *Digital sport for performance enhancement and competitive evolution: Intelligent gaming technologies* (pp. 36–62). Hershey, PA: IGI Global. doi:10.4018/978-1-60566-406-4.ch003

Pratt, J. G. (2009). Falling behind: A case study in uncritical assessment. In Godara, V. (Ed.), *Risk assessment and management in pervasive computing: Operational, legal, ethical, and financial perspectives* (pp. 102–133). Hershey, PA: IGI Global.

Price, M. (2008). A bio-psycho-social review of usability methods and their applications in healthcare. In Kushniruk, A., & Borycki, E. (Eds.), *Human, social, and organizational aspects of health information systems* (pp. 23–48). Hershey, PA: IGI Global. doi:10.4018/978-1-59904-792-8.ch002

Qi, Y., Song, M., Yoon, S., & deVersterre, L. (2011). Combining supervised learning techniques to key-phrase extraction for biomedical full-text. *International Journal of Intelligent Information Technologies, 7*(1), 33–44. doi:10.4018/jiit.2011010103

Raïevsky, C., & Michaud, F. (2009). Emotion generation based on a mismatch theory of emotions for situated agents. In Vallverdú, J., & Casacuberta, D. (Eds.), *handbook of research on synthetic emotions and sociable robotics: New applications in affective computing and artificial intelligence* (pp. 247–266). Hershey, PA: IGI Global. doi:10.4018/978-1-60566-354-8.ch014

Raikes, H. (2011). Corpus Corvus: Stereoscopic 3D mixed reality dance performance. *International Journal of Art, Culture and Design Technologies, 1*(2), 44–58. doi:doi:10.4018/IJACDT.2011070105

Rajalakshmi, M., Purusothaman, T., & Pratheeba, S. (2010). Collusion-free privacy preserving data mining. *International Journal of Intelligent Information Technologies, 6*(4), 30–45. doi:10.4018/jiit.2010100103

Ramos, C. (2009). Ambient intelligence environments. In Rabuñal Dopico, J., Dorado, J., & Pazos, A. (Eds.), *Encyclopedia of artificial intelligence* (pp. 92–98). Hershey, PA: IGI Global.

Ramos, C., Marreiros, G., & Santos, R. (2011). A survey on the use of emotions, mood, and personality in ambient intelligence and smart environments. In Chong, N., & Mastrogiovanni, F. (Eds.), *Handbook of research on ambient intelligence and smart environments: Trends and perspectives* (pp. 88–107). Hershey, PA: IGI Global. doi:10.4018/978-1-61692-857-5.ch006

Ramos Corchado, F. F., Orozco Aguirre, H. R., & Razo Ruvalcaba, L. A. (2009). Artificial emotional intelligence in virtual creatures. In Vallverdú, J., & Casacuberta, D. (Eds.), *Handbook of research on synthetic emotions and sociable robotics: New applications in affective computing and artificial intelligence* (pp. 350–378). Hershey, PA: IGI Global. doi:10.4018/978-1-60566-354-8.ch018

Rani, C., & Deepa, S. N. (2011). An intelligent operator for genetic fuzzy rule based system. *International Journal of Intelligent Information Technologies, 7*(3), 28–40. doi:10.4018/jiit.2011070103

Rapaport, W. J. (2012). Semiotic systems, computers, and the mind: How cognition could be computing. *International Journal of Signs and Semiotic Systems, 2*(1), 32–71. doi:doi:10.4018/ijsss.2012010102

Razak, A. A., Abidin, M. I., & Komiya, R. (2008). Voice driven emotion recognizer mobile phone: Proposal and evaluations. *International Journal of Information Technology and Web Engineering, 3*(1), 53–69. doi:10.4018/jitwe.2008010104

Reese, D. (2010). Introducing Flowometer : A CyGaMEs assessment suite tool. In Van Eck, R. (Ed.), *Gaming and cognition: Theories and practice from the learning sciences* (pp. 227–254). Hershey, PA: IGI Global. doi:10.4018/978-1-61520-717-6.ch011

Reese, D. D. (2009). GaME design for intuitive concept knowledge. In Ferdig, R. (Ed.), *Handbook of research on effective electronic gaming in education* (pp. 1104–1126). Hershey, PA: IGI Global.

Rigi, M. A., & Khoshalhan, F. (2011). Eliciting user preferences in multi-agent meeting scheduling problem. *International Journal of Intelligent Information Technologies, 7*(2), 45–62. doi:10.4018/jiit.2011040103

Rockland, R., Kimmel, H., Carpinelli, J., Hirsch, L. S., & Burr-Alexander, L. (2012). Medical robotics in k-12 education. In Barker, B., Nugent, G., Grandgenett, N., & Adamchuk, V. (Eds.), *Robots in k-12 education: A new technology for learning* (pp. 120–140). Hershey, PA: IGI Global. doi:10.4018/978-1-4666-0182-6.ch006

Rodríguez, S. J., Herrero, P., & Rodríguez, O. J. (2009). A cognitive appraisal based approach for emotional representation. In Vallverdú, J., & Casacuberta, D. (Eds.), *Handbook of research on synthetic emotions and sociable robotics: New applications in affective computing and artificial intelligence* (pp. 228–246). Hershey, PA: IGI Global. doi:10.4018/978-1-60566-354-8.ch013

Rosen, J., Stillwell, F., & Usselman, M. (2012). Promoting diversity and public school success in robotics competitions. In Barker, B., Nugent, G., Grandgenett, N., & Adamchuk, V. (Eds.), *Robots in k-12 education: A new technology for learning* (pp. 326–342). Hershey, PA: IGI Global. doi:10.4018/978-1-4666-0182-6.ch016

Russell, S., & Yoon, V. Y. (2009). Agents, availability awareness, and decision making. *International Journal of Intelligent Information Technologies, 5*(4), 53–70. doi:10.4018/jiit.2009080704

Saad, G. (2010). Using the Internet to study human universals. In Lee, I. (Ed.), *Encyclopedia of e-business development and management in the global economy* (pp. 719–724). Hershey, PA: IGI Global. doi:10.4018/978-1-61520-611-7.ch071

Saari, T., Turpeinen, M., & Ravaja, N. (2010). Technological and psychological fundamentals of psychological customization systems: An example of emotionally adapted games. In Mourlas, C., & Germanakos, P. (Eds.), *Mass customization for personalized communication environments: Integrating human factors* (pp. 182–214). Hershey, PA: IGI Global.

Sadri, F., & Stathis, K. (2009). Ambient intelligence. In Rabuñal Dopico, J., Dorado, J., & Pazos, A. (Eds.), *Encyclopedia of artificial intelligence* (pp. 85–91). Hershey, PA: IGI Global.

Salam, A. (2008). Semantic supplier contract monitoring and execution DSS architecture. *International Journal of Intelligent Information Technologies, 4*(3), 1–26. doi:10.4018/jiit.2008070101

Sánchez, E., & Lama, M. (2009). Artificial intelligence and education. In Rabuñal Dopico, J., Dorado, J., & Pazos, A. (Eds.), *Encyclopedia of artificial intelligence* (pp. 138–143). Hershey, PA: IGI Global.

Santofimia, M. J., del Toro, X., Villanueva, F. J., Barba, J., Moya, F., & Lopez, J. C. (2012). A rule-based approach to automatic service composition. *International Journal of Ambient Computing and Intelligence, 4*(1), 16–28. doi:doi:10.4018/jaci.2012010102

Santofimia, M. J., Moya, F., Villanueva, F. J., Villa, D., & López, J. C. (2012). How intelligent are ambient intelligence systems? In Curran, K. (Ed.), *Innovative applications of ambient intelligence: Advances in smart systems* (pp. 65–70). Hershey, PA: IGI Global. doi:10.4018/978-1-4666-0038-6.ch006

Saville, M. J. (2010). Robotics as a vehicle for multiliteracies. In Pullen, D., & Cole, D. (Eds.), *Multiliteracies and technology enhanced education: Social practice and the global classroom* (pp. 209–229). Hershey, PA: IGI Global.

Saxon, A., Walker, S., & Prytherch, D. (2009). Whose questionnaire is it, anyway? *International Journal of Information Technology and Web Engineering, 4*(4), 1–21. doi:10.4018/jitwe.2009100101

Saxon, A., Walker, S., & Prytherch, D. (2011). Measuring the unmeasurable?: Eliciting hard to measure information about the user experience. In Alkhatib, G. (Ed.), *Web Engineered Applications for Evolving Organizations: Emerging Knowledge* (pp. 256–277). Hershey, PA: IGI Global. doi:10.4018/978-1-60960-523-0.ch015

Scheutz, M. (2011). Architectural roles of affect and how to evaluate them in artificial agents. *International Journal of Synthetic Emotions, 2*(2), 48–65. doi:10.4018/jse.2011070103

Schiffel, J. A. (2009). Using organizational semiotics and conceptual graphs in a two-step method for knowledge management process improvement measurement. *International Journal of Intelligent Information Technologies, 5*(2), 48–67. doi:10.4018/jiit.2009040104

Sedig, K. (2012). Importance of interface design in e-Learning tools. In Jia, J. (Ed.), *Educational stages and interactive learning: From kindergarten to workplace training* (pp. 49–71). Hershey, PA: IGI Global. doi:10.4018/978-1-4666-0137-6.ch004

Sedig, K., & Parsons, P. (2012). Interactivity of information representations in e-learning environments. In Wang, H. (Ed.), *Interactivity in e-learning: Case studies and frameworks* (pp. 29–50). Hershey, PA: IGI Global. doi:10.4018/978-1-61350-441-3.ch002

Seiffertt, J., & Wunsch, D. C. II. (2009). Higher order neural network architectures for agent-based computational economics and finance. In Zhang, M. (Ed.), *Artificial higher order neural networks for economics and business* (pp. 79–93). Hershey, PA: IGI Global. doi:10.4018/978-1-59904-897-0.ch004

Serenko, A. (2009). User perceptions and employment of interface agents for e-mail notification: An inductive approach. *International Journal of Intelligent Information Technologies*, *5*(3), 55–83. doi:10.4018/jiit.2009070103

Shahdi, A., & Sirouspour, S. (2012). Adaptive control of bilateral teleoperation with time delay. *International Journal of Intelligent Mechatronics and Robotics*, *2*(1), 1–27. doi:doi:10.4018/ijimr.2012010101

Sharkey, A. J. (2009). Swarm robotics. In Rabuñal Dopico, J., Dorado, J., & Pazos, A. (Eds.), *Encyclopedia of artificial intelligence* (pp. 1537–1542). Hershey, PA: IGI Global.

Sieck, W. R., Rasmussen, L. J., & Smart, P. (2010). Cultural network analysis: A cognitive approach to cultural modeling. In Verma, D. (Ed.), *Network science for military coalition operations: Information exchange and interaction* (pp. 237–255). Hershey, PA: IGI Global. doi:10.4018/978-1-61520-855-5.ch011

Sikder, I. U., & Misra, S. K. (2008). Semantic interoperability of geospatial services. *International Journal of Intelligent Information Technologies*, *4*(1), 31–51. doi:10.4018/jiit.2008010102

Silveira, R. A., & Carvalho da Silva, J. M. (2008). Building intelligent learning environments using intelligent learning objects. In Viccari, R., Jaques, P., & Verdin, R. (Eds.), *Agent-based tutoring systems by cognitive and affective modeling* (pp. 19–42). Hershey, PA: IGI Global. doi:10.4018/978-1-59904-768-3.ch002

Singh, R. (2007). A multi-agent decision support architecture for knowledge representation and exchange. *International Journal of Intelligent Information Technologies*, *3*(1), 37–60. doi:10.4018/jiit.2007010103

Slater, S., & Burden, D. (2012). Enhancing characters for virtual worlds and interactive environments through human-like enhancements. In Yang, H., & Yuen, S. (Eds.), *Handbook of research on practices and outcomes in virtual worlds and environments* (pp. 19–33). Hershey, PA: IGI Global. doi:10.4018/978-1-60960-762-3.ch002

Smart, P. R., Engelbrecht, P. C., Braines, D., Strub, M., & Giammanco, C. (2010). The network-extended mind. In Verma, D. (Ed.), *Network science for military coalition operations: Information exchange and interaction* (pp. 191–236). Hershey, PA: IGI Global. doi:10.4018/978-1-61520-855-5.ch010

Smith, J. M. (2009). The open learning initiative, scientifically designed and feedback driven eLearning. In Rogers, P., Berg, G., Boettcher, J., Howard, C., Justice, L., & Schenk, K. (Eds.), *Encyclopedia of distance learning* (2nd ed., pp. 1534–1540). Hershey, PA: IGI Global. doi:10.4018/978-1-60566-198-8.ch224

Sommer, S., Schieber, A., Heinrich, K., & Hilbert, A. (2012). What is the conversation about?: A topic-model-based approach for analyzing customer sentiments in Twitter. *International Journal of Intelligent Information Technologies*, *8*(1), 10–25. doi:doi:10.4018/jiit.2012010102

Sridevi, U. K., & Nagaveni, N. (2011). An ontology based model for document clustering. *International Journal of Intelligent Information Technologies*, *7*(3), 54–69. doi:10.4018/jiit.2011070105

Stahl, B. C., Heersmink, R., Goujon, P., Flick, C., van den Hoven, J., & Wakunuma, K. (2010). Identifying the ethics of emerging information and communication technologies: An essay on issues, concepts and method. *International Journal of Technoethics*, *1*(4), 20–38. doi:10.4018/jte.2010100102

Stubbs, K., Casper, J., & Yanco, H. A. (2012). Designing evaluations for k-12 robotics education programs. In Barker, B., Nugent, G., Grandgenett, N., & Adamchuk, V. (Eds.), *Robots in k-12 education: A new technology for learning* (pp. 31–53). Hershey, PA: IGI Global. doi:10.4018/978-1-4666-0182-6.ch002

Sudeikat, J., & Renz, W. (2008). Building complex adaptive systems: On engineering self-organizing multi-agent systems. In Shan, Y., & Yang, A. (Eds.), *Applications of complex adaptive systems* (pp. 229–256). Hershey, PA: IGI Global. doi:10.4018/978-1-59904-962-5.ch009

Swan, R. H. (2010). Feedforward as an essential active principle of engagement in computer games. In Van Eck, R. (Ed.), *Gaming and cognition: Theories and practice from the learning sciences* (pp. 108–136). Hershey, PA: IGI Global. doi:10.4018/978-1-61520-717-6.ch005

Takác, M. (2009). Construction of meanings in biological and artificial agents. In Trajkovski, G., & Collins, S. (Eds.), *Handbook of research on agent-based societies: Social and cultural interactions* (pp. 139–157). Hershey, PA: IGI Global. doi:10.4018/978-1-60566-236-7.ch010

Tamilselvi, P. R., & Thangaraj, P. (2012). A modified watershed segmentation method to segment renal calculi in ultrasound kidney images. *International Journal of Intelligent Information Technologies*, *8*(1), 46–61. doi:doi:10.4018/jiit.2012010104

Tapia, D. I., Alonso, R. S., & Corchado, J. M. (2011). Improving an ambient intelligence based multi-agent system for alzheimer health care using wireless sensor networks. In Curran, K. (Ed.), *Ubiquitous developments in ambient computing and intelligence: Human-centered applications* (pp. 17–30). Hershey, PA: IGI Global. doi:10.4018/978-1-60960-549-0.ch002

Thangamani, M., & Thangaraj, P. (2011). Effective fuzzy ontology based distributed document using non-dominated ranked genetic algorithm. *International Journal of Intelligent Information Technologies*, *7*(4), 26–46. doi:10.4018/jiit.2011100102

Thomas, D. I., & Vlacic, L. B. (2009). Toward societal acceptance of artificial beings. In Khosrow-Pour, M. (Ed.), *Encyclopedia of information science and technology* (2nd ed., pp. 3778–3783). Hershey, PA: IGI Global.

Thomas, M. A., Yoon, V. Y., & Redmond, R. (2007). Extending loosely coupled federated information systems using agent technology. *International Journal of Intelligent Information Technologies*, *3*(3), 1–20. doi:10.4018/jiit.2007070101

Tiberio, L., Scopelliti, M., & Giuliani, M. V. (2011). Attitudes toward intelligent technologies: Elderly people and caregivers in nursing homes. In Soar, J., Swindell, R., & Tsang, P. (Eds.), *Intelligent technologies for bridging the grey digital divide* (pp. 231–252). Hershey, PA: IGI Global.

Traynor, D., Xie, E., & Curran, K. (2012). Context-awareness in ambient intelligence. In Curran, K. (Ed.), *Innovative applications of ambient intelligence: Advances in smart systems* (pp. 13–23). Hershey, PA: IGI Global. doi:10.4018/978-1-4666-0038-6.ch002

Tripathi, A., Gupta, P., Trivedi, A., & Kala, R. (2011). Wireless sensor node placement using hybrid genetic programming and genetic algorithms. *International Journal of Intelligent Information Technologies*, *7*(2), 63–83. doi:10.4018/jiit.2011040104

Tsadiras, A. (2009). Using prolog for developing real world artificial intelligence applications. In Khosrow-Pour, M. (Ed.), *Encyclopedia of information science and technology* (2nd ed., pp. 3960–3964). Hershey, PA: IGI Global. doi:10.4018/978-1-60566-026-4.ch631

Tscholl, M., & Dowell, J. (2010). Collaborative knowledge construction: examples of distributed cognitive processing. In Ertl, B. (Ed.), *E-collaborative knowledge construction: learning from computer-supported and virtual environments* (pp. 74–90). Hershey, PA: IGI Global. doi:10.4018/978-1-61520-729-9.ch004

Tsianos, N., Lekkas, Z., Germanakos, P., & Mourlas, C. (2010). Individual learning and emotional characteristics in Web-based communities of practice. In Karacapilidis, N. (Ed.), *Web-based learning solutions for communities of practice: Developing virtual environments for social and pedagogical advancement* (pp. 113–127). Hershey, PA: IGI Global. doi:10.4018/978-1-60566-711-9.ch009

Tun, N. N., & Tojo, S. (2008). EnOntoModel: A semantically-enriched model for ontologies. *International Journal of Intelligent Information Technologies*, *4*(1), 1–30. doi:10.4018/jiit.2008010101

Tynjala, T. (2007). Supporting demand supply network optimization with petri nets. *International Journal of Intelligent Information Technologies*, *3*(4), 58–73. doi:10.4018/jiit.2007100104

Ugurlu, B., & Kawamura, A. (2012). Prototyping and real-time implementation of bipedal humanoid robots: Dynamically equilibrated multimodal motion generation. In Sobh, T., & Xiong, X. (Eds.), *Prototyping of robotic systems: Applications of design and implementation* (pp. 146–181). Hershey, PA: IGI Global. doi:10.4018/978-1-4666-0176-5.ch006

ul-Asar, A., Ullah, M. S., Wyne, M. F., Ahmed, J., & ul-Hasnain, R. (2009). Traffic responsive signal timing plan generation based on neural network. *International Journal of Intelligent Information Technologies*, *5*(3), 84-101. doi:10.4018/jiit.2009070104

van der Aalst, W. M., & Nikolov, A. (2008). Mining e-mail messages: Uncovering interaction patterns and processes using e-mail logs. *International Journal of Intelligent Information Technologies*, *4*(3), 27–45. doi:10.4018/jiit.2008070102

van Hoof, J., Wouters, E. J., Marston, H. R., Vanrumste, B., & Overdiep, R. A. (2011). Ambient assisted living and care in The Netherlands: The voice of the user. *International Journal of Ambient Computing and Intelligence*, *3*(4), 25–40. doi:10.4018/jaci.2011100103

Veeramalai, S., & Kannan, A. (2011). Intelligent information retrieval using fuzzy association rule classifier. *International Journal of Intelligent Information Technologies*, *7*(3), 14–27. doi:10.4018/jiit.2011070102

Villanueva, F. J., Moya, F., Santofimia, F. R., Villa, D., Barba, J., Rincon, F., & Lopez, J. C. (2011). A comprehensive solution for ambient intelligence: From hardware to services. In Curran, K. (Ed.), *Ubiquitous developments in ambient computing and intelligence: Human-centered applications* (pp. 56–70). Hershey, PA: IGI Global. doi:10.4018/978-1-60960-549-0.ch005

Vincenti, G., & Braman, J. (2009). Hybrid emotionally aware mediated multiagency. In Trajkovski, G., & Collins, S. (Eds.), *Handbook of research on agent-based societies: Social and cultural interactions* (pp. 199–214). Hershey, PA: IGI Global. doi:10.4018/978-1-60566-236-7.ch014

Wang, B., & Willard, R. L. (2011). Dynamic ambient networks with middleware. In Chong, N., & Mastrogiovanni, F. (Eds.), *Handbook of research on ambient intelligence and smart environments: Trends and perspectives* (pp. 239–247). Hershey, PA: IGI Global. doi:10.4018/978-1-61692-857-5.ch013

Wang, G., Yang, Y., & He, K. (2010). A robust facial feature tracking method based on optical flow and prior measurement. *International Journal of Cognitive Informatics and Natural Intelligence, 4*(4), 62–75. doi:10.4018/jcini.2010100105

Wang, Y. (2008). Cognitive informatics. In Tomei, L. (Ed.), *Encyclopedia of information technology curriculum integration* (pp. 104–111). Hershey, PA: IGI Global. doi:10.4018/978-1-59904-881-9.ch017

Wang, Y. (2009). On abstract intelligence: Toward a unifying theory of natural, artificial, machinable, and computational intelligence. *International Journal of Software Science and Computational Intelligence, 1*(1), 1–17. doi:10.4018/jssci.2009010101

Wang, Y. (2011). A cognitive informatics reference model of autonomous agent systems (AAS). In Wang, Y. (Ed.), *Transdisciplinary advancements in cognitive mechanisms and human information Processing* (pp. 1–16). Hershey, PA: IGI Global. doi:10.4018/978-1-60960-553-7.ch001

Wang, Y. (2011). Towards the synergy of cognitive informatics, neural informatics, brain informatics, and cognitive computing. *International Journal of Cognitive Informatics and Natural Intelligence, 5*(1), 75-93. Hershey, PA: IGI Global. doi:10.4018/jcini.2011010105

Wang, Y., Berwick, R. C., Haykin, S., Pedrycz, W., Kinsner, W., & Baciu, G. (2011). Cognitive informatics and cognitive computing in year 10 and beyond. *International Journal of Cognitive Informatics and Natural Intelligence, 5*(4), 1–21. doi:10.4018/jcini.2011100101

Wang, Y., Bhatti, M. W., & Guan, L. (2010). Neural networks for language independent emotion recognition in speech. In Wang, Y. (Ed.), *Discoveries and breakthroughs in cognitive informatics and natural intelligence* (pp. 461–484). Hershey, PA: IGI Global. doi:10.4018/978-1-60566-902-1.ch025

Wang, Y., Widrow, B. C., Zhang, B., Kinsner, W., Sugawara, K., & Sun, F. (2011). Perspectives on the field of cognitive informatics and its future development. *International Journal of Cognitive Informatics and Natural Intelligence, 5*(1), 1–17. doi:10.4018/jcini.2011010101

Wang, Y. D. (2009). Trust in B2C e-commerce interface. In Khosrow-Pour, M. (Ed.), *Encyclopedia of information science and technology* (2nd ed., pp. 3826–3830). Hershey, PA: IGI Global.

Wang, Y. D., & Emurian, H. H. (2007). Inducing online trust in e-commerce: Empirical investigations on Web design factors. In Khosrow-Pour, M. (Ed.), *Utilizing and managing commerce and services online* (pp. 74–100). Hershey, PA: IGI Global. doi:10.4018/978-1-59140-932-8.ch005

Weber, J. (2008). Human-robot interaction. In Kelsey, S., & St.Amant, K. (Eds.), *Handbook of research on computer mediated communication* (pp. 855–867). Hershey, PA: IGI Global. doi:10.4018/978-1-59904-863-5.ch061

Werner, L., & Böttcher, S. (2007). Supporting text retrieval by typographical term weighting. *International Journal of Intelligent Information Technologies, 3*(2), 1–16. doi:10.4018/jiit.2007040101

Wiberg, M. (2009). Designing interactive architecture: Lessons learned from a multi-professional approach to the design of an ambient computing environment. *International Journal of Ambient Computing and Intelligence, 1*(3), 1–18. doi:10.4018/jaci.2009070101

Wiedermann, J. (2012). A high level model of a conscious embodied agent. In Wang, Y. (Ed.), *Breakthroughs in software science and computational intelligence* (pp. 65–82). Hershey, PA: IGI Global. doi:10.4018/978-1-4666-0264-9.ch005

Wijekumar, K. K. (2009). Using intelligent tutoring technologies to enhance online learning environments. In Rogers, P., Berg, G., Boettcher, J., Howard, C., Justice, L., & Schenk, K. (Eds.), *Encyclopedia of distance learning* (2nd ed., pp. 2246–2251). Hershey, PA: IGI Global. doi:10.4018/978-1-60566-198-8.ch332

Williams, H., Tansley, C., & Foster, C. (2009). HRIS project teams skills and knowledge: A human capital analysis. In Bondarouk, T., Ruel, H., Guiderdoni-Jourdain, K., & Oiry, E. (Eds.), *Handbook of research on e-transformation and human resources management technologies: Organizational outcomes and challenges* (pp. 135–152). Hershey, PA: IGI Global. doi:10.4018/978-1-60566-304-3.ch008

Williams, R., & Kitchen, P. J. (2009). Involvement, elaboration and the sources of online trust. *International Journal of Technology and Human Interaction, 5*(2), 1–22. doi:10.4018/jthi.2009040101

Woletz, J. D. (2008). Digital storytelling from artificial intelligence to YouTube. In Kelsey, S., & St.Amant, K. (Eds.), *Handbook of research on computer mediated communication* (pp. 587–601). Hershey, PA: IGI Global. doi:10.4018/978-1-59904-863-5.ch042

Wood-Bradley, G. (2009). A new framework for interactive entertainment technologies. In Pagani, M. (Ed.), *Encyclopedia of multimedia technology and networking* (2nd ed., pp. 1061–1065). Hershey, PA: IGI Global. doi:10.4018/978-1-60566-014-1.ch143

Woolf, B. P., & Aïmeur, E. (2007). Portal for artificial intelligence in education. In Tatnall, A. (Ed.), *Encyclopedia of portal technologies and applications* (pp. 737–742). Hershey, PA: IGI Global. doi:10.4018/978-1-59140-989-2.ch121

Xu, K. S., Wang, W., Ren, J., Xu, J. S., Liu, L., & Liao, S. (2011). Classifying consumer comparison opinions to uncover product strengths and weaknesses. *International Journal of Intelligent Information Technologies, 7*(1), 1–14. doi:10.4018/jiit.2011010101

Yang, Y., & Wang, G. (2011). A novel emotion recognition method based on ensemble learning and rough set theory. *International Journal of Cognitive Informatics and Natural Intelligence, 5*(3), 61-72. Hershey, PA: IGI Global. doi:10.4018/IJCINI.2011070104

Yao, Z., & Choi, B. (2007). Clustering Web pages into hierarchical categories. *International Journal of Intelligent Information Technologies, 3*(2), 17–35. doi:10.4018/jiit.2007040102

Yousfi-Monod, M., & Prince, V. (2007). Knowledge acquisition modeling through dialogue between cognitive agents. *International Journal of Intelligent Information Technologies, 3*(1), 60–78. doi:10.4018/jiit.2007010104

Zaharakis, I. D., & Kameas, A. D. (2008). Engineering emergent ecologies of interacting artefacts. In Lumsden, J. (Ed.), *Handbook of research on user interface design and evaluation for mobile technology* (pp. 364–384). Hershey, PA: IGI Global. doi:10.4018/978-1-59904-871-0.ch023

Zappi, P., Lombriser, C., Benini, L., & Tröster, G. (2012). Collecting datasets from ambient intelligence environments. In Curran, K. (Ed.), *Innovative applications of ambient intelligence: Advances in smart systems* (pp. 113–127). Hershey, PA: IGI Global. doi:10.4018/978-1-4666-0038-6.ch009

Zhang, Y., & Bhattacharyya, S. (2010). Information sharing strategies in business-to-business e-hubs: An agent-based study. *International Journal of Intelligent Information Technologies*, *6*(2), 1–20. doi:10.4018/jiit.2010040101

Zhou, J., Wang, G., & Yang, Y. (2011). Important attributes selection based on rough set for speech emotion recognition. In Wang, Y. (Ed.), *Transdisciplinary advancements in cognitive mechanisms and human information processing* (pp. 262–271). Hershey, PA: IGI Global. doi:10.4018/978-1-60960-553-7.ch016

Zurloni, V., Mantovani, F., Mortillaro, M., Vescovo, A., & Anolli, L. (2008). Addressing emotions within e-learning systems. In Kidd, T., & Song, H. (Eds.), *Handbook of research on instructional systems and technology* (pp. 803–816). Hershey, PA: IGI Global. doi:10.4018/978-1-59904-865-9.ch057

About the Contributors

Jordi Vallverdú, B.Phil, P. Mus, MSc, Ph.D., is Lecturer Professor at UAB (Catalonia, Spain), where he teaches Philosophy and History of Science and Computing. His research is dedicated to the epistemological and cognitive aspects of Philosophy of Computing and Science. He is Editor-in-Chief of the *International Journal of Synthetic Emotions* (IJSE), and as researcher is member of the EuCogIII and the Convergent Science Network of Biomimetic and Biohybrid Systems Net. He has written several books on computer epistemology and artificial emotions. Very recently, he won a Japanese JSPS fellowship for his studies on HRI at Nishidalab (Kyoto University).

* * *

Joost Broekens received a MSc degree in computer science at the University of Delft, The Netherlands, in 2001. In December 2007 he received his PhD in computer science at the University of Leiden, The Netherlands, in the area of computational modelling of emotion in relation to learning processes. He has published in the area of computational models of emotion (ranging from theoretical approaches to more applied ones), developed a master-level course on the topic, and has given several invited lectures as well as less formal talks for the larger public related to affective computing. His most recent interests include reinforcement learning, affective computing, human-robot and human-computer interaction, and gaming research.

Joanna J. Bryson studies the structure of both natural and artificial cognitive systems. She holds degrees in behavioural science, psychology and artificial intelligence from Chicago (BA), Edinburgh (MSc and MPhil), and MIT (PhD). Since 2002 she has been a lecturer (assistant professor) at the University of Bath where she founded Artificial Models of Natural Intelligence. She has over sixty peer-reviewed publications in AI, Biology, Cognitive Science and Philosophy, and serves as en expert consultant on cognitive systems for the European commission. From 2007-2009 she served as pursued a sabbatical fellowship at the Konrad Lorenz Institute for Evolution & Cognition Research in Altenberg, Austria, studying the biological evolution of cultural evolution. Her main engineering interest is in broadening access to artificial intelligence by making it easier to design and develop.

Hatice Gunes received the PhD degree in computing sciences from the University of Technology Sydney (UTS), Australia, in 2007. From 2006 to 2008, she was a postdoctoral research associate at UTS, where she worked on an Australian research council–funded Linkage Project for UTS and iOmniscient Pty Ltd. She is currently a postdoctoral research associate at the HCI2 Group, Visual Information Processing

Section, Imperial College London, U.K. working on a European Commission (EC-FP7) project, and is also an honorary associate of UTS. Gunes has published over 30 technical papers in the areas of video analysis and pattern recognition, with applications to video surveillance, human-computer interaction, emotion recognition and affective computing. She is a member of the IEEE and the ACM.

Seiji Inokuchi was born at Hiroshima, Japan, in 1940. He received a PhD from Osaka University in 1969. He joined the Faculty of Engineering Science, Osaka University. From 1985 to 2003 he was professor of the Department of Systems Engineering of Osaka University. At a retirement age he was given the title of Emeritus from Osaka University. From 2003 to 2005, He was professor of human and social environment, Hiroshima International University. Currently he is professor of the Faculty of Media Content, Takarazuka University of Arts and Design. He held the post of director in the Laboratories of Image Information Science and Technologies, 1995-2005. His main research interests include pattern recognition, 3D image processing and Kansei information processing. He is the author of *Three-dimensional image measurement*, and *Kansei information processing*. In 1999, he was the president, the IEICE Information and Systems Society of Japan.

Neha Khetrapal is currently a graduate level researcher at the Indian Institute of Information Technology located at India (IIIT), Allahabad. Before joining IIIT, she was at the Centre of Excellence "Cognitive Interaction Technology" (CITEC) and the Faculty of Psychology and Sport Sciences, University of Bielefeld investigating the interaction of spatial processes and language and was supported by Deutsche Forschungsgemeinschaft (DFG) grant managed through the Graduate School of CITEC, Germany. She has been a holder of various prestigious awards and has the honor of earning an important recognition from the Marquis Who's Who in the World for 2009 for scientific contributions in the developing world. She has also published in high profile journals like the European Journal of Cognitive Psychology, Philosophical Psychology, Empirical Musicology Review and the Australian Journal of Psychology to name a few.

Tatsuya Nomura received the M.S. degree in mathematics from Osaka University, Osaka, Japan, in 1989, and the D.E. degree in engineering from Kyoto University, Kyoto, Japan, in 1998. From 1989 to 2000, he was with the Corporate Research and Development Group at Sharp Corporation. From 2000 to 2004, he was with Hannan University, Osaka, Japan. He is currently an Associate Professor in the Department of Media Informatics, Ryukoku University, Otsu, Japan, and a Researcher in the Advanced and Technology (ATR) Intelligent Robotics and Communication Laboratories, Japan. His current research interests include human factors in interaction with computers and robots. He is a member the Japanese Psychological Association, the Japanese Cognitive Science Society, and the Mathematical Society of Japan.

Maja Pantic received her MSc and PhD degrees in computer science from Delft University of Technology, the Netherlands, in 1997 and 2001, respectively. Until 2006, she was an assistant and then an associate professor at the same university. In 2006, she joined Imperial College London, UK, Computing Department, where she is reader in Multimodal HCI, and University of Twente, the Netherlands, Department of Computer Science, where she is professor of affective and behavioral computing. She is the editor in chief of *Image and Vision Computing Journal* and an associate editor for the IEEE Transactions on Systems, Man, and Cybernetics, Part B. In 2008, she received European research council starting grant, as one of 2.5% of the best young researchers in Europe in any scientific discipline. Her research interests include computer vision and machine learning applied to face and body gesture recognition, multimodal HCI, and affective computing. She has published more than 90 technical papers in these areas and she has more than 1500 citations to her work. She is a senior member of the IEEE and a member of the ACM.

Karla Parussel graduated with a BSc(HONS) in computer science from the University of Kent at Canterbury in 1997 and an MSc in evolutionary and adaptive systems from Sussex University the following year. She graduated at Stirling University in 2007 after studying for a PhD researching the functionality of emotions by emulating and applying neuromodulation to artificial neural networks. She was later employed as a research fellow on the Humaine project at the University of Hertfordshire and then as a research assistant for the Inter-life project back at Stirling University. Her career has also involved several years experience in industry as a senior software engineer in research and development.

Kazuma Saeki received the B.S. degree from Ryukoku University, Otsu, Japan, in 2009. From 2008 to 2009, he was with the laboratory managed by Nomura in Ryukoku University. His research interests include human-robot interaction and behavior design of robots. He is currently with Amagasaki Shinkin Bank, Osaka, Japan.

Emmanuel Tanguy completed his PhD in June 2006 under the supervision of professor Phil Willis as his first supervisor and Joanna J. Bryson as his second supervisor, working in the field of facial animation and synthetic emotions with the developement of a dynamic emotion representation model. The title of his PhD thesis is *Emotions: the Art of Communication Applied to Virtual Actors*. Currently, he is developing research on the influences of emotions on synthetic facial expressions and their effects on people's perception of embodied virtual agents. He developed an Emotionally Expressive Facial Animation System (EE-FAS: e-face) for embodied virtual agents, integrating a dynamic emotion representation inspired by natural models and psychological studies of human emotions.

Index

F

G

H

I

K

L

M

N

O

P

R

S

T

W